James
Patho

Difficult Diagnoses in Breast Pathology

Difficult Diagnoses in Breast Pathology

EDITED BY

Juan P. Palazzo, MD

Department of Pathology
Thomas Jefferson University
Philadelphia, Pennsylvania

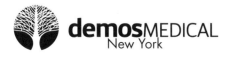
New York

ISBN: 978-1-933864-79-2
eBook ISBN: 978-1-935281-30-6

Acquisitions Editor: Richard Winters
Production Editor: Dana Bigelow
Compositor: Manila Typesetting Company
Printer: SCI

Visit our website at www.demosmedpub.com

Medicine is an ever-changing science. Research and clinical experience are continually expanding our knowledge, in particular our understanding of proper treatment and drug therapy. The authors, editors, and publisher have made every effort to ensure that all information in this book is in accordance with the state of knowledge at the time of production of the book. Nevertheless, the authors, editors, and publisher are not responsible for errors or omissions or for any consequences from application of the information in this book and make no warranty, express or implied, with respect to the contents of the publication. Every reader should examine carefully the package inserts accompanying each drug and should carefully check whether the dosage schedules mentioned therein or the contraindications stated by the manufacturer differ from the statements made in this book. Such examination is particularly important with drugs that are either rarely used or have been newly released on the market.

Library of Congress Cataloging-in-Publication Data
Difficult diagnoses in breast pathology / edited by Juan P. Palazzo.
    p. ; cm.
    Includes bibliographical references and index.
    ISBN 978-1-933864-79-2
  1. Breast—Diseases—Diagnosis. 2. Tumor markers. I. Palazzo, Juan P.
  [DNLM: 1. Breast—pathology. 2. Biopsy, Fine-Needle. 3. Breast Diseases—diagnosis.
4. Tumor Markers, Biological. WP 840]
  RG493.D547 2011
  618.1′9—dc22
                                                2011008921

Made in the United States of America
11 12 13 14 15   5 4 3 2 1

Contents

Preface

The goal of this book is to provide pathologists with a reference guide to use in the diagnosis and differential diagnosis of common and uncommon breast diseases.

The role of the pathologist has become very important in the diagnosis and management of patients with breast diseases. Pathologists are frequently asked to make diagnosis in small samples and are faced with difficult decisions in their daily practice.

The book is organized into chapters devoted to the challenges in the diagnosis of breast diseases using core biopsies and chapters dedicated to specific epithelial and mesenchymal lesions, lymphoid proliferations, and immunohistochemistry.

This is a book that primarily emphasizes the diagnostic morphologic features. The text highlights the most important aspects of each entity with a particular focus in the diagnostic criteria, differential diagnosis, immunohistochemical findings, and management. Tables and key points are included in each chapter to summarize the most important findings.

I was very fortunate to have worked with such an outstanding group of experts in the field. Without their great dedication and effort this book would not have been possible. Each chapter reflects the authors, own experience in practice and the best guide to solve problem cases from their own perspective.

My hope is that this book provides information that will help pathologists with the interpretation of breast biopsies and will also be a source of education for residents and fellows, as well as other physicians interested in breast disorders.

I want to thank all my colleagues from the Department of Pathology of Jefferson University for sharing breast cases with me. Mr. Richard Winters from Demos Medical Publishing for his patience and valuable advice and Christopher Braster from Jefferson University for help with the photographs. My entire family for the relentless support in all my endeavors.

Juan P. Palazzo

Contributors

Edi Brogi, MD, PhD
Associate Professor of Pathology
Weill Cornell Medical College
Associate Attending Pathologist
Memorial Sloan-Kettering Cancer Center
New York, New York

John S. J. Brooks, MD, FRCPath
Professor of Pathology and Laboratory Medicine
University of Pennsylvania Health System
Chair, Department of Pathology
Pennsylvania Hospital
Philadelphia, Pennsylvania

José Palacios Calvo, MD, PhD
Department of Pathology
Virgen del Rocio University Hospital and
Institute for Biomedical Research of Seville (IBIS)
Seville, Spain

Joan F. Cangiarella, MD
Associate Professor of Pathology
Vice-Chair of Clinical Operations
Department of Pathology
New York University School of Medicine
New York, New York

Adriana D. Corben, MD
Assistant Attending Pathologist
Memorial Sloan-Kettering Cancer Center
New York, New York

Judith A. Ferry, MD
Associate Professor of Pathology
Harvard Medical School
Director of Hematopathology
The James Homer Wright Pathology Laboratories
Massachusetts General Hospital
Boston, Massachusetts

Felipe C. Geyer, MD
The Breakthrough Breast Cancer Research Centre
Institute of Cancer Research
London, United Kingdom

Dilip Giri, MD, FACP
Associate Attending Pathologist
Memorial Sloan Kettering Cancer Center
New York, New York

Cansu Karakas, MD
Experimental Radiation Oncology
The University of Texas MD Anderson Cancer Center
Houston, Texas

Magali Lacroix-Triki, MD
The Breakthrough Breast Cancer Research Centre
Institute of Cancer Research
London, United Kingdom

Melinda F. Lerwill, MD
Assistant Professor of Pathology
Harvard Medical School
The James Homer Wright Pathology Laboratories
Massachusetts General Hospital
Boston, Massachusetts

Melissa P. Murray, DO
Assistant Attending Pathologist
Memorial Sloan-Kettering Cancer Center
New York, New York

Juan P. Palazzo, MD
Professor
Department of Pathology
Thomas Jefferson University
Philadelphia, Pennsylvania

Jorge S. Reis-Filho, MD, PhD, MRCPath
Professor of Molecular Pathology, Team Leader
Molecular Laboratory
The Breakthrough Breast Cancer Research Centre
Institute of Cancer Research
London, United Kingdom

Erika Resetkova, MD, PhD
Associate Professor
Department of Pathology
The University of Texas MD Anderson Cancer Center
Houston, Texas

Aysegul A. Sahin, MD
Professor
Department of Pathology
The University of Texas MD Anderson Cancer Center
Houston, Texas

Aylin Simsir, MD
Associate Professor of Pathology
Director of Cytopathology
Department of Pathology
New York University School of Medicine
New York, New York

Melinda E. Sanders, MD
Assistant Professor of Pathology
Vanderbilt Breast Consultation Service
Department of Pathology
Vanderbilt University
Nashville, Tennessee

Difficult Diagnoses in Breast Pathology

1

The Diagnostic Challenges of Core Needle Biopsy Interpretation

AYLIN SIMSIR

JOAN F. CANGIARELLA

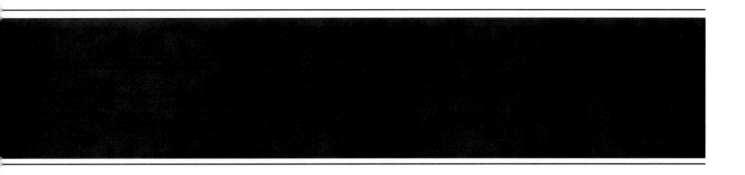

Percutaneous core needle biopsy (CNB) is a safe, accurate, and cost-effective diagnostic method. Over the last few decades, there has been a marked growth in its use for the diagnosis of palpable and nonpalpable mammary lesions. Radiologic guidance, including stereotactic guidance, ultrasonography, and magnetic resonance imaging, has significantly enhanced the ability to sample lesions by CNB. With the introduction of vacuum-assisted biopsy (VAB) and the use of larger needles, the amount of tissue obtained by CNB has also increased. Despite these advances, diagnostic challenges in the pathologic interpretation and controversies in the management of certain lesions diagnosed by percutaneous CNB still remain.

A key component to the success of a CNB program is the mandatory use of the triple test with effective communication among members of the multidisciplinary team. There must be knowledge of the clinical and radiologic findings and confidence that the lesion targeted for biopsy is adequately sampled and that the pathologic results are concordant with the imaging and clinical findings. Discordance among the clinical, radiologic, or pathologic findings warrants excision. Pathologists must be effective communicators and should not interpret a CNB without knowledge of the clinical and radiologic findings.

The challenges for pathologists in the interpretation of percutaneous core biopsies are two-fold. First, there exists a variety of lesions that are diagnostically difficult to interpret in CNB due to an overlap of pathologic features with other entities. These lesions are uncommon in CNB, and the small amount of tissue obtained by percutaneous CNB makes classification of these lesions diagnostically difficult. The second issue is that some lesions when identified in percutaneous CNB often create uncertainty with regard to proper clinical management. These lesions include atypical ductal hyperplasia (ADH), papillary lesions, atypical lobular hyperplasia (ALH) and lobular carcinoma in situ (LCIS), fibroepithelial lesions, radial scars, and mucinous lesions.

■ ATYPICAL DUCTAL HYPERPLASIA

Atypical ductal hyperplasia is a proliferative lesion of the breast epithelium that fulfills some, but not all, of the criteria of a low-grade, non–comedo-type ductal carcinoma in situ (DCIS). Microcalcifications are the most common mammographic presentation of ADH. When ADH is encountered in CNB, one must consider whether the radiologic findings correlate with the pathologic findings. Sampling error by core remains a potential problem. In many cases of DCIS identified at surgical excision, DCIS is found in the central portion of the lesion, and foci of ADH are found at the periphery (1). If the CNB samples the peripheral areas only, ADH will be present on the core specimen, but DCIS may be identified at surgical excision. Although the diagnostic features of ADH in a CNB are similar to those of a surgical excision specimen, one should not overinterpret the findings in small CNB samples. When debating between a diagnosis of usual ductal hyperplasia (UDH) and ADH in core, the impact of the diagnosis must be considered since only a diagnosis of ADH warrants surgical excision. If debating between ADH and DCIS, preference is given to diagnosing the lesion as an ADH and rendering a definitive diagnosis on the excision specimen.

Pathologic Features

One of the most difficult challenges for the pathologist in the interpretation of breast biopsies is distinguishing ADH from usual duct hyperplasia and DCIS. Distinguishing ADH from low-grade DCIS or from florid ductal epithelial hyperplasia is even more challenging in the limited tissue sample obtained by CNB. Microscopically, 3 components to the diagnosis of ADH include architectural pattern, cytology, and extent (2,3). These components may be difficult to evaluate in small samples. Interobserver

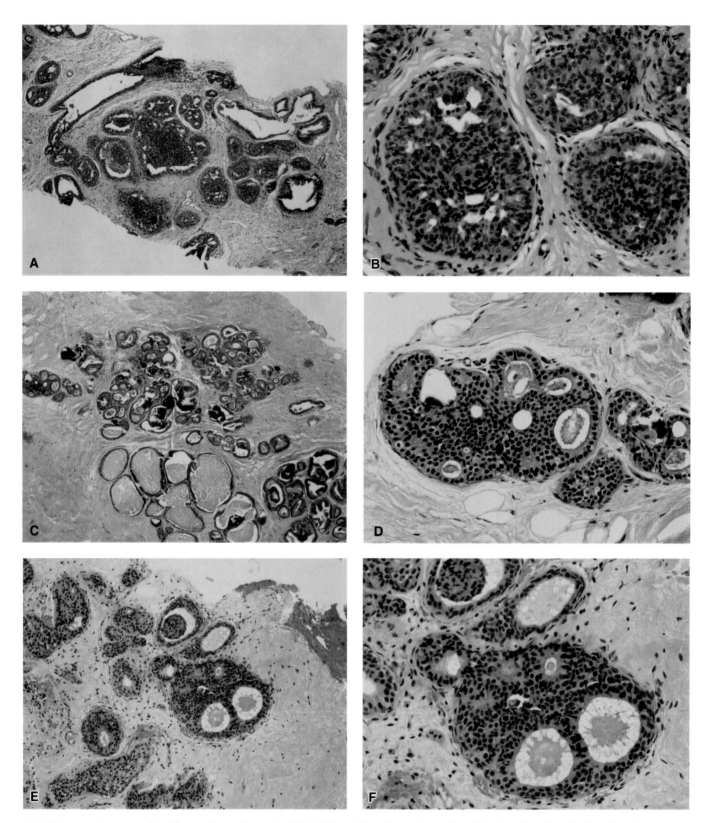

FIGURE 1.1 Spectrum of proliferative breast lesions in CNB. (A) Florid ductal hyperplasia. A proliferation of epithelial cells within ductal spaces leading to the formation of irregular slit-like spaces is noted. (B) Florid ductal hyperplasia. Higher magnification shows a heterogeneous population of cells with streaming and irregular, peripheral secondary lumens. (C) Ductal carcinoma in situ, cribriform type. A cribriform proliferation is noted with evenly placed, rounded "punched-out" spaces. (D) Ductal carcinoma in situ, cribriform type. Higher magnification shows cells with distinct cell membranes and minimal overlapping. There is cytologic monotony and uniformity. The spaces are round and uniform. (E) Atypical ductal hyperplasia. Atypical ductal hyperplasia meets some, but not all, of the criteria of DCIS. The proliferation involves only 1 duct, and the spaces appear more regular than that seen in florid ductal hyperplasia. (F) Atypical ductal hyperplasia. Higher magnification shows some cells with nuclear enlargement at the periphery, but the cells in the central portion of the duct show streaming of nuclei.

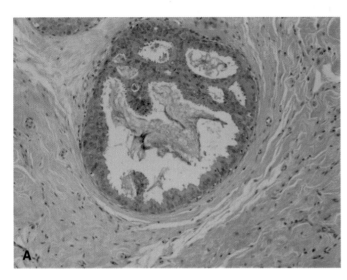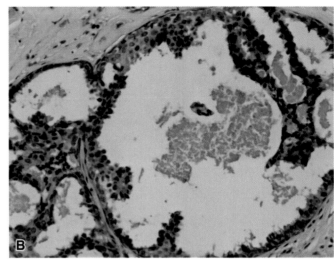

FIGURE 1.2 Difficulty in distinguishing ADH from DCIS in core biopsy. In core biopsy, the small amount of tissue obtained can make distinguishing ADH from DCIS challenging. Proliferations shown here that involve only 1 duct but show tufts (A) and micropapillae (B) are especially challenging.

variability in the pathologic diagnosis of ADH is widely recognized (4). The pathologic findings in UDH to DCIS occur on a spectrum with patterns that may overlap. Usual ductal hyperplasia has a heterogeneous population of cells, with cells streaming and secondary lumina that are irregular, slit-like, and often arranged at the periphery (Figure 1.1A, B). In DCIS, spaces are round and regular with a monotonous cell population (Figure 1.1C, D). Atypical ductal hyperplasia falls in the middle, with either uniform cells with irregular cell spaces or regular spaces

■ **Table 1.1** Comparative pathologic features among florid ductal hyperplasia, ADH, and low-grade DCIS

	Florid Ductal Epithelial Hyperplasia	ADH	Low-Grade DCIS
Definition	Increase in the number of cells above the normal 2 cell layer	Meets some but not all of the criteria of low-grade, non–comedo-type DCIS	Meets all of the criteria of low-grade, non–comedo-type DCIS
Architectural pattern	Streaming of nuclei, solid, papillary, bridging, and fenestrated patterns	Cribriform, micropapillary, papillary, columnar cell	Solid, cribriform, micropapillary
Cell placement	Uneven nuclear spacing, irregular peripherally placed spaces in a duct, parallel arrangements	Evenly spaced; second cell population of polarized columnar cells adjacent to the basement membrane	Evenly spaced; rigid bars with long axis of cells perpendicular to the long axis of the bar
Characteristic of spaces	Peripherally placed, irregular spaces in a duct	Bar crossing an entire space or 6–7 cells across	Rigid bars, secondary lumina with rounded, "punched out" spaces
Cytology	Irregularly shaped nuclei, nuclear overlap, inconspicuous nucleoli, infrequent mitotic figures, indistinct cell membranes	Uniform, regular oval, and round nuclei; cytologic uniformity and monotony or cytologic atypia with nuclear enlargement, hyperchromasia, and the presence of nucleoli; more prominent cell membranes	Cytologic uniformity and monotony, minimal overlapping of nuclei, distinct cell membranes
Extent		Involvement of only 1 duct that meets the criteria of low-grade DCIS	Involvement of 2 or more ducts
Size		<2 mm	≥2 mm

with heterogeneous cells (Figures 1.1E-F and 1.2A-B). The pathologic features distinguishing florid hyperplasia, atypical ductal carcinoma, and DCIS are summarized in Table 1.1.

Immunohistochemistry

The routine distinction of ADH from UDH and DCIS relies on the microscopic study of hematoxylin and eosin (H&E) stains without the use of immunohistochemistry. Although immunohistochemical staining may distinguish florid hyperplasia from ADH or DCIS, it has not been shown to be useful in distinguishing ADH from DCIS. Immunohistochemical staining with cytokeratin 5/6 (high-molecular-weight cytokeratin) shows positivity in the luminal epithelial cells in the majority of UDH (88%) but negativity in ADH (92%) (5). Caution must be exercised in the interpretation of this stain because apocrine metaplasia and columnar alterations also show a negative reaction.

Management Issues

Atypical ductal hyperplasia is encountered in percutaneous CNB in only 2% to 15% (6,7) of core biopsies. Surgical excision is the recommended management because 7% to 56% (8,9) of the cases diagnosed as ADH in CNB will be upgraded to DCIS or invasive carcinoma after excision. Underestimation is related to sampling error and is directly associated with the amount of tissue removed at biopsy. Underestimation rates are lower for 11-gauge VAB (10%–27%) (10,11) as compared with 14-gauge automated CNB (44%–56%) (12,13) due to the significant increase in volume of tissue obtained by using larger needles and vacuum assistance. Most cases of carcinoma found at excision are DCIS, with invasive carcinoma representing approximately 30%. Factors related to the underestimation of carcinoma in cases diagnosed as ADH in CNB are summarized in Table 1.2.

Key Points

- The pathologic diagnosis of ADH in CNB is difficult due to an inability to distinguish these lesions from low-grade DCIS in a limited sample obtained by core.
- Strict criteria should be followed to accurately diagnose ADH in CNB and avoid underdiagnosis or overdiagnosis.
- In a CNB in which the diagnosis falls between UDH and ADH, discussion of the cases at an intradepartmental conference or review by a second pathologist is also helpful, as surgical excision will not be recommended for diagnoses of UDH.

■ **Table 1.2** Factors related to the underestimation of carcinoma at surgical excision in cases diagnosed as ADH on percutaneous CNB

Size of core needle (smaller size needles [larger gauge] associated with greater underestimation)

Method of biopsy (automated vs VAB) (automated biopsy associated with greater underestimation)

No. of foci of ADH (2 or more associated with greater underestimation)

Incomplete removal of lesion by VAB

Larger lesion size (inadequate sampling due to large lesion size leads to greater underestimation)

Lower number of cores obtained at biopsy (inadequate sampling leads to underestimation)

Presence of a mass by palpation or on ultrasound

Personal history of breast cancer

- The finding of ADH in CNB warrants surgical excision, as the underestimation rate of carcinoma at surgical excision ranges from 7% to 56%.
- Immunohistochemical stains may be applied to differentiate these lesions in some cases; however, the diagnosis should be based primarily on the features identified on H&E stains.

■ PAPILLARY LESIONS

There are numerous challenges for the pathologist in diagnosing papillary lesions in general and specifically in CNB. Papillary lesions represent a spectrum of changes ranging from benign papillomas to atypical papillomas, to intraductal papillary carcinoma, and to invasive papillary carcinoma. Papillomas are often easily recognized by pathologists due to their fibrovascular cores lined by 2 cell layers: the inner myoepithelial cell layer and the outer layer of cuboidal or columnar epithelial cells (Figure 1.3A-D). Papillomas are single in approximately 50% of cases and present with nipple discharge in about 30%. Papillomas appear radiographically as an architectural distortion, as a density, or as a mass with or without associated microcalcification. Papillomas with atypia have an increased risk for the development of invasive breast cancer, similar to or even greater than those with ADH within the parenchyma of the breast (14).

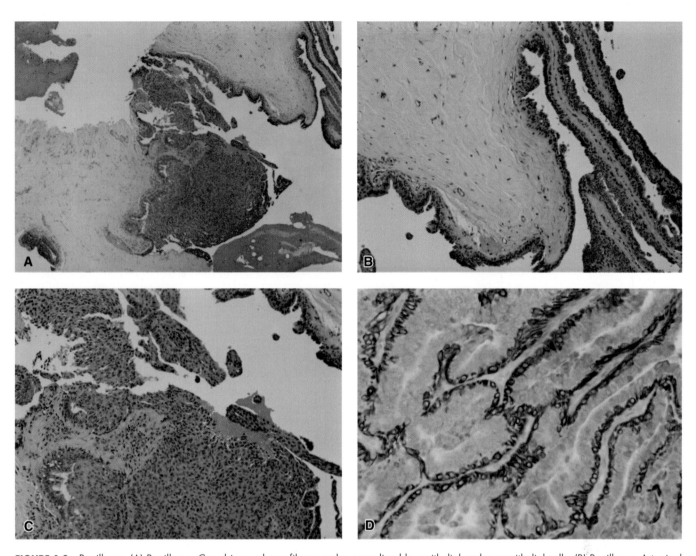

FIGURE 1.3 Papilloma. (A) Papilloma. Core biopsy shows fibrovascular cores lined by epithelial and myoepithelial cells. (B) Papilloma. A typical fibrovascular core is noted. (C) Papilloma with hyperplasia. Areas of hyperplasia become more complex and crowded; however, the cells are heterogeneous and lack atypia. (D) Papilloma (cytokeratin 5/6 stain). Immunohistochemical stain for cytokeratin 5/6 highlights the epithelial proliferation in this benign papilloma.

Pathologic Features

Core biopsies frequently represent a limited sample of the entire lesion. Difficulties arise in the categorization of papillary lesions as benign, atypical, or malignant. The pathologic features of the spectrum of papillary lesions are summarized in Table 1.3. Some papillomas have epithelial proliferations that fulfill the cytologic and architectural features of ADH or DCIS. Atypical papillomas show a monotonous cell population usually with a cribriform architecture. Ductal carcinoma in situ involving a papilloma is usually low grade and of the solid, cribriform, or micropapillary types (Figure 1.4A, B). Distinguishing a papilloma with ADH from one with DCIS can be demanding. Size and extent are used to distinguish atypical papillomas from papillomas with DCIS. On a sample obtained by core, size and extent are difficult to evaluate. Papillary lesions frequently fragment in CNB,

making interpretation difficult. Another issue is related to sampling; does the lesion diagnosed in core represent the most worrisome area in a papillary lesion? In papillomas with ADH, the foci of ADH comprise less than 25% of the papilloma, and thus, sampling by CNB is a concern (14). Another interpretative problem in papillary lesions in CNB is the potential confusion with invasive carcinoma, which can occur in both sclerosing and infarcted papillomas. In sclerosing papillomas, the fibrovascular cores may undergo sclerosis and distortion leading to entrapment of the epithelium that mimics a pseudoinvasive pattern (15) (Figure 1.5A, B). The presence of a myoepithelial layer (Figure 1.5C), a lack of cytologic atypia in the entrapped tubules, and the absence of invasion into interlobular fat help to distinguish this lesion from a carcinoma. In infarcted papillomas, fibrosis at the periphery of the lesion can also simulate invasive

■ Table 1.3 Comparative pathologic features among benign papilloma, atypical papilloma, papilloma with DCIS, and papillary DCIS

	Benign Papilloma	Atypical Papilloma	Papilloma With DCIS	Papillary DCIS
Architectural pattern	Papillary	Architectural pattern of ADH or DCIS (≤3 mm in size) or atypical population comprises between 10% and <33% of the lesion	Architectural pattern of DCIS (>3 mm in size) or atypical population involves at least a third but <90% of the lesion	
Presence of fibrovascular cores	Yes	Yes	Yes	Yes; may be obscured
Cellular components	Epithelial and myoepithelial; epithelial hyperplasia may be present	Epithelial; myoepithelial layer may be lost; focal ADH with monotonous cell proliferation	Epithelial; typically loss of myoepithelial cell layer	Epithelial only; no evidence of a preexisting benign papilloma
Atypia	Absent	Present; can be focal	Usually present; varying degrees	Usually present
Necrosis	Absent	Usually absent	May be present	May be present
				Single cell population with a uniform appearance; columnar cells with degrees of stratification; uniform cells in solid, cribriform or micropapillary patterns
Cytology	Heterogeneous	Monotonous	Monotonous	Monotonous
Myoepithelial cell layer	Present	Present in area of benign papilloma; reduced or absent in atypical area	Usually absent	Usually absent
Immunohistochemistry	CK 5/6 positive (Figure 1.3D)	Usually CK 5/6 negative in ADH	Usually CK 5/6 negative	CK 5/6 negative

carcinoma. The presence of clusters of squamous metaplastic cells surrounded by fibrotic tissue can also mimic an infiltrative process. The preservation of the papillary architecture in the areas of ischemic necrosis (necrosis in carcinomas usually lacks underlying architectural detail) and the lack of cytologic atypia within the entrapped ductules help in making the correct diagnosis (16). The careful attention to the histologic features and the use of myoepithelial cell markers aid in distinguishing these lesions from a carcinoma. Pathologic features distinguishing sclerotic and infarcted papillomas from invasive carcinomas are presented in Table 1.4.

Immunohistochemistry

The use of a panel that includes myoepithelial cells markers, high-molecular-weight cytokeratins, and neuroendocrine markers that have been shown to distinguish benign from malignant papillary proliferations (17) is summarized in Table 1.5.

Management Issues

The risk of the development of carcinoma has been shown to be largely local, in the region of the original papilloma supporting the recommendation of excision of all atypical

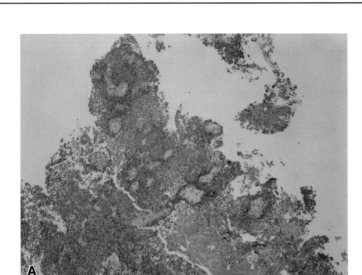
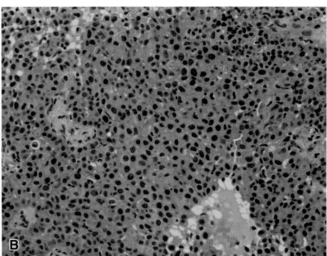

FIGURE 1.4 Papilloma with DCIS. (A) Papilloma with DCIS. A papillary proliferation is seen by the presence of fibrovascular cores. The epithelial proliferation shows a solid pattern of growth. Fragmentation of the cores is evident. (B) Papilloma with DCIS. Higher magnification shows the presence of fibrovascular cores surrounded by a solid proliferation of epithelial cells with nuclear atypia.

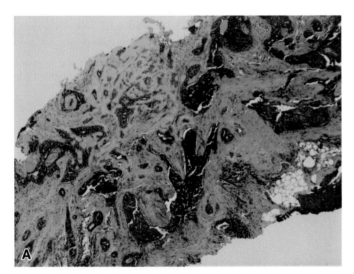
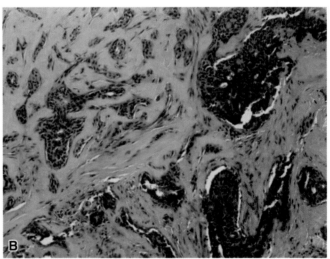
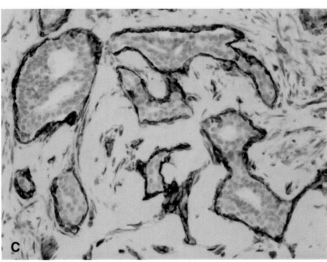

FIGURE 1.5 Distinguishing a sclerotic papilloma from invasive carcinoma. (A) Sclerosing papilloma. A sclerotic papilloma shows fibrovascular and fibrotic central cores that have entrapment of tubules making distinction from invasive carcinoma difficult. (B) Sclerosing papilloma. The entrapped tubules are embedded in poorly cellular stroma and contain a myoepithelial cell layer. (C) Sclerosing papilloma (calponin stain). A stain for calponin highlights the myoepithelial cell layer of the entrapped tubules and can be used to distinguish a sclerotic papilloma from an invasive carcinoma.

■ **Table 1.4** Comparative features to distinguish sclerosing papillomas and infarcted papillomas from invasive carcinomas

	Sclerosing Papilloma	Infarcted Papilloma
Architecture	Central fibrotic core with entrapment of distorted ductules; at the periphery, the sclerotic process merges with a benign papillary process	Ischemic necrosis is seen; however, outlines of the papilloma is preserved; peripheral area usually spared from ischemia
Stroma	Poorly cellular, sclerotic, hyalinized stroma; hemosiderin-laden macrophages and mononuclear cells may be present	Fibroblastic and collagenous proliferation with entrapment of compressed and distorted ductules
Ductules	Entrapped ductules contain a myoepithelial cell layer and lack atypia; ductules are confined to the core of the papilloma and extension of ductules into fat is not seen	Epithelium may show squamous metaplasia; hyperchromatic nuclei may be present but usually lacks cytologic atypia or mitotic figures
Myoepithelial cell marker	Positive in entrapped ductules	Positive in entrapped ductules

■ **Table 1.5** Immunohistochemical stains that aid in distinguishing benign from malignant papillary lesions

Cell Type	Cell Marker	Use
Myoepithelial cell marker	Smooth muscle actin, p63, calponin, S100 protein, CD10	Highlights myoepithelial cell layer in benign papillomas; decreased or absent in atypical papillomas and papillary carcinomas
Epithelial cell marker	High-molecular-weight cytokeratin, CK5/6, 34bE12, CK14	Positive in epithelial proliferations in benign papillomas; lacking in atypical papillomas and papillary DCIS
Neuroendocrine marker	Chromogranin A and synaptophysin	Negative in benign papillomas

- The presence of infarction and sclerosis should be considered before making a diagnosis of carcinoma.
- A panel of immunohistochemical stains utilizing myoepithelial markers, high-molecular-weight cytokeratins, and neuroendocrine markers can be used in the classification of papillary lesions.
- Atypical papillary lesions and papillary carcinoma in CNB warrant excision.
- Management of benign papillomas in CNB is controversial, but most studies recommend surgical excision.

papillomas. Multiplicity also increases the risk. Papillary lesions are encountered in percutaneous CNB, ranging from 0.01% to 8.1% of all core biopsies. Although the accepted recommendation for atypical papillary lesions and papillary carcinoma diagnosed in percutaneous CNB is excision, the management of benign papillary lesions remains controversial. The concern is that if excision is not performed, focal areas of ADH or DCIS may be missed in the small sample obtained by CNB. The literature pertaining to the diagnosis of benign papillary lesions in percutaneous CNB is limited; however, the incidence of carcinoma found after biopsy of a benign papillary lesion is wide, ranging from 0% to 29% (18,19). Most studies recommend excision of all papillary lesions diagnosed at percutaneous CNB due to the small but definite risk of malignancy at excision.

Key Points

- Papillary lesions in core biopsies are difficult to diagnose due to the tissue fragmentation and the sampling limitations.

■ LOBULAR LESIONS

Introduction

Both ALH and LCIS are considered risk factors for the development of carcinoma. The risk for the development of breast cancer is 4 to 5 times that of the general population for ALH and approximately 11 times for LCIS (20, 21). Lobular carcinoma in situ is often bilateral and multifocal and associated with an increased risk of invasive carcinoma of either breast. Recent genetic and molecular evidence have challenged the notion of LCIS as a risk factor but suggested that ALH and LCIS may be indolent precursors. Since most cases of LCIS are discovered as an incidental finding with no associated clinical or radiologic findings, the presence of LCIS rarely accounts for the primary histologic diagnosis after CNB. A multidisciplinary approach with radiologic correlation is critical when a diagnosis of LCIS or ALH is made in percutaneous CNB.

Pathologic Findings

Lobular carcinoma in situ consists of an intralobular proliferation of small uniform cells in which the abnormal cells must comprise all of the cells in the lobular unit with no intercellular spaces between cells and at least 50% of the acini in the lobular unit are distorted or expanded (Figure 1.6A, B). Atypical lobular hyperplasia has less than 50% of the affected lobule with the cytologic appearance of LCIS (Figure 1.6C). Classical and pleomorphic forms of LCIS are described in Table 1.6. The main difficulty for the pathologist is to distinguish pleomorphic LCIS from DCIS and to distinguish low-grade DCIS with cancerization of lobules from LCIS. Marked cellular pleomorphism in pleomorphic LCIS along with the presence of necrosis and calcification makes distinction from DCIS difficult. Radiographic correlation does not help in the distinction because the pleomorphic LCIS can be indistinguishable from DCIS. Cancerization of lobules, or spread of DCIS into lobules, creates lobular expansion and confusion with LCIS. The cells in LCIS are usually more dyscohesive and lack any microacinar pattern. The presence of intracytoplasmic vacuoles, although not specific, may be a clue to the diagnosis of LCIS. Pathologic features that can be used to distinguish low-grade DCIS from LCIS are summarized in Table 1.7. The distinction of LCIS from DCIS is critical because management of the patient with regard to the need to obtain negative margins at surgical excision (important for DCIS but not for LCIS) and

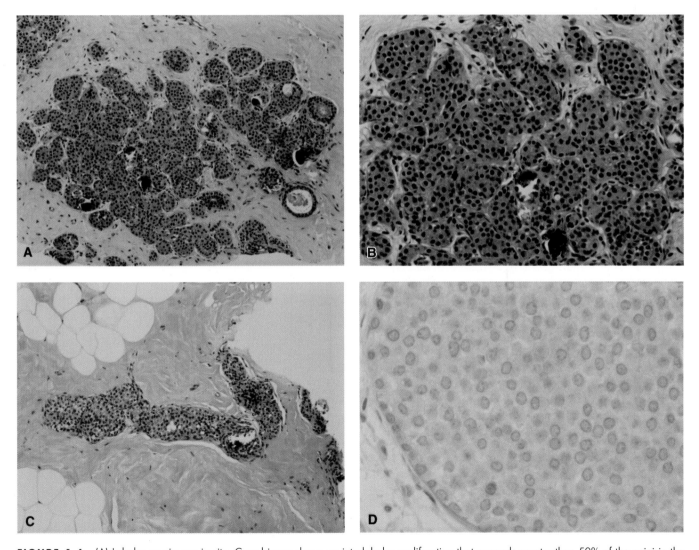

FIGURE 1.6 (A) Lobular carcinoma in situ. Core biopsy shows an intralobular proliferation that expands greater than 50% of the acini in the lobular unit. (B) Lobular carcinoma in situ. The intralobular proliferation is composed of small uniform cells with round nuclei and eosinophilic cytoplasm. (C) Atypical lobular hyperplasia. Atypical lobular hyperplasia shows a similar proliferation, but less than 50% of the acini in the lobular unit are distorted or expanded. (D) Lobular carcinoma in situ (E-cadherin stain). E-cadherin is negative in LCIS.

■ **Table 1.6** Comparative pathologic features between classical LCIS and pleomorphic LCIS (see Figure 1.7)

	Classical LCIS	Pleomorphic LCIS
Cell size	Small	Large
Nuclei	Uniform; round to oval	Pleomorphic; atypical
Cytoplasm	Small amount of clear to lightly eosinophilic	Abundant; eosinophilic, granular
Nucleoli	Inconspicuous	Conspicuous and large
Necrosis	Absent	Present
Microcalcification	Usually absent	Present
E-cadherin reactivity	Negative	Negative

■ **Table 1.7** Comparative features between LCIS and low-grade DCIS (see Figure 1.8)

	LCIS	Low-grade DCIS
Pattern	Mainly involves lobules; can involve ducts in a pagetoid fashion	Mainly involves ducts; can involve lobules (cancerization of lobules)
Cohesiveness of cells	Discohesive	Cohesive
Architecture	Mosaic pattern; solid	Microacinar pattern; cribriform, micro-papillary, solid
Cellular characteristics	Monotonous; intracyto-plasmic vacuoles common	Monotonous; more variability as compared with LCIS
Immunohistochemistry	E-cadherin negative	E-cadherin positive

the use of radiotherapy differs. Distinguishing DCIS from LCIS by microscopy alone can be extremely challenging, but fortunately, the use of E-cadherin immunohistochemistry (DCIS positive, LCIS negative) resolves most cases (Figure 1.6D).

Immunohistochemistry

The use of E-cadherin, a transmembrane glycoprotein involved in cell adhesion, is useful to distinguish DCIS from LCIS, as loss of expression is noted in LCIS and invasive lobular carcinomas. Although this marker has been shown to be extremely useful in distinguishing LCIS from DCIS in most cases, aberrant expression in LCIS has been described (22).

Management Issues

A diagnosis of ALH or LCIS in percutaneous CNB accounts for less than 2% of core biopsies in most series. Although ALH and LCIS identified at surgical excision are managed conservatively by clinical and radiologic follow-up, management guidelines for ALH and LCIS diagnosed at percutaneous CNB remain more controversial. Some studies find excision to be unnecessary, whereas most studies recommend surgical excision. There is a significant risk of approximately 13% for ALH and 20% for LCIS for finding carcinoma at surgical excision after a diagnosis of either ALH or LCIS in CNB (23). One study recommended excision if there was radiologic-pathologic discordance, if there was another high-risk lesion diagnosed by the CNB, or if there were overlapping pathologic features with DCIS (24). Most

retrospective studies comparing CNB diagnosis of ALH or LCIS and subsequent excision show selection bias, as surgery was not performed for all cases. Pleomorphic LCIS should be approached similar to DCIS. The finding of pleomorphic LCIS in core is associated with a much higher percentage (33%–60%) of invasive cancer at surgical excision (25).

Key Points

- A diagnosis of ALH or LCIS in most core biopsies is an incidental finding. Radiologic correlation with the pathologic findings is necessary to avoid missing a significant lesion.
- Distinguishing LCIS from ALH can be subjective because these lesions represent a continuum. This is less problematic in CNB because the management is the same.
- Pathologists must be able to distinguish LCIS with pagetoid spread from DCIS with cancerization of lobules in percutaneous CNB because management differs. Dyscohesive cells in a mosaic pattern and the presence of intracytoplasmic vacuoles should point toward a diagnosis of LCIS. E-cadherin immunohistochemistry can be particularly helpful in this distinction.

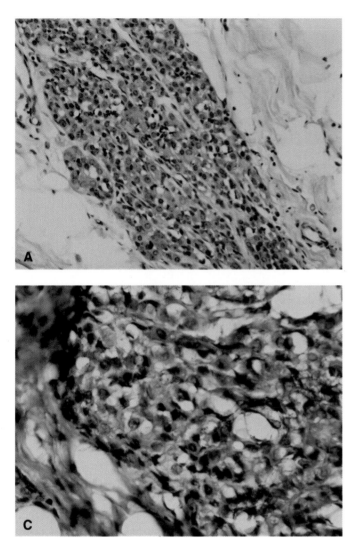

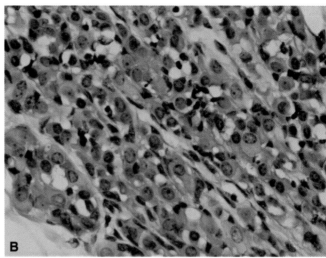

FIGURE 1.7 Pleomorphic LCIS. (A) Pleomorphic LCIS. This intralobular proliferation is composed of larger cells with pleomorphic nuclei and should be distinguished from DCIS. (B) Pleomorphic LCIS. Pleomorphic nuclei with large, conspicuous nucleoli are noted. (C) Pleomorphic LCIS (E-cadherin). An E-cadherin stain is negative, confirming LCIS.

- Pleomorphic LCIS can be confused with DCIS. It is important to recognize this variant due to its more aggressive course and differing treatment. Distinguishing DCIS from pleomorphic LCIS may be impossible by microscopy alone and may require E-cadherin staining for definitive diagnosis.
- Immunohistochemical staining with E-cadherin can be used to help distinguish DCIS (positive) from LCIS (negative).
- Most studies recommend surgical excision after a diagnosis of ALH or LCIS in CNB, as the underestimation rate of carcinoma is 13% and 20%, respectively (mean).

■ FIBROEPITHELIAL LESIONS

Pathologic Findings

Although there should be no difficulty separating a malignant phyllodes tumor (PT) from a fibroadenoma,

the distinction of low-grade phyllodes tumor from fibroadenoma in CNB can be problematic due to overlapping histologic features. The histologic distinction of a phyllodes tumor from a fibroadenoma is based on the evaluation of several parameters noted in Table 1.8: stromal cellularity, infiltrative/pushing borders, presence of a leaf-like pattern with stromal overgrowth, atypia, mitotic figures, pleomorphism, and necrosis; these may all be lacking in CNB. Pathologists often encounter problems in separating cellular fibroadenoma from phyllodes tumor due to a variety of issues noted in Table 1.9. Stromal overgrowth (×10 field with no epithelium), fragmentation of the cores, and adipose tissue within stroma are helpful in distinguishing a phyllodes tumor from a fibroadenoma in CNB (26).

Immunohistochemistry

There are no reliable immunohistochemical stains to distinguish a phyllodes tumor from a fibroadenoma. Ki-67 has been used to show proliferative activity and usually

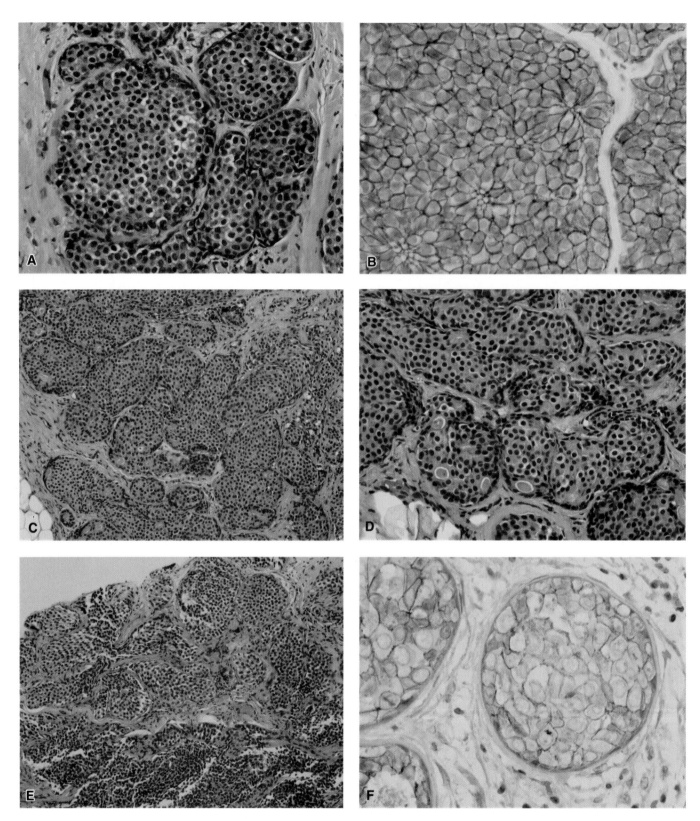

FIGURE 1.8 Distinguishing LCIS from DCIS. (A) Low-grade DCIS. In this core biopsy, there is an intralobular proliferation of discohesive uniform cells that mimic LCIS. (B) Low-grade DCIS (E-cadherin). Membranous positivity for E-cadherin categorizes this lesion as DCIS, solid type. (C) Low-grade DCIS. A monotonous proliferation distends ducts and acini. (D) Low-grade DCIS. Focally, a microacinar pattern is seen, a feature indicative of low-grade DCIS. (E) DCIS. Cancerization of lobules by DCIS can mimic LCIS. (F) DCIS (E-cadherin). Membranous positivity for E-cadherin categorizes this lesion as DCIS.

■ **Table 1.8** Comparative pathologic features between cellular fibroadenomas and phyllodes tumors (Figure 1.9)

	Cellular Fibroadenoma	Low-Grade Phyllodes Tumors
Margins on microscopy	Well circumscribed	More often circumscribed than infiltrative
Stromal atypia	None	Minimal
Stromal proliferation	Yes	Yes (×10 field with no epithelium)
Epithelial lined clefts—epithelium at edge of tissue fragments	Usually absent or less prominent	Present
Stromal cellularity	Heterogeneous	Heterogeneous; periductal condensation
Mitotic activity	Absent	Minimal to none

has higher proliferation indices in phyllodes tumor as compared with fibroadenoma (27).

Management Issues

A definitive diagnosis of phyllodes tumor should rarely be made in CNB. In a series of 23 patients with a phyllodes tumor at surgical excision, the CNB diagnosis was fibroadenoma in 3 or benign in 6 (28), giving a false-negative rate of 39%. Fifty-two percent were diagnosed as equivocal for phyllodes tumor, and only 9% were definitively diagnosed as phyllodes tumor in core. In summary, fibroepithelial lesions with increased stromal cellularity in percutaneous CNB should be excised to exclude a phyllodes tumor.

Key Points

- The definitive diagnosis of phyllodes tumors should rarely be made in CNB.

  It is best to diagnose these lesions as fibroepithelial lesions with cellular stroma and recommend excision.
- The heterogeneous nature of the stromal cellularity, the lack of atypia and mitotic figures, and the absence of infiltrating margins in core biopsy make distinguishing benign phyllodes tumors from cellular fibroadenomas in core biopsy difficult.

■ **Table 1.9** Problems in distinguishing benign phyllodes tumors from fibroadenomas in CNB

- Fragmentation of cores with cystic spaces between cores mimicking leaf-like architecture
- Stromal hypercellularity is heterogeneous and variable and may be missed by sampling
- Lack of atypia and mitotic activity in low-grade phyllodes tumors
- Lack of distinguishing radiographic features

■ RADIAL SCAR

Pathologic Findings

Radial scar (RS) is characterized histologically by a fibroelastotic core surrounded by radiating ducts and lobules with various amounts of ectasia, epithelial hyperplasia, and adenosis. Radiographically and pathologically, it is difficult to distinguish a radial scar from a carcinoma due to its stellate configuration. Some data suggest that radial scar may be an independent risk factor for the development of breast carcinoma (29). One study that looked at carcinomas in radial scars showed that the carcinoma was most often found at the periphery of the radial scar at excision, an important issue to consider when sampling by CNB (30). Core needle biopsy for these lesions is problematic due to the potential for sampling error and the possible confusion with invasive carcinoma on the histologic assessment of limited samples. The presence of tubules surrounded by areas of fibrosis can also be seen in tubular carcinoma and all types of adenosis, especially sclerosing adenosis. The ductules of a radial scar are entrapped in the fibroelastotic core and may simulate invasive carcinoma, especially tubular carcinoma. Sclerosing adenosis should also be included in the differential. Sclerosing adenosis shows a disordered proliferation of acinar and ductal epithelial cells, myoepithelial cells, and intralobular stroma that result in expansion and distortion of lobules. The lobulocentric nature of the process is helpful in making the correct diagnosis. Pathologic features that aid in distinguishing radial scar, tubular carcinoma, and sclerosing adenosis are summarized in Table 1.10.

Immunohistochemistry

The presence of a myoepithelial cell layer either on H&E stain or by immunohistochemistry (p63, calponin, or smooth muscle actin (SMA)) should help to exclude a tubular carcinoma. Myoepithelial markers can also highlight the myoepithelial cell layer in sclerosing adenosis.

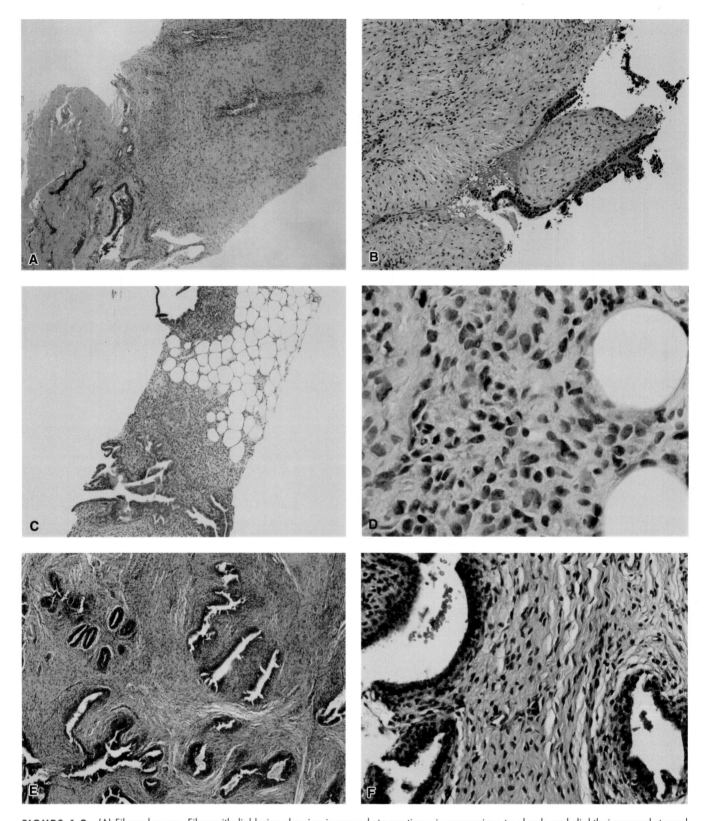

FIGURE 1.9 (A) Fibroadenoma. Fibroepithelial lesion showing increased stroma tissue in comparison to glands and slightly increased stromal cellularity. This lesion was thought to be a phyllodes tumor (PT) in core biopsy. Excisional biopsy showed fibroadenoma. (B) Fibroadenoma. Higher power shows detached stromal fragment with a leaf-like architecture. (C) Phyllodes tumor. This phyllodes tumor displays cellular stroma infiltrating fat. (D) Phyllodes tumor. The stromal cells are mild to moderately atypical, and rare mitotic figures are seen. (E) Cellular fibroadenoma. Cellular fibroadenoma displaying increased stromal cellularity. (F) Cellular fibroadenoma. On higher power, stromal cells do not display any atypia or mitosis.

■ **Table 1.10** Comparative pathologic features among radial scar, tubular carcinoma, and sclerosing adenosis

	Radial Scar (Figure 1.10A-C)	Tubular Carcinoma (Figure 1.11A-C)	Sclerosing Adenosis (Figure 1.11D-F)
Pattern	Infiltrative	Infiltrative	Lobulocentric
Tubules	Elongated flattened tubules with slit-like spaces	Angulated tubules with wide lumina; teardrop in shape	Distorted acini and tubules with compressed lumina
Tubule lining	Lined by normal appearing ductal epithelial cells	Lining epithelial cells are larger than normal ductal cells with apocrine snouts	Lined by normal appearing ductal cells
Stroma	Fibroelastotic; sclerotic	Desmoplastic	Sclerotic
Myoepithelial cell layer	Present	Absent	Present

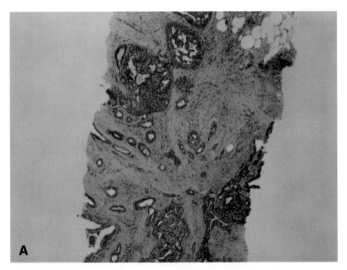

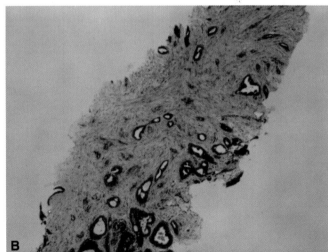

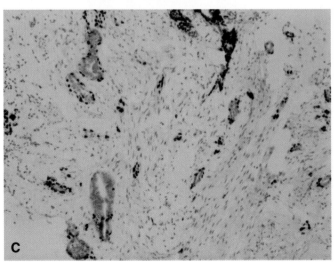

FIGURE 1.10 (A) Radial scar. A radial scar shows a fibroelastotic core surrounded by radiating ducts. Some ducts show epithelial hyperplasia. (B) Radial scar. Entrapment of tubules with the fibroelastotic stroma can cause confusion with invasive carcinoma. (C) Radial scar (p63, ×20). A p63 stain highlights the myoepithelial cell layer and distinguishes this lesion from an invasive carcinoma.

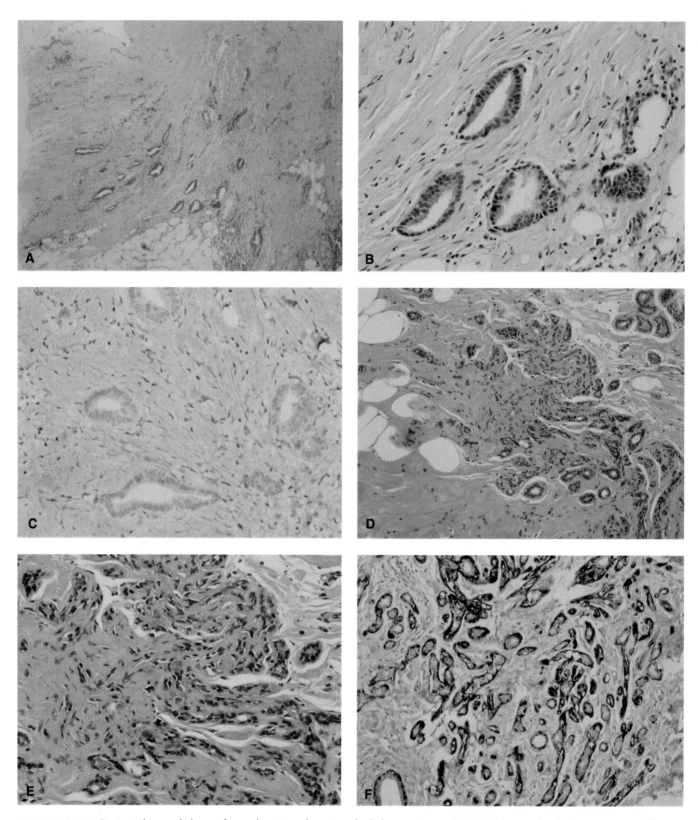

FIGURE 1.11 Distinguishing radial scars from sclerosing adenosis and tubular carcinoma. (A) Radial scar with tubular carcinoma. Infiltrative angulated glands are embedded in desmoplastic stroma. Note the central fibrotic scar. (B) Tubular carcinoma. The angulated tubules show wide lumina and show lining epithelial cells with apocrine snouts. (C) Tubular carcinoma (calponin stain). Calponin staining shows a lack of myoepithelial cells. (D) Sclerosing adenosis. Distorted tubules and acini are arranged in a lobulocentric pattern. (E) Sclerosing adenosis. Distorted tubules, many with compressed lumina, are embedded in a sclerotic stroma. (F) Sclerosing adenosis (calponin stain). Calponin staining highlights the myoepithelial cell layer surrounding the tubules.

■ **Table 1.11** Differential diagnosis of CNB with extravasated mucin (Figure 1.12)

	Fibrocystic Change	Benign Mucocele-Like Lesion	Mucinous Carcinoma
Epithelial component	Dilated ducts and cysts	Multiple cysts lined by flattened or cuboidal epithelium	Well-differentiated tumor cells (low grade) with lack of myoepithelial cells
Mucinous component	Cysts contain mucin; may have extravasation into stroma	Extravasated mucin into stroma; usually acellular mucin; may contain macrophages	Epithelial cells floating in mucin; thin walled capillaries can be noted

Management Issues

Most authors recommend surgical excision when the imaging findings are compatible with a radial scar, and thus, there are only a limited number of studies pertaining to the use of CNB in the diagnosis of radial scars. Up to 40% of the cases diagnosed as radial scar at percutaneous biopsy in one series (31) showed carcinoma at excision. Another study (32) evaluated 43 lesions diagnosed as radial scar by CNB and found, at surgical excision, radial scar in 63%, radial scar with ADH in 18%, radial scar associated with carcinoma in 12%, and only carcinoma in 7%. Although a recent study suggested that mammographic follow-up was possible for radial scars diagnosed in CNB provided there was no associated ADH, DCIS, or LCIS (33), the paucity of the data makes this recommendation controversial. The standard current recommended management is surgical excision for radial scars diagnosed by percutaneous CNB.

Key Points

- Difficulty in diagnosis in CNB is due to sampling error and inability to distinguish from invasive carcinoma.
- The use of a panel of myoepithelial markers may help distinguish radial scar (RS) from other lesions including invasive carcinoma.
- It is important to examine the periphery of RS for the presence of an associated lesion.
- Most studies recommend surgical excision for cases diagnosed as radial scar in CNB due to the small but significant chance of finding carcinoma at excision.

■ MUCINOUS LESIONS

Pathologic Findings

The presence of mucin can be seen in a variety of breast lesions from fibrocystic change, to mucocele-like lesions, to colloid carcinoma highlighted in Table 1.11. Mucocele-like lesions are characterized by multiple cystic spaces lined by flattened nonatypical epithelium and spillage of mucin into the stroma (34). Mucocele-like lesions need to be distinguished from mucinous carcinoma especially when epithelial cells are seen floating within the mucin. This may be difficult on the limited material obtained in CNB. Another issue is the finding of extravasated mucin only in CNB. In this situation, surgical excision is warranted to rule out a mucinous carcinoma. Mucinous carcinomas with a micropapillary pattern have been described with poor prognosis.

Management Issues

Only a few series have studied mucinous lesions in CNB (35–38). Most indicate that mucinous lesions can be accurately diagnosed by CNB; however, given the limited data, the exact role for surgical excision remains controversial. The mucocele-like lesions are more problematic due to their known association with ADH or carcinoma at excision (39) and the potential for sampling error with CNB. Surgical excision is the current recommended management for mucocele-like lesions diagnosed in percutaneous CNB. It is unclear what the recommended management should be when extravasted mucin is identified in core from ruptured cysts in cases of fibrocystic change.

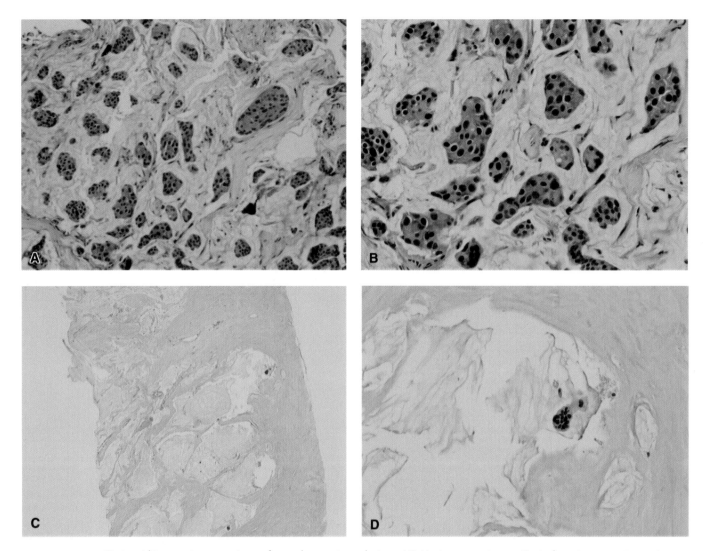

FIGURE 1.12 Distinguishing mucinous carcinoma from other mucinous lesions. (A) Mucinous carcinoma. Typical mucinous carcinoma in core biopsy shows tumor cells floating in mucin. (B) Mucinous carcinoma. The tumor cells are usually well differentiated with small nuclei and prominent nucleoli. (C) Mucinous carcinoma. Some mucinous carcinomas show a predominance of mucin in core biopsy. (D) Mucinous carcinoma. Rare cohesive clusters of malignant cells may be seen but could be missed by core biopsy sampling.

Key Points

- Extracellular mucin can be noted in percutaneous CNB in fibrocystic change, mucocele-like lesions, and mucinous carcinoma.
- It is prudent to recommend surgical excision for the finding of extracellular mucin and mucocele-like lesions in CNB.

of these lesions is also difficult due to the small series reported in the literature and the retrospective nature of most studies. Prospective studies are needed to clearly evaluate the true significance of these lesions in percutaneous CNB. Until then, surgical excision must be recommended for any lesion diagnosed in percutaneous CNB that has even a remote chance of finding carcinoma at surgical excision.

■ CHAPTER SUMMARY

The above-described lesions can be difficult to diagnose by CNB due to the limited sample obtained and the overlapping of features with other entities. The management

■ REFERENCES

1.   Lennington WJ, Jensen RA, Dalton LW, et al. Ductal carcinoma in situ of the breast: heterogeneity of individual lesions. Cancer. 1994;73:118–124.

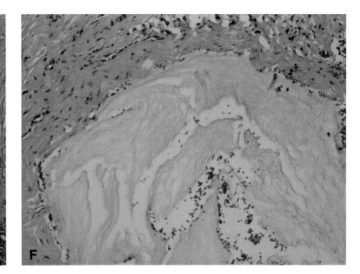

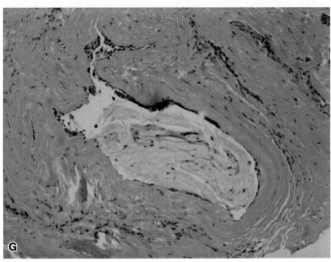

FIGURE 1.12 *(Continued)* (E) Mucocele-like lesion. Mucocele-like lesions show dilated spaces filled with extravasated mucin. (F) Mucocele-like lesion. The spaces may lack an epithelial lining. (G) Mucin extravasation in fibrocystic change. This case shows both extravasted mucin and a dilated cyst with a flattened or low cuboidal epithelial layer filled with mucin. Excisional biopsy showed only fibrocystic changes.

2. Page DL, Rogers LW. Combined histologic and cytologic criteria for the diagnosis of mammary atypical ductal hyperplasia. *Hum Pathol.* 1992;23:1095–1097.

3. Tavassoli FA, Norris HJ. A comparison of the results of long-term follow-up for atypical intraductal hyperplasia and intraductal hyperplasia of the breast. *Cancer.* 1990;65:518–529.

4. Schnitt SJ, Connelly JL, Tavassoli FA, et al. Interobserver variability in the diagnosis of ductal proliferative breast lesions using standardized criteria. *Am J Surg Pathol.* 1992;16:1133–1143.

5. Otterbach F, Bankfalvi A, Bergner S, et al. Cytokeratin 5/6 immunohistochemistry assists the differential diagnosis of atypical proliferations of the breast. *Histopathology.* 2000;37:232–240.

6. Ko E, Han W, Lee JW, et al. Scoring system for predicting malignancy in patients diagnosed with atypical ductal hyperplasia at ultrasound-guided core needle biopsy. *Breast Cancer Res Treat.* 2008;112:189–195.

7. Eby PR, Ochsner JE, DeMartini WB, Allison KH, Peacock S, Lehman CD. Is surgical excision necessary for focal atypical ductal hyperplasia found at stereotactic vacuum assisted breast biopsy? *Ann Surg Oncol.* 2008;15:545–550.

8. Sneige N, Lim SC, Whitman GJ, et al. Atypical ductal hyperplasia diagnosis by directional vacuum-assisted stereotactic biopsy of breast microcalcifications. Considerations for surgical excision. *Am J Clin Pathol.* 2003;119:248–253.

9. Meyer JE, Smith DN, Lester SC, et al. Large-needle CNB: nonmalignant breast abnormalities evaluated with surgical excision or repeat CNB. *Radiology.* 1998;206:717–720.

10. Liberman L, Smolkin JH, Dershaw DD, et al. Calcification retrieval at stereotactic, 11-gauge,

directional, vacuum-assisted breast biopsy. *Radiology.* 1998;208:251–260.

11. Plantade R, Hammou JC, Fighiera M, et al. Underestimation of breast carcinoma with 11-gauge stereotactically guided directional vacuum-assisted biopsy. *J Radiol.* 2004;85:391–401.

12. Darling ML, Smith DN, Lester SC, et al. Atypical ductal hyperplasia and ductal carcinoma in situ as revealed by large-core needle breast biopsy: results of surgical excision. *AJR Am J Roentgenol.* 2000;175:1341–1346.

13. Jackman RJ, Nowels KW, Shepard MJ, et al. Stereotaxic large-core needle biopsy of 450 nonpalpable breast lesions with surgical correlation in lesions with cancer or atypical hyperplasia. *Radiology.* 1994;193:91–95.

14. Page DL, Salhany KE, Jensen RA, et al. Subsequent breast carcinoma risk after biopsy with atypia in a breast papilloma. *Cancer.* 1996;78:258–266.

15. Fenoglio C, Lattes R. Sclerosing papillary proliferations in the female breast. A benign lesion often mistaken for carcinoma. *Cancer.* 1974;63:691–700.

16. Flint A, Oberman HA. Infarction and squamous metaplasia of intraductal papilloma: a benign breast lesion that may simulate carcinoma. *Hum Pathol.* 1984;15:764–767.

17. Moritani S, Ichihara S, Kushima R, et al. Myoepithelial cells in solid variant of intraductal papillary carcinoma of the breast: a potential diagnostic pitfall and a proposal of an immunohistochemical panel in the differential diagnosis with intraductal papilloma with usual ductal hyperplasia Virchows Arch. 2007;450:539–547.

18. Bazzocchi M, Berra I, Francescutti GE, et al. Papillary lesions of the breast: diagnostic imaging and contribution of percutaneous needle biopsy with 14 g needle. *Radiol Med.* 2001;101:424–431.

19. Tseng HS, Chen YL, Chen ST, et al. The management of papillary lesion of the breast by core needle biopsy. Eur J Surg Oncol. 2009;35:21–24.

20. Page DL, Kidd TE Jr, Dupont WD, et al. Lobular neoplasia of the breast: higher risk for subsequent invasive cancer predicted by more extensive disease. *Hum Pathol.* 1991;22:1232–1239.

21. Page DL, Dupont WD, Rogers LW, et al. Atypical hyperplastic lesions of the female breast: a long-term follow-up study of cancer risk. Cancer. 1985;55:2698–2708.

22. Da Silva L, Parry S, Reid L, et al. Aberrant expression of E-cadherin in lobular carcinomas of the breast. *Am J Surg Pathol.* 2008;32:773–783.

23. Cangiarella J, Guth A, Axelrod D, et al. Is surgical excision necessary for the management of atypical lobular hyperplasia (ALH) and lobular carcinoma in-situ (LCIS) diagnosed on core needle biopsy? A report of 38 cases and review of the literature. *Arch Pathol Lab Med.* 2008;132:979–983.

24. Liberman L, Sama M, Susnik B, et al. Lobular carcinoma in situ at percutaneous breast biopsy: surgical biopsy findings. *AJR Am J Roentgenol.* 1999;173:291–299.

25. Lavoue V, Graesslin O, Classe JM, et al. Management of lobular neoplasia diagnosed by core needle biopsy: study of 52 biopsies with follow-up surgical excision. *Breast.* 2007;16:533–539.

26. Lee AH, Hodi Z, Ellis IO, et al. Histological features useful in the distinction of phyllodes tumour and fibroadenoma on needle CNB of the breast. *Histopathology.* 2007;51:336–344.

27. Yohe S, Yeh IT. "Missed" diagnoses of phyllodes tumor on breast biopsy: pathologic clues to its recognition. *Int J Surg Pathol.* 2008;16:137–142.

28. Dillon MF, Quinn CM, McDermott EW, et al. Needle CNB in the diagnosis of phyllodes neoplasm. *Surgery.* 2006;140:779–784.

29. Jacobs TW, Byrne C, Colditz G, et al. Radial scars in benign breast biopsy specimens and the risk of cancer. *N Engl J Med.* 1999;340:430–436.

30. Sloane JP, Mayers MM. Carcinoma and atypical hyperplasia in radial scars and complex sclerosing lesions: importance of lesion size and patient age. *Histopathology.* 1993;23:225–231.

31. Jackman RJ, Kowels KW, Rodriguez-Soto J, et al. Stereotactic, automated large-core needle biopsy of non-palpable breast lesions: false negative and histologic underestimation rates after long term follow-up. *Radiology.* 1999;210:799–805.

32. Lopez-Medina A, Cintora E, Mugica B, et al. Radial scars diagnosed at stereotactic core-needle biopsy: surgical biopsy findings. *Eur Radiol.* 2006;16:1803–1810.

33. Cawson JN, Malara F, Kavanagh A, et al. Fourteen gauge needle CNB of mammographically evident radial scars. Is excision necessary? *Cancer.* 2003;97:345–351.

34. Rosen PP. Mucocele-like tumors of the breast. *Am J Surg Pathol.* 1986;10:464–469.

35. Renshaw AA. Can mucinous lesions of the breast be reliably diagnosed by core needle biopsy? *Am J Clin Pathol.* 2002;118:82–84.

36. Wang J, Simsir A, Mercado C, Cangiarella J. Can core biopsy reliably diagnose mucinous lesions of the breast? *Am J Clin Pathol.* 2007;127:124–127.

37. Carder PJ, Murphy CE, Liston JC. Surgical excision is warranted following a core biopsy diagnosis of mucocele-like lesion of the breast. *Histopathology.* 2004;45:148–154.

38. Lam WW, Chu WC, Tse GM, Ma TK, Tang AP. Role of fine needle aspiration and tru cut biopsy in diagnosis of mucinous carcinoma of breast—from a radiologist's perspective. *Clin Imaging.* 2006;30:6–10.

39. Ro JY, Sneige N, Sahin AA, et al. Mucocelelike tumor of the breast associated with atypical ductal hyperplasia or mucinous carcinoma: a clinicopathologic study of seven cases. *Arch Pathol Lab Med.* 1991;115:137–140.

2

Morphologic Precursors of Mammary Carcinoma and Their Mimics

EDI BROGI

ADRIANA D. CORBEN

MELISSA P. MURRAY

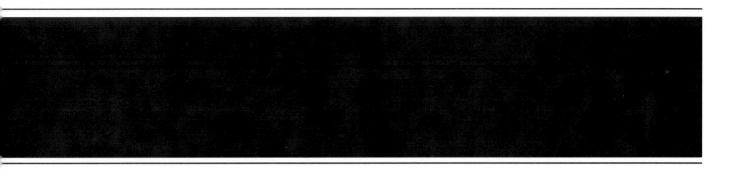

It is well established that ductal carcinoma in situ (DCIS) and atypical ductal hyperplasia (ADH) are nonobligate morphologic precursors of invasive mammary carcinoma. Lobular carcinoma in situ (LCIS) and atypical lobular hyperplasia (ALH), together referred to as lobular neoplasia (LN), have been traditionally regarded as high-risk lesions, but current evidence indicates that they also constitute nonobligate precursors of invasive breast carcinoma. Unusual variants of LCIS characterized by necrosis and/or marked cytologic atypia have been identified recently. They are also regarded as precursors of invasive carcinoma, but more aggressive than classic LN. Clinical follow-up information on these tumors is very limited, and their management is not standardized.

In this chapter, we review the above-mentioned precursors of invasive mammary carcinoma and highlight features helpful in the differential diagnosis with their morphologic mimics. We also discuss briefly the clinical implications of these lesions for patient management.

■ ATYPICAL DUCTAL HYPERPLASIA

Morphology

The diagnosis of ADH is essentially a diagnosis of exclusion rather than based on positive criteria and designates a proliferation with many, but not all, of the features of low-grade DCIS (LG-DCIS) (Figure 2.1). The atypical cells are slightly enlarged compared with normal ductal cells and have more abundant cytoplasm, which is often pale pink or amphophilic. Cell borders are well defined. Nuclei are also slightly enlarged compared with those of normal ductal cells and have a smooth and regular outline, with pale, homogeneous, and fine chromatin. Nucleoli are usually absent or punctiform. Most of the cells are polarized and show minimal to no maturation across the duct, from its periphery toward the lumen. The atypical proliferation does not involve the entire cross section of the duct, but displays only focal architectural complexity, with formation of abortive cribriform spaces, trabecular bars, and Roman arches or micropapillae. Cytologically, the cells comprising ADH and LG-DCIS are very similar to identical, and the distinction between the two lesions rests for most part on quantitative criteria, including number of involved ducts (ADH is limited to one or two) (1) and size (ADH spans <2 mm) (2). Interobserver variability in the diagnosis of ADH versus LG-DCIS has been reported (3),

but following specific diagnostic criteria has been shown to greatly improve diagnostic consistency (4). As a rule of thumb, when the differential diagnosis of ADH and DCIS is considered, the former should be favored (5).

Differential Diagnosis of ADH

Low-Grade DCIS

The distinction between ADH and LG-DCIS is based on extent of the lesion. Low-grade DCIS involves the entire cross section of a few ducts and shows complex and regular architecture. The neoplastic cells uniformly display low-grade nuclear atypia, with regularly arranged monotonous nuclei and finely granular chromatin. (Table 1.1 in the core biopsy chapter summarizes some of the morphologic features that can be useful in the differential diagnosis of ADH and LG-DCIS. See also paragraph and images of LG-DCIS in this chapter.)

Usual Ductal Hyperplasia

Usual ductal hyperplasia (UDH) consists of a haphazard and cohesive non-neoplastic ductal epithelial proliferation and can be part of fibrocystic changes or involve other lesions such as papilloma or radial scar. The UDH cells variably fill the duct lumen, which is often reduced to few peripheral cleft-like fenestrations lined by nonpolarized

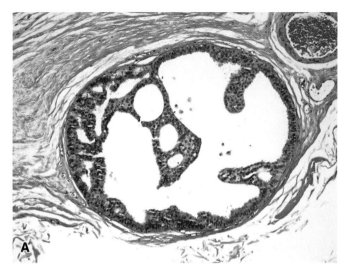
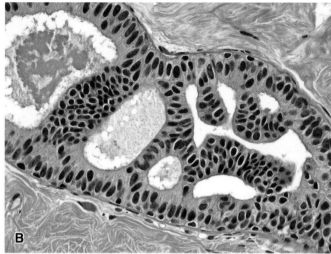

FIGURE 2.1 Atypical ductal hyperplasia. (A) An atypical ductal proliferation consists of fairly monotonous cells showing slight cytologic atypia and focal complex and regular architecture but does not occupy the full cross section of involved ducts. (B) Polarized cells line the neoformed lumina.

ductal cells. In florid UDH, the ductal lumen is occupied by a solid proliferation that can rarely show central necrosis in the context of a radial sclerosing lesion, nipple duct adenoma, or juvenile papillomatosis. UDH cells are haphazardly arranged and tightly cohesive with indistinct cell borders ("syncytial" aggregates) (Figure 2.2). The cells located toward the center of the duct lumen are nonpolarized, flattened, and spindled, with a central nucleus that abuts the duct lumen. Cells located in the center of the duct often line up parallel to one another along its length (so called "streaming"). The micropapillae of UDH are stubby and have a jagged and irregular outline, features that help to differentiate them from the micropapillae of ADH/LG-DCIS (see Table 2.1). The nuclei of UDH vary slightly in size and shape and do not show specific orientation. The nuclear membrane is slightly irregular and often shows longitudinal grooves, indentations, and intranuclear inclusions. As UDH cells "mature" from the periphery of a duct toward its center, they become smaller, with scant dense cytoplasm and darker and indistinct nuclear chromatin.

Myoepithelial cells are typically scattered throughout UDH. Their presence among ductal cells supports the diagnosis of UDH in benign but morphologically ambiguous ductal proliferations that simulate DCIS. The use of immunoperoxidase stains for basal cytokeratins (CK5/6 and 34βE12) can also help in the differential diagnosis of UDH from ADH and LG-DCIS; however, results of

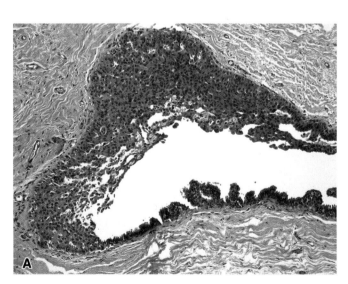
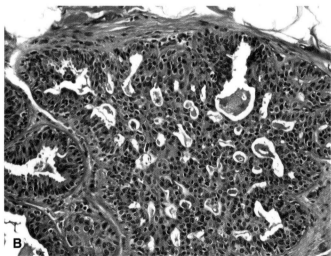

FIGURE 2.2 Usual ductal hyperplasia. Hyperplastic ductal cells are haphazardly arranged. Cell borders are indistinct and the nuclei are small with dense chromatin. (A) The micropapillae of UDH show cell maturation from the periphery toward the lumen of the duct. (B) The pseudocribriform fenestrations of UDH are lined by nonpolarized cells.

■ **Table 2.1** UDH with micropapillae versus micropapillary LG-DCIS

	UDH	MP-DCIS, Low Grade
Micropapillae		
Spacing along the duct	Irregular	Regular
Outline	Frayed and irregular	Smooth
Symmetry	Asymmetric	Symmetric
Base	Wide	Narrow
Club shape	Absent	Common
Height/width ratio	1:2	3:1 or more
Cell maturation	Present	Absent
Fibrovascular cores	Absent to focally present	Absent (by definition)
Adjacent DCIS (often cribriform)	Not present	May be present
Adjacent columnar cell changes with or without atypia	Not characteristic	Common
Cytology		
Cytoplasm	Normal to scant	Slightly abundant
Nuclear/ cytoplasmic ratio	Normal or low	Increased
Nuclear size	×1–×1.5 red blood cell	×1.5–×2.5 red blood cell
Nuclear chromatin	Irregular, indistinct	Homogenous to dense
Nuclear hyperchromasia	Absent	Present
Nucleoli	Small, inconspicuous	Absent to rare

immunoperoxidase studies should be used only to support a morphologic impression and can never replace it (see also chapter on immunohistochemistry).

Partial Involvement of Acini or UDH by LN Can Mimic ADH or UDH

Partial involvement of acini by LN is uncommon. In this scenario, lobular neoplastic cells surround a preserved acinar lumen lined by native polarized ductal cells. In another scenario, a focus of UDH is peripherally infiltrated by lobular neoplastic cells. These arrangements can be misinterpreted as ADH because low-grade nuclear atypia is present in some of the cells, or can be overlooked as focal UDH showing maturation toward the center of the acinus/duct. The correct diagnostic interpretation rests on the identification of two admixed cell populations. The UDH cells show no cytologic atypia and are usually crowded in the center of the duct, whereas LN cells show low-grade atypia, are round to ovoid, nonpolarized, and have a central nucleus. LN cells are located at the periphery of the duct/acini, and few can grow admixed with the native epithelium; however, they do not line the lumen of ducts and acini (Figures 2.3 and 2.4).

Management

ADH is found in about 2% to 8% of benign breast biopsies (6,7). Its diagnosis confers a 4- to 5-fold risk of subsequent carcinoma, which can involve both breasts with similar frequency (6).

Based on its morphologic, immunophenotypic, and genetic features, ADH represents a minute focus of LG-DCIS, but management of the two lesions differs greatly.

ADH in a breast excision specimen prompts no additional surgery or need for adjuvant radiotherapy, and its relation to a margin is not reported. Incidental ADH near a margin, however, could constitute peripheral sampling of a more severe lesion, and reexcision should be considered, especially if ADH is associated with calcifications and post-excision imaging shows residual breast calcifications.

The diagnosis of focal DCIS arising in a background of ADH is managed as DCIS is. If ADH is present in core biopsy material, surgical excision of the area is performed. The excision specimen is entirely submitted or extensively sampled, with special attention to the area adjacent to the biopsy site. If no obvious carcinoma is found in the excision specimen, excision and core biopsy slides should be reviewed together, whenever possible, to ensure that the atypical ductal proliferation is evaluated in its entirety.

The rate of upgrade of ADH found in a core biopsy ranges from 15% to 30%, depending on the number and size of the cores. Excision of ADH can yield DCIS or, less often, invasive carcinoma (see also core biopsy chapter). Many investigators have tried to establish criteria that could help determine which core biopsies with ADH do not require excision, but such attempts have been inconclusive.

Chemopreventive hormonal therapy with tamoxifen reduces the risk of subsequent carcinoma in women with

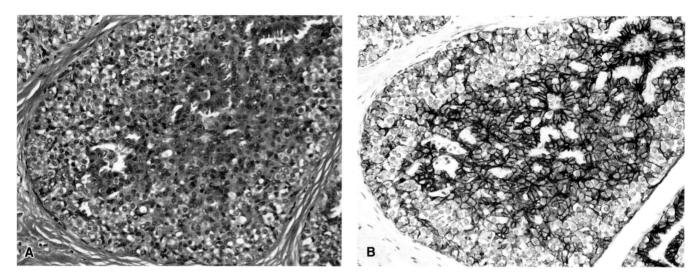

FIGURE 2.3 Lobular neoplasia involving UDH mimics ADH or UDH with maturation. (A) Atypical lobular cells infiltrate the periphery of a duct involved by UDH; the latter consists of cells with indistinct borders and dense nuclear chromatin located in the center of the duct. This pattern can be mistaken as ADH because some of the cells show low-grade atypia or as UDH with maturation. (B) Lack of membranous reactivity for E-cadherin highlights the atypical lobular cells.

ADH. Aromatase inhibitors are prescribed instead of tamoxifen in postmenopausal women.

Key Points

Atypical Ductal Hyperplasia

- ADH is a proliferation of polarized cells with low-grade atypia, similar to LG-DCIS.
- ADH is characterized by limited extent and involves 1 or 2 ducts and spans less than 2 mm.
- The diagnosis of ADH applies only to cases for which the differential diagnosis of LG-DCIS is also considered.

- A ductal proliferation with unequivocal intermediate or high-grade nuclear atypia qualifies as intermediate/high-grade DCIS (HG-DCIS) independent of size.
- Generally speaking, if the differential diagnosis includes LG-DCIS and ADH, the latter should be favored.
- Focal ductal proliferations with unusual morphology do not qualify as ADH and should not be reported as such, but their presence in a core biopsy should prompt excision.
- ADH in core biopsy material warrants surgical excision.
- In general, presence of ADH near a margin is not reported, as ADH does not require additional surgery.

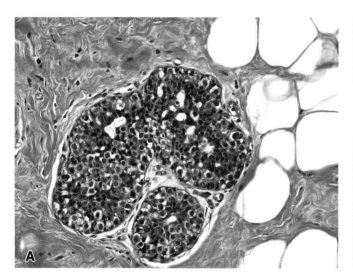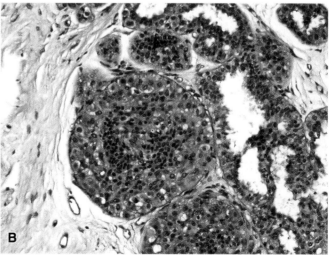

FIGURE 2.4 Partial acinar involvement by LN mimics ADH or UDH with maturation. (A and B) Atypical lobular cells partially involve few acini, and undermine the luminal epithelium without replacing it entirely. The luminal cells retain polarized morphology.

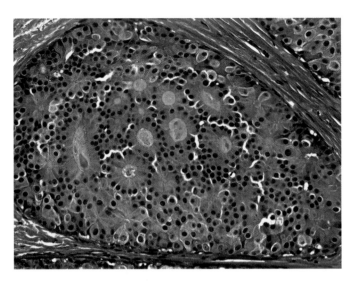

FIGURE 2.5 Cribriform LG-DCIS. Monotonous polarized neoplastic cells with abundant amphophilic cytoplasm line neoformed glandular lumina. Nuclei are slightly enlarged with fine homogeneous chromatin.

Mention of ADH near a margin is appropriate when incidental ADH could represent peripheral sampling of DCIS, such as when ADH is associated with calcifications and post-excision imaging shows residual calcium.

■ DUCTAL CARCINOMA IN SITU

Low-Grade DCIS

Low-grade DCIS consists of ductal cells with low-grade nuclear atypia forming complex architectural arrangements. The neoplastic cells are larger than those of UDH and have more abundant cytoplasm, which is pale pink or gray-purple and amphophilic, and sharply defined cell borders. No cell maturation is observed across involved ducts and acini.

Low-grade DCIS cells are polarized and have a basally located nucleus and an apical cytoplasmic compartment. Polarized cells are the building blocks of the various architectural patterns of LG-DCIS. Cribriform spaces consist of self-enclosed, neo-formed glandular lumina, which do not connect with one another and are not in continuity with the native lumen of the duct in which they reside. The cribriform spaces are identical in size and shape and are evenly distributed (Figure 2.5). Micropapillary LG-DCIS has slender and filiform micropapillae with smooth contour. The micropapillae have a bulbous tip, with diameter wider than the base. The micropapillae often bend slightly to one side, forming incomplete Roman arches. The cells show no maturation across the length of the micropapillae, with no variation in nuclear size and chromatin quality. Cell polarity is evident throughout, including at the tip of the micropapillae. Micropapillary LG-DCIS often arises in a background of columnar cell changes with atypia/flat epithelial atypia (8) (Figure 2.6). Other architectural patterns of LG-DCIS include solid and/or papillary, but no flat (clinging) LG-DCIS is recognized at present (9) (see also chapter on flat epithelial atypia).

The nuclei of LG-DCIS are round to ovoid, slightly enlarged (×1.5–×2.5 red blood cell), and show smooth and regular nuclear membrane, finely dispersed chromatin, and small inconspicuous nucleoli, which often abut the nuclear membrane. Mitoses are rare to absent, and necrosis is uncommon. Small concentric lamellar calcifications are frequently associated with LG-DCIS, either embedded in the neoplastic epithelium or located within the neo-formed glandular lumina. In contrast to the pleomorphic calcifications found in DCIS with high nuclear grade, the calcifications of LG-DCIS rarely associate with necrosis.

Low-grade DCIS often arises in association with other low-grade lesions, such as classic LCIS (C-LCIS)/ALH,

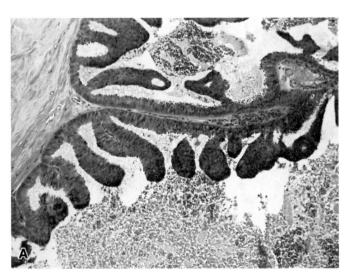
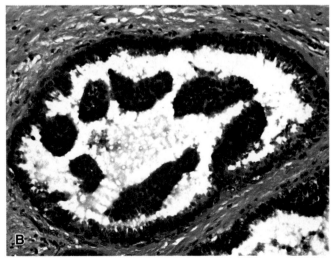

FIGURE 2.6 Low-grade micropapillary DCIS. (A and B) The neoplastic micropapillae are regularly distributed along the duct wall and show smooth and regular outline. They are composed of monotonous polarized cells with enlarged nuclei and fine to dark chromatin with no maturation. Luminal necrosis is sometimes present.

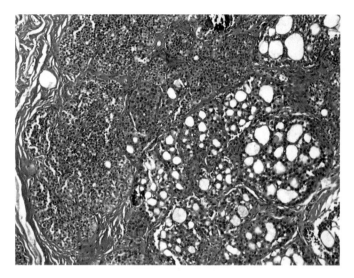

FIGURE 2.7 LCIS involving collagenous spherulosis simulates low-grade cribriform DCIS. Lobular neoplasia is adjacent to and admixed with collagenous spherulosis. On a superficial examination, the translucent collagenous spherules simulate cribriform spaces. Calcifications within the collagenous spherule often prompt stereotactic biopsy.

ADH, and columnar cell changes without and with atypia/flat epithelial atypia, or with well-differentiated invasive ductal carcinoma, tubular carcinoma, and invasive lobular carcinoma, classic type. Abdel-Fatah et al (10,11) and Aulmann et al (12) have noted that all these lesions share similar genetic alterations and have proposed a unifying concept of low-grade mammary neoplasia that encompasses all these processes.

Differential Diagnosis of LG-DCIS

The differential diagnosis of LG-DCIS with ADH and UDH is discussed in the previous paragraphs (ADH section) (see also Chapter 1).

Other lesions in the differential diagnosis of LG-DCIS include:

LCIS Involving Collagenous Spherulosis

Collagenous spherulosis consists of globules of extracellular matrix deposited by myoepithelial cells. The globules are either densely eosinophilic or delicately translucent. They are encircled by a refractive layer of basement membrane, which is in turn surrounded by myoepithelial cells. Lobular carcinoma in situ often grows admixed with collagenous spherulosis, in a pattern that can closely mimic LG-DCIS, especially on quick low-power examination (Figure 2.7). Globules composed of translucent basement membrane can mimic pseudoglandular lumina. In contrast to cribriform spaces, however, the globules of collagenous spherulosis tend to vary in size, are not lined by polarized cells, and are surrounded by basement membrane and flattened myoepithelial cells. The basement membrane surrounding the spherules sometimes detaches from the myoepithelium, collapsing into the pseudoglandular lumen with a characteristic "chord" sign (Figure 2.8A). Correct diagnosis rests on recognizing that the atypical cells are nonpolarized (and thus they are not ductal cells) and do not line the pseudoglandular lumina, which in turn are not empty, but filled by delicate fibrillary material (13). Results of immunoperoxidase stains for myoepithelial markers and/or E-cadherin are helpful to support the diagnosis (Figure 2.8B).

DCIS and LCIS Coexisting in the Same Lobule

DCIS and LCIS rarely coexist in the same lobule or duct. When this happens, the two neoplastic populations appear quite distinct and do not merge with one another. DCIS consists of polarized cells with low nuclear grade and

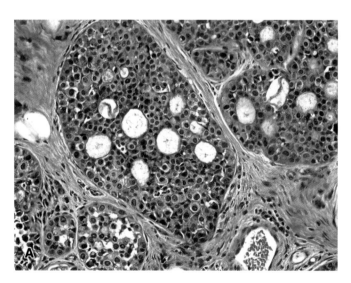
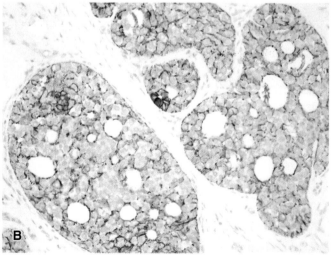

FIGURE 2.8 Lobular carcinoma in situ involving collagenous spherulosis simulates low-grade cribriform DCIS. (A) Lobular neoplasia involves collagenous spherulosis. The pseudoglandular spaces contain delicate fibrillary material, are not lined by polarized cells (compare and contrast with Figure 2.5), and surrounded by basement membrane and myoepithelium. (B) The atypical lobular cells lack membranous immunoreactivity for E-cadherin, whereas the myoepithelium displays a granular dot-like linear staining pattern for the same antigen.

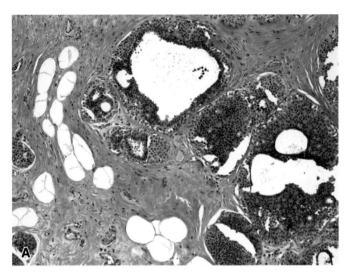
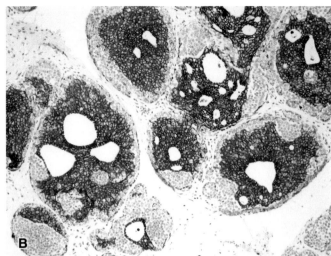

FIGURE 2.9 Low-grade DCIS and LCIS rarely coexist in the same lobule(s). (A) Dyshesive LCIS undermines cribriform DCIS. Neoplastic ductal and lobular cells are distinct but show similar low–nuclear-grade atypia. (B) The cells of LCIS show no membranous immunoreactivity for E-cadherin.

minimal to no necrosis. The cells of LCIS are dyshesive cells, with "fried egg" morphology, and undermine the neoplastic ductal cells. In problematic cases, immunostaining for E-cadherin is helpful to distinguish the two neoplastic populations (Figure 2.9).

Low-grade DCIS and C-LCIS often coexist in the same breast, and finding one should always prompt careful examination for the other.

Micropapillary UDH

The micropapillae of low-grade micropapillary DCIS (MP-DCIS) have a smooth outline and are regularly spaced along the wall of a duct. They are symmetric and slender, filiform or club shaped, taller than wide; they have a narrow base and a wider tip, and consist of polarized cells.

Low-grade MP-DCIS is often adjacent to cribriform DCIS or arises in a background of columnar cell changes with atypia/flat epithelial atypia. In contrast, the micropapillae of UDH are irregularly scattered along the wall of a duct and are asymmetric with frayed edges, variable height and width, broad base and tapering tips. Micropapillary UDH consists of nonpolarized cells that mature from the base of the micropapillae to their tip. Features helpful in the differential diagnosis between micropapillary UDH and low-grade MP-DCIS are summarized in Table 2.1 (Figures 2.2A and 2.6) (see also core biopsy chapter).

Invasive Cribriform Carcinoma

Invasive cribriform carcinoma is a rare low-grade variant of invasive carcinoma (14). It consists of large cribriform nests that invade with only minimal stromal reaction. The

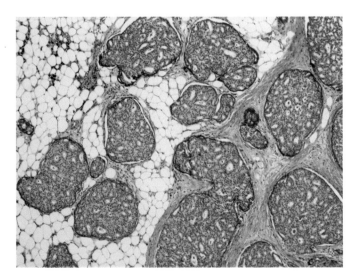

FIGURE 2.10 Invasive cribriform ductal carcinoma. Large cribriform nests of ductal carcinoma infiltrate into adipose tissue. They vary in size and shape and have an irregular outline. Cleft-like spaces separate the invasive tumor from the stroma, with no evidence of basement membrane and myoepithelium.

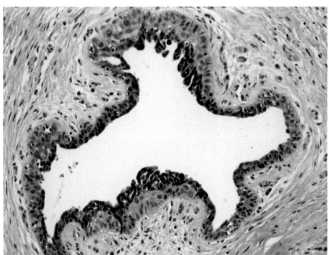

FIGURE 2.11 Gynecomastia. The epithelium of ducts involved by gynecomastia shows UDH, often of micropapillary type, with maturation. The ducts are typically surrounded by cellular stroma, which is absent around ducts involved by low grade DCIS.

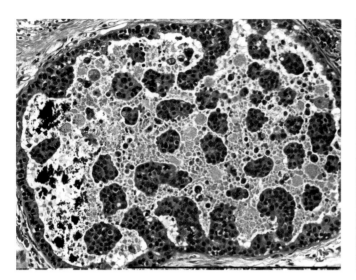

FIGURE 2.12 High-grade micropapillary DCIS. The micropapillae of HG-DCIS are irregular, dyshesive, and often admixed with abundant necrosis. The neoplastic cells show marked nuclear atypia.

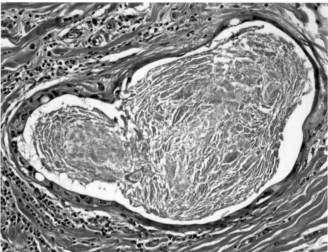

FIGURE 2.13 High-grade flat-type DCIS can be inconspicuous. Flat DCIS with high nuclear grade grows in abnormally dilated acini and ducts filled with amorphous and/or necrotic debris. The neoplastic cells are flattened or cuboidal and have enlarged nuclei and evident nucleoli. Periductal stromal fibrosis and inflammation are common.

nests vary in size and shape and have irregular outlines. The neoplastic glands are usually separated from the adjacent stroma by a cleft-like space (Figure 2.10), in contrast to DCIS, that is contiguous with the duct wall and surrounded by myoepithelium, basement membrane, and few periductal blood vessels. Cribriform invasive ductal carcinoma has indolent prognosis and is regarded as an indolent variant of invasive carcinoma, similar to tubular carcinoma (14).

Gynecomastia

DCIS arising in the male breast usually has low nuclear grade, cribriform architecture, and very limited to absent necrosis. In contrast, gynecomastia resembles micropapillary UDH and is almost invariably associated with periductal stromal desmoplasia (Figure 2.11). In its florid phase, gynecomastia can be mitotically active. The criteria for the diagnosis of ADH and DCIS in the male breast are the same as for ADH and DCIS in the female breast. DCIS in the male breast usually shows low-grade cytologic atypia and a rigid architecture and lacks the periductal stromal desmoplasia characteristically present in gynecomastia.

High-Grade DCIS

High-grade DCIS is characterized by severe nuclear atypia and rarely poses a diagnostic challenge. The architectural patterns of HG-DCIS are similar to those of LG-DCIS, with solid and micropapillary growth being more common and cribriform less frequent. The micropapillae of HG-DCIS are haphazardly scattered along the duct wall, show an irregular outline, and tend to vary in height, width, and contour. The neoplastic cells have marked nuclear atypia and are loosely adherent to the duct wall

(Figure 2.12). Flat (clinging) HG-DCIS can sometimes be relatively inconspicuous. On low-power examination, involved ducts and acini are overtly distended compared to normal and are lined by a flat layer of only one or two cells. This appearance can be overlooked, especially if only limited material is available (Figure 2.13). Cell polarity is not a characteristic feature of HG-DCIS cells. The neoplastic cells are usually large and have pleomorphic and hyperchromatic nuclei with prominent nucleoli, which are often irregular and sometimes multiple. Mitotic activity is easily appreciated. Central necrosis is common, ranging from focal to extensive. Comedonecrosis occupies most of the cross section of a duct, and only a residual

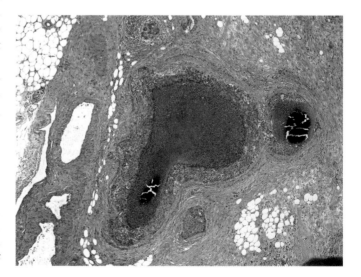

FIGURE 2.14 High-grade solid DCIS with extensive central necrosis (comedonecrosis) harboring calcifications. The coarse calcifications associated with HG-DCIS are detected mammographically as pleomorphic calcifications with linear branching distribution.

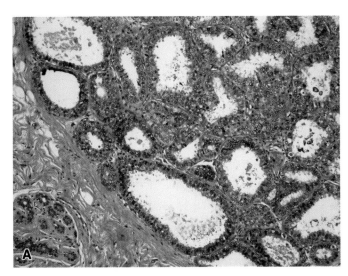
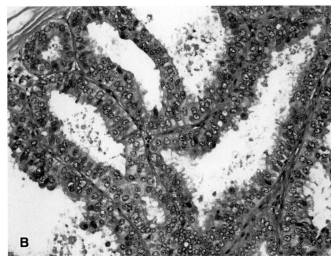

FIGURE 2.15 Intermediate–nuclear-grade DCIS, flat type. (A) Flat DCIS with intermediate nuclear grade consists of cells with enlarged nuclei and evident nucleoli. (B) The cells are columnar and grow as a one- to two-cell layer in dilated acini and ducts. Mitoses are easily observed.

peripheral rim of neoplastic epithelium is evident in some cases. Necrosis often harbors coarse calcifications, which are linearly distributed along the involved ducts, enabling mammographic detection (Figure 2.14). Extensive calcifications sometimes nearly obliterate the neoplastic epithelium, which is usually unveiled in deeper-level sections.

Periductal desmoplasia and inflammatory infiltrate are common. Capillaries around ducts involved by HG-DCIS are also prominent and can mimic microinvasive carcinoma (see chapter on microinvasion).

Intermediate-Grade DCIS

Intermediate-grade DCIS (IG-DCIS) shows morphologic features in between LG-DCIS and HG-DCIS. The neoplastic cells have intermediate nuclear atypia and usually show a prominent nucleolus. Nuclear size is increased, but the nuclei still have similar shape and size. The diagnosis of

intermediate-grade DCIS is usually not problematic, except for flat IG-DCIS. The latter grows as a layer of one or two cells, raising the differential diagnosis of flat epithelial atypia (see Chapter 4 on flat epithelial atypia). In these cases, it is good to compare the nuclear features of the atypical proliferation with those of the adjacent normal epithelium for reference. Extent of the lesion is also important in assigning the diagnosis of flat IG-DCIS (Figure 2.15).

■ DUCTAL CARCINOMA IN SITU WITH UNUSUAL MORPHOLOGY

Spindle Cell DCIS

On low-power examination, spindle cell DCIS fills the entire duct lumen, with no residual peripheral spaces or

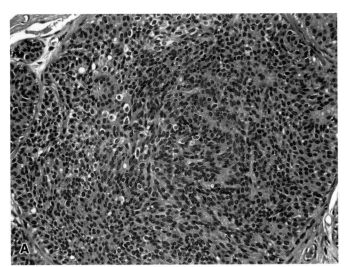
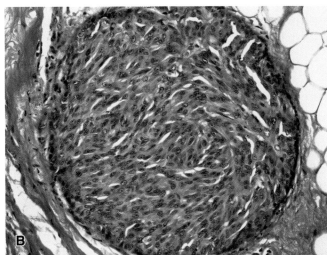

FIGURE 2.16 Spindle cell DCIS, with low nuclear grade. (A and B) Low-grade spindle cell DCIS consists of elongated cells with enlarged nuclei and inconspicuous nucleoli. The cells fill the entire duct and show no maturation.

fenestrations. The neoplastic nuclei are spindled and can form short swirling fascicles, somewhat reminiscent of the streaming of UDH (Figure 2.16). The neoplastic nuclei show intermediate- or high-grade nuclear atypia, but nuclear atypia is low in spindle cell DCIS associated with solid and papillary carcinoma. Central necrosis, or at least focal apoptosis, and mitoses are present. Continuity with other architectural patterns of DCIS, such as cribriform or micropapillary, is a common and helpful diagnostic feature. Spindle cell DCIS often shows positive immunoreactivity for neuroendocrine markers (chromogranin and/or synaptophysin) (15).

Differential Diagnosis of Spindle Cell DCIS

Usual Ductal Hyperplasia

In contrast to UDH, spindle cell DCIS shows nuclear atypia, does not have peripheral fenestrations, and displays no maturation of the epithelium toward the center of the duct lumen (see also Table 2.2).

Myoepitheliosis

Myoepitheliosis is a rare florid proliferation of myoepithelial cells with spindled and globoid cytoplasm, usually admixed with basement membrane material. The hyperplastic myoepithelial cells undermine the native ductal epithelium (Figure 2.17). Positive immunoreactivity for myoepithelial markers, such as calponin, 4A4/p63, and actin, supports the diagnosis of myoepitheliosis in problematic cases.

Apocrine DCIS

Apocrine DCIS often involves sclerosing lesions and causes expansion of the sclerosed ducts and lobules, which is best appreciated by comparison with the adjacent sclerotic breast parenchyma uninvolved by carcinoma. Apocrine DCIS can have a cribriform, solid, micropapillary, or flat architecture.

Apocrine DCIS with high nuclear grade (Figure 2.18) consists of large cells with abundant vacuolated cytoplasm and large irregular nuclei with coarse or smudged chromatin. Variation in nuclear size of at least three-fold is a helpful diagnostic feature. Necrosis is common and often harbors coarse calcifications. Nucleoli are large, sometimes multiple, and can be irregular. The cytoplasm is abundant and densely eosinophilic, but can show a gray-blue tinge indicative of intracytoplasmic mucin accumulation. Mucin extravasation can sometimes be found adjacent to atypical/neoplastic apocrine cells. Mitotic activity in an atypical apocrine proliferation strongly supports the diagnosis of DCIS, which however always requires expansion of the atypical epithelial component.

■ **Table 2.2** Spindle cell DCIS versus UDH

	UDH	Spindle Cell DCIS
Architectural features		
Peripheral fenestrations	Present	Absent
Cell maturation	Present	Not present
Syncytial growth	Present	Not characteristic
Adjacent cribriform or micropapillary DCIS	Absent	Often present
Cytology		
Nuclear/cytoplasmic ratio	Normal or low	Increased
Nuclear chromatin	Irregular, clumped	Finely granular (low nuclear grade) to more coarse (intermediate and high nuclear grade)
Nuclear hyperchromasia	Absent	Present
Nucleoli	Small, inconspicuous	Absent to inconspicuous in low and intermediate nuclear grade; evident in high nuclear grade
Mitoses	Uncommon	Common
Necrosis	Uncommon	Common

Apocrine DCIS with low nuclear grade is uncommon and closely resembles apocrine metaplasia. It consists of cells with eosinophilic cytoplasm and nuclei slightly larger than those of apocrine metaplasia, with only minimal atypia. Monotonous apocrine cytology in an expansive apocrine proliferation with rigid and complex architecture and slight nuclear atypia supports the diagnosis of apocrine DCIS (Figure 2.19).

Apocrine DCIS with intermediate nuclear grade is difficult to recognize and can be confused with IG-DCIS of

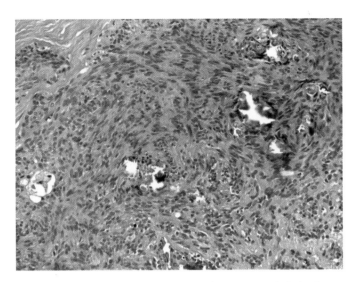

FIGURE 2.17 Myoepitheliosis. Hyperplastic myoepithelial cells are closely admixed with basement membrane-like material. Nuclear atypia is absent, and palisading of the nuclei can be observed.

no special type, from which it differs because of the ample eosinophilic cytoplasm.

Apocrine DCIS shows nuclear positivity for androgen receptor, but is negative for estrogen and progesterone receptors. One study found that about 50% of apocrine DCIS are HER2-positive (16).

Differential Diagnosis of Apocrine DCIS

Apocrine Metaplasia

Apocrine metaplasia is a part of fibrocystic changes, although it shows genetic alterations and may constitute a focal clonal proliferation (17). Apocrine metaplasia is also common in the context of sclerosing lesions. It usually constitutes a limited and focal proliferation, but

often affects different areas of the same breast. Apocrine metaplasia often lines cysts, and sometimes shows fairly complex micropapillary projections into the cyst lumen. Apocrine metaplastic cells tend to be dyshesive, display abundant eosinophilic cytoplasm, and have enlarged round nuclei with prominent nucleoli. The myoepithelium underlying apocrine metaplasia is usually reduced or absent. Translucent calcium oxalate crystals are often present within apocrine cysts (Figure 2.20). The differential diagnosis of apocrine metaplasia versus low-grade apocrine DCIS can be very challenging. An expansive and monotonous apocrine proliferation, with uniform nuclear atypia, rigid and complex architecture, and scattered mitotic activity, is diagnostic of low-grade apocrine DCIS.

Apocrine Pleomorphic LCIS

Apocrine pleomorphic LCIS (P-LCIS) is a rare and unusual variant of LCIS and shows morphologic and immunohistochemical overlap with apocrine DCIS of intermediate nuclear grade. The two can sometimes occur in continuity in the same breast. Apocrine DCIS consists of cohesive, polygonal, and for the most part polarized cells, whereas the cells of apocrine P-LCIS are dyshesive, with ovoid to plasmacytoid shape, and often merge with adjacent C-LCIS. Positive immunoreactivity for E-cadherin highlights apocrine DCIS, whereas no membranous staining is detected in apocrine P-LCIS (see P-LCIS paragraph and figures).

Apocrine Atypia

Apocrine atypia often involves foci of adenosis (apocrine adenosis) and sclerosis. Compared with apocrine metaplasia, the atypical cells have abundant cytoplasm and enlarged nuclei. They often show intracytoplasmic vacuoles

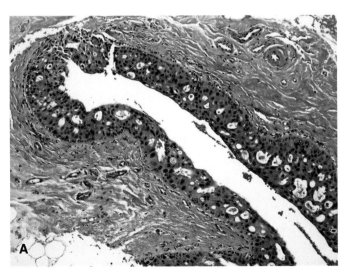

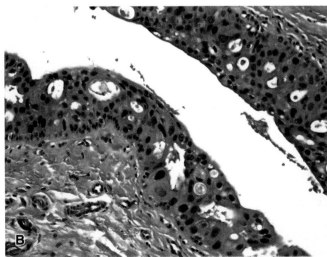

FIGURE 2.18 High-grade apocrine DCIS. (A) The neoplastic cells show marked nuclear atypia. (B) The cytoplasm is abundant and densely eosinophilic with few mucin-filled vacuoles.

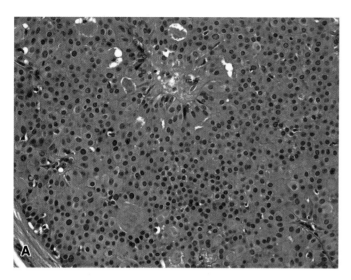
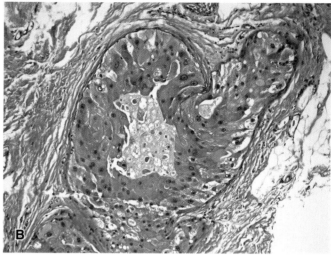

FIGURE 2.19 (A and B) Low-grade apocrine DCIS. Low-grade apocrine DCIS has abundant eosinophilic cytoplasm and slightly enlarged round nuclei with a visible nucleolus.

of different size or have gray-blue cytoplasm, indicative of intracytoplasmic mucin accumulation. Chromatin tends to be coarse, and nucleoli are evident and enlarged. Apocrine atypia is limited in extent and shows no epithelial expansion; mitoses and necrosis are absent (Figure 2.21).

Non-apocrine DCIS

The differential diagnosis of intermediate and high nuclear grade apocrine DCIS includes their non-apocrine counterparts. Apocrine differentiation does not carry specific prognostic significance.

Radiation Changes

Radiation-induced alterations of the breast parenchyma include lobular atrophy, thickening of the basement membrane, and cytologic alterations in stromal cells and

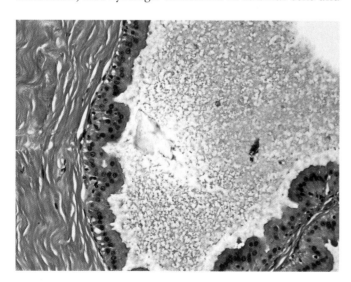

FIGURE 2.20 Apocrine metaplasia. Cysts lined by apocrine metaplasia often contain translucent oxalate crystals.

epithelium. The luminal epithelium affected by radiation shows abundant cytoplasm, intracytoplasmic vacuolization, enlarged nuclei and nucleoli, bi/multinucleation, and smudged chromatin. These changes can be associated with scattered dystrophic calcifications, which often trigger biopsy. Changes encountered a few years after radiation are usually limited to scattered epithelial cells (Figure 2.22). In contrast, alterations encountered shortly (6–18 months) after radiation can be quite extensive and very difficult to distinguish from apocrine atypia or DCIS. Focal necrosis can be present for a few months after radiotherapy has been completed and should not be overestimated. In such cases, finding epithelial hyperplasia and mitotic activity will favor a neoplastic process. Obtaining information about prior radiation treatment and the time interval since it was completed, as well as comparison with the prior carcinoma, are all critical steps for accurate interpretation of these challenging biopsies (Figure 2.23).

Basal-Like DCIS

Gene array analysis has identified a subgroup of poorly differentiated invasive breast carcinoma with "basal-like" gene profile. These tumors usually are triple-negative and positive for CK5/6 and/or epidermal growth factor receptor (EGFR). Investigators have identified DCIS with the same immunophenotype and speculated that it could represent the morphologic precursor of basal-like invasive carcinoma. Basal-like DCIS is not a morphologic entity, but is defined as DCIS that is triple negative and positive for CK5/6 and/or EGFR (18,19). So defined, basal-like DCIS constitutes less than 10% of all DCIS in two separate series (18,19). It usually shows solid growth and high-grade cytology, with enlarged hyperchromatic nuclei and evident nucleoli or high-grade, neuroendocrine-type chromatin. It can be associated with a dense lymphocytic

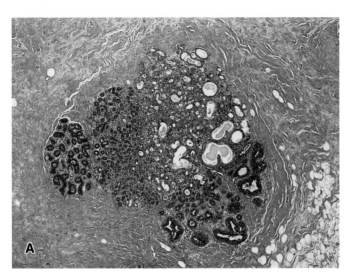 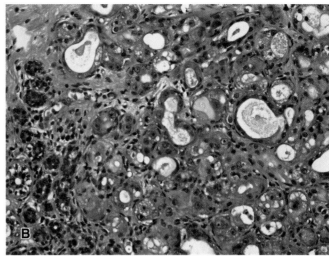

FIGURE 2.21 Apocrine atypia (apocrine adenosis). (A) Apocrine atypia often involves adenosis or sclerosing lesions. (B) Apocrine atypia consists of cells with abundant vacuolated cytoplasm, enlarged nuclei, and prominent nucleoli. The proliferation has limited extent and shows no epithelial expansion, mitoses, or necrosis.

infiltrate (Figure 2.24). At present, the diagnosis of basal-like DCIS has only academic interest, and the term should not be used in diagnostic reports, as the clinical behavior of basal-like DCIS is unclear and its management does not differ from the management of any other DCIS types (20,21). Basal-like DCIS is mentioned here only for academic interest and completeness sake.

Clear Cell DCIS

Clear cell DCIS consists of cells with sharp cell borders and conspicuous clear cytoplasm, but it can also show areas with

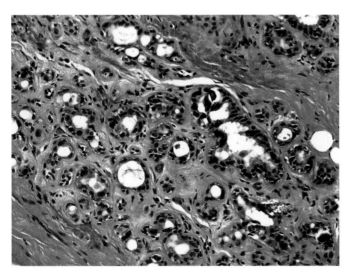

FIGURE 2.22 Radiation changes. Scattered enlarged cells show nuclei with smudged chromatin and prominent nucleoli, but no epithelial proliferation is present. Identification of a thick basement membrane around the atrophic acini with changes suggestive of apocrine atypia should always raise the possibility of prior radiation and prompt clinical correlation.

more eosinophilic cytoplasm. It displays all architectural patterns, including solid, flat, micropapillary, and cribriform. The tumor cells have a central enlarged and hyperchromatic nucleus, often with a prominent nucleolus. Nuclear grade is usually intermediate to high. Necrosis is common and can harbor calcifications (Figure 2.25). Adjacent ducts may show neoplastic clear cells admixed with DCIS with more common morphology or in association with "glycogen-rich" carcinoma.

Differential Diagnosis of Clear Cell DCIS

Clear Cell Changes

Clear cell changes usually involve one or few adjacent lobules and consist of bland cells with clear cytoplasm and small nuclei. This alteration is usually focal and has no known specific clinical implication (Figure 2.26).

Classic LCIS

Clear cell DCIS involving lobules can superficially resemble LCIS. In clear cell DCIS the clear spaces are sharply defined and located within the cell outline, whereas the clearing associated with LCIS is secondary to cell dyshesion and is distributed in between, not within, the cells. Cell cohesion and focal cell polarity support the diagnosis of DCIS. Immunoperoxidase stain for E-cadherin can be used in difficult cases (see differential diagnosis of LCIS).

Lactation/Secretory Changes

Lobules involved by secretory changes have enlarged acini lined by flattened, cuboidal, or columnar cells with finely vacuolated cytoplasm. The nuclei have open chromatin

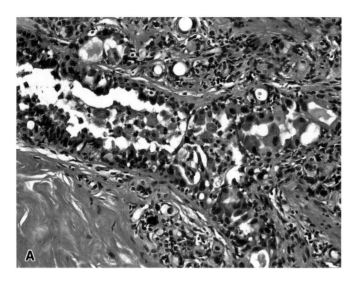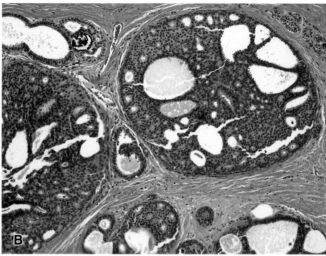

FIGURE 2.23 Early radiation changes (within 6 months to 1 year postradiation). (A) A core biopsy obtained 6 months postradiation to sample residual mammographic calcifications shows extensive radiation changes closely mimicking apocrine DCIS. Note that no epithelial expansion is evident, supporting radiation atypia over carcinoma. A subsequent excision showed no evidence of carcinoma. Extreme caution and a conservative approach are recommended in similar cases. Comparison with the prior carcinoma is extremely helpful to avoid overdiagnosis. (B) The original DCIS had low nuclear grade and cribriform architecture.

and a smooth outline, with evident nucleoli. Binucleation is common. No cell proliferation is evident (Figure 2.27).

Cystic Hypersecretory DCIS

Cystic hypersecretory DCIS is a rare form of DCIS with a unique morphology (20,21). It usually arises in a background of cystic hypersecretory hyperplasia with and without atypia and typically shows intermediate nuclear grade. Micropapillary and solid patterns are most common, but cribriform architecture can also be seen. Mitoses are frequent, whereas necrosis is less

common. Acini and ducts involved by cystic hypersecretory DCIS are expanded and almost entirely filled by the neoplastic cells and therefore contain very little to none of the colloid-like homogeneous eosinophilic secretions characteristic of cystic hypersecretory hyperplasia. The neoplastic cells do not contain intracytoplasmic mucin. The nuclei of cystic hypersecretory lesions are enlarged, irregular, and hyperchromatic. They are frequently elongated and can show longitudinal grooves and intranuclear inclusion. The overall morphology of the carcinoma is somewhat reminiscent of papillary thyroid carcinoma (Figure 2.28).

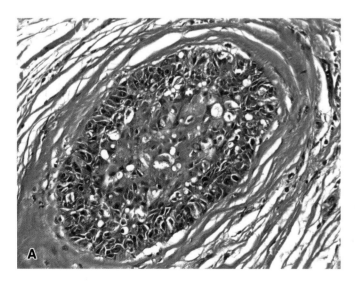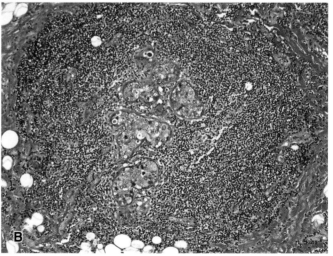

FIGURE 2.24 Basal-like DCIS. Basal-like DCIS does not constitute a morphologic variant of DCIS, and it carries no clinical significance at present. It is defined immunohistochemically as ER-, PR-, and HER2-negative (triple negative) and positive for CK5/6 and/or EGFR. (A) Morphologically, it usually shows solid architecture and high nuclear grade. (B) Basal-like DCIS can be associated to a dense lymphocytic infiltrate.

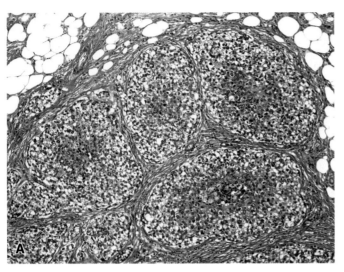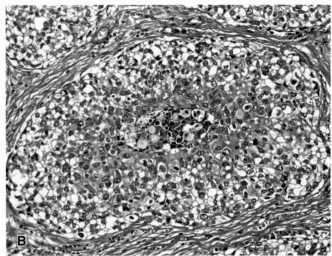

FIGURE 2.25 Clear cell DCIS. (A and B) Clear cell DCIS often shows solid growth. It consists of polygonal cells with clear or sometimes more eosinophilic cytoplasm. Cell borders are sharp. Central necrosis is common and can show associated calcifications.

Differential Diagnosis of Cystic Hypersecretory DCIS

Atypical Cystic Hypersecretory Hyperplasia

Atypical cystic hypersecretory hyperplasia is a proliferation of cells with vacuolated cytoplasm, enlarged and hyperchromatic nuclei, with cytologic atypia. Nuclear grooves and intracytoplasmic vacuoles can be seen. Involved lobules have distended acini filled with homogeneous eosinophilic secretions, which show the characteristic "venetian blinds" shattering artifact (20) (Figure 2.29).

Cystic Hypersecretory Hyperplasia/Change

Cystic hypersecretory hyperplasia/change consists of cells with abundant vacuolated delicate cytoplasm and bland

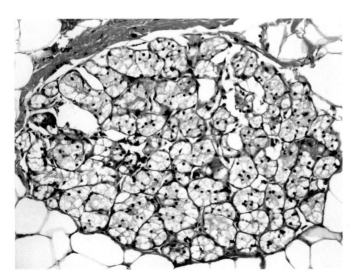

FIGURE 2.26 Clear cell changes. Clear cell changes are typically limited to one or two lobules. The cells are bland with abundant clear cytoplasm, sharp cell borders, and small nuclei.

nuclei. Involved lobules are composed of distended acini filled with colloid-like homogeneous eosinophilic secretions with "venetian blinds" shattering artifact. The epithelium lining the acini is usually cuboidal to flattened and inconspicuous (Figure 2.30). Calcifications can be encountered and may lead to biopsy (22).

Secretory/Lactational Changes

Secretory/lactational change can occur outside of pregnancy/lactation. It is usually a very focal change and consists of cells with abundant vacuolated, frothy, and delicate cytoplasm. Nuclei are enlarged, with smooth outline, open chromatin, and often evident nucleoli; binucleation can occur (Figure 2.27). Calcifications can be encountered and may lead to biopsy (23). Shin and Rosen have reported proximity of secretory/lactational changes and atypical cystic hypersecretory hyperplasia/cystic hypersecretory carcinoma (22,23).

DCIS With Mucinous Features

DCIS with mucinous features is present in the breast parenchyma surrounding mucinous carcinoma in 30% to 75% of cases. In most cases, the DCIS is low to intermediate grade and has a micropapillary or cribriform pattern. Neuroendocrine differentiation has been described. The neoplastic cells often have pale or blue-gray cytoplasm (Figure 2.31).

Differential Diagnosis of DCIS Versus Lymphovascular Invasion

Disruption of DCIS from the duct wall due to trauma or poor tissue preservation can mimic lymphovascular invasion (LVI). Vice versa, occlusive intravascular tumor emboli

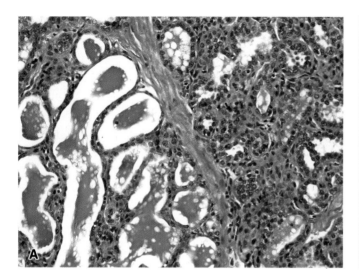
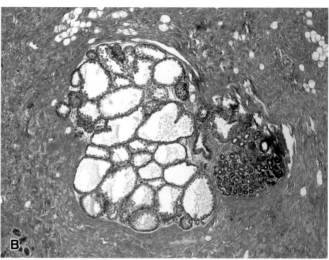

FIGURE 2.27 Lactation/secretory changes. (A) Secretory changes during pregnancy/lactation involve the entire breast. The cells have abundant vacuolated and frothy cytoplasm. Nuclei are enlarged but have a smooth outline and pale chromatin. Nucleoli are prominent, and binucleation is common. The acinar lumen is often distended by eosinophilic secretions. (B) Idiopathic secretory changes are usually limited to few scattered lobules.

can sometimes be misdiagnosed as DCIS (Figure 2.32). Identification of flattened cells lining empty and distended space has limited value in distinguishing LVI from DCIS, as endothelium cannot be reliably differentiated from myoepithelium based on morphology alone in such cases.

Presence of ducts uninvolved by DCIS within the area of concern favors LVI. Similarly, finding adjacent intravascular tumor emboli in perivascular and/or periductal distribution supports LVI over DCIS.

Ductal carcinoma in situ disrupted from the duct wall shows a jagged and irregular outline, and few DCIS cells can remain anchored to the duct wall, whereas tumor emboli suspended in a fluid medium are spherical and have a smooth outline. Periductal stromal desmoplasia,

inflammatory cells, and prominent capillaries are common around DCIS, but absent around LVI. Red blood cells are often admixed with intravascular tumor emboli, but they are absent or not as abundant around disrupted DCIS (Figure 2.33). Although rarely, necrosis, calcifications, and pseudo-cribiform architecture can occur in intravascular tumor emboli.

In problematic cases, immunoperoxidase stains for myoepithelial (calponin and p63/4A4) and vascular (CD31, D2-40) markers help solve the differential diagnosis (see also chapter on immunoperoxidase stains).

Distinguishing between DCIS and LVI is of critical significance in the evaluation of margin status. DCIS close/ at a margin will prompt additional surgery, whereas the

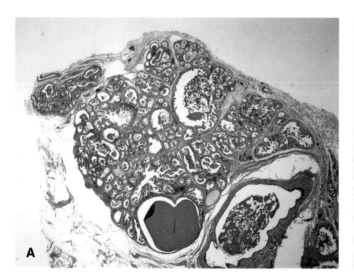
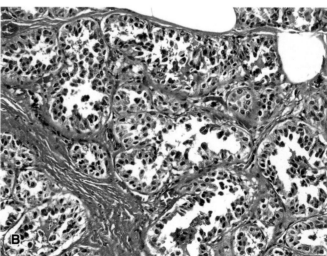

FIGURE 2.28 (A and B) Cystic hypersecretory DCIS. Cystic hypersecretory DCIS fills and expands the acini with dyshesive micropapillae. The colloid-like eosinophilic secretion characteristic of cystic hypersecretory lesions is scant.

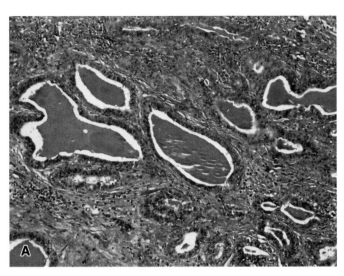
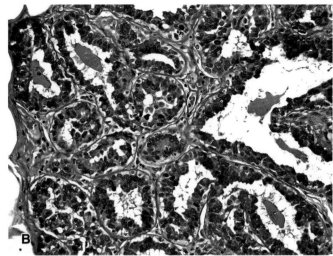

FIGURE 2.29 Atypical cystic hypersecretory hyperplasia. (A) Lobules involved by atypical cystic hypersecretory hyperplasia are expanded and have acini filled by dense eosinophilic secretions, reminiscent of thyroid colloid. (B) Some of the cells show elongated nuclei with longitudinal grooves, reminiscent of papillary thyroid carcinoma.

relation of LVI to a margin is not reported. Misdiagnosis of extensive and occlusive LVI as DCIS in a core biopsy could erroneously prompt surgical excision instead of additional radiologic workup and possible neoadjuvant chemotherapy before definitive surgery is performed.

Management of DCIS

DCIS is a very heterogenous disease, and our knowledge of its local recurrence, subsequent invasion, and response to therapy still remains limited. Young age at initial diagnosis, clinical presentation as a mass, high nuclear grade, extensive necrosis, and close resection margins are among the factors associated with local recurrence of DCIS and progression to invasive carcinoma (24,25).

The current treatment of DCIS is similar to that of invasive ductal carcinoma and consists of either mastectomy or surgical excision with negative margins followed by radiotherapy. The latter significantly reduces the risk of local recurrence in patients treated with breast conservation. The overall rate of local recurrence of DCIS in prospective randomized trials (NASBP-B-17 and EORTC-10853) was about 30% in women who did not receive radiation and only about 12% to 15% in those who did (26,27). Locally recurrent disease after breast conservation in patients with DCIS consists of invasive carcinoma in about half of the cases. Radiotherapy for conservative management of DCIS is likely not required for all patients and carries a low risk of postradiation sarcoma, especially angiosarcoma, which tends to be very aggressive.

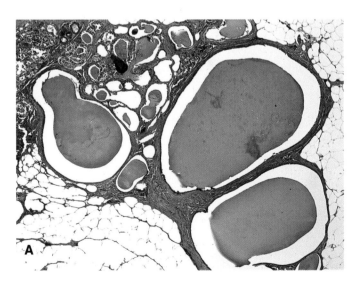
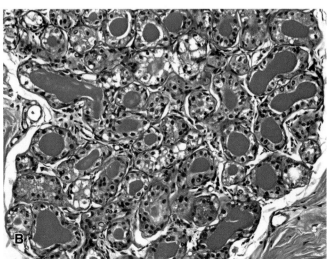

FIGURE 2.30 Cystic hypersecretory change/hyperplasia. (A) Lobules involved by cystic hypersecretory change/hyperplasia are expanded and have acini filled by dense eosinophilic secretions, reminiscent of thyroid colloid. (B) Few pale glycogenated nuclei are evident.

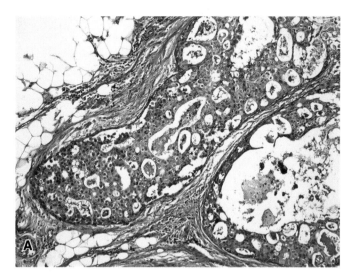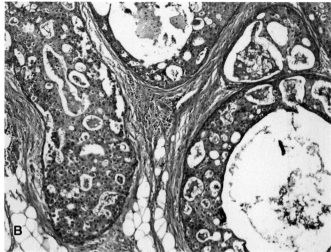

FIGURE 2.31 Ductal carcinoma in situ with mucinous features. (A and B) Ductal carcinoma in situ with mucinous features often consists of pale cells with distinct cell borders. The cytoplasm is usually abundant and can show a gray-blue color. Mucin is often present within the lumen.

Nonetheless, even LG-DCIS with a margin clearance of 1 cm or greater shows an unacceptably high recurrence rate without radiotherapy (28). Few studies indicate that a wider clear margin is associated with reduced rate of local recurrence (24,29), but the margin width required for optimal breast conservation remains uncertain. The combined local and distant recurrence rate of DCIS after mastectomy ranges from 1% to 2%.

Hormonal therapy is recommended for all patients with DCIS who undergo either breast conservation or ipsilateral mastectomy, as it reduces by half the risk of ipsilateral recurrence as shown in the NASBP-24 trial (30). Hormonal therapy also significantly reduces the risk of contralateral breast carcinoma. Unpublished data suggest that the beneficial effect of tamoxifen is dependent on the level of estrogen and progesterone receptor positivity of

DCIS. An ongoing trial (NSABP-37) is comparing the use of aromatase inhibitors versus tamoxifen in patients with DCIS.

The use of sentinel lymph node biopsy in the staging of patients with DCIS is also controversial. About 5% of patients with DCIS can show sentinel lymph node involvement. In one study, 43 of 470 women with high-risk DCIS had sentinel lymph node involvement, including 3 (7%) of 43 with pN1, 4 (9%) of 43 with pN1mi, and 36 (84%) of 43 with pN0(i+) (31). At present, some surgeons perform sentinel lymph node biopsy in patients with mass-forming HG-DCIS, in patients with DCIS suggestive of microinvasion, and in patients undergoing mastectomy (31,32).

Management of special variants of DCIS, such as apocrine, spindle cell, basal-type DCIS, and others, is the same

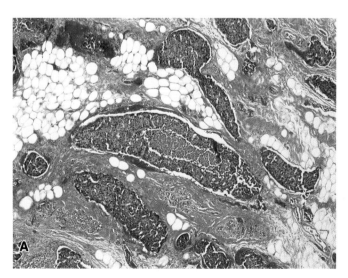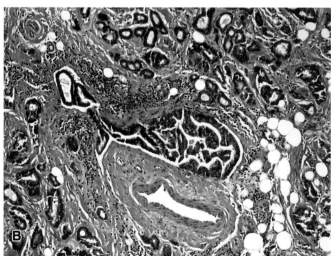

FIGURE 2.32 Lymphovascular invasion mimicking DCIS. (A) Nearly occlusive tumor emboli with central necrosis distend vascular spaces mimicking DCIS. Note that the tumor emboli are surrounded by abundant red blood cells. (B) Tumor emboli have a pseudocribriform architecture. Note that the tumor emboli occupy perivascular lymphatics. The stroma around vessels filled by tumor emboli shows no reactive changes.

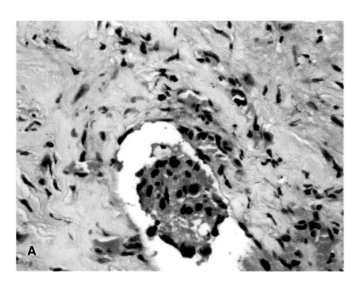
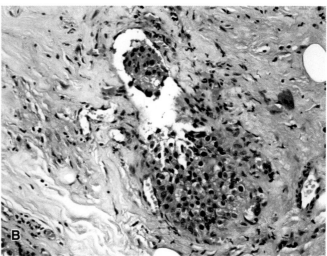

FIGURE 2.33 Ductal carcinoma in situ mimicking LVI. (A) A cluster of carcinoma in a clear space closely mimics LVI but actually represents a detached fragment of DCIS. (B) Note the reactive changes and prominent feeding capillaries in the stroma around the DCIS.

as for any DCIS type, although hormonal therapy is likely not as effective in DCIS that is negative for estrogen and progesterone receptors. A prospective study (NASBP-43) is currently evaluating the benefit of trastuzumab in women with HER2-positive DCIS.

Key Points

Ductal Carcinoma In Situ

- Low-grade DCIS is often associated with other low-grade lesions, such as ADH, LN, tubular carcinoma, well-differentiated low-grade ductal carcinoma, and invasive lobular carcinoma.
- Some of the morphologic variants of DCIS can mimic a benign proliferation, such as UDH.
- Assessment of nuclear atypia is critical in the evaluation of any ductal proliferation.
- At present, DCIS is managed with breast conservation (surgical excision with clear margins followed by adjuvant radiotherapy) or mastectomy.
- Hormonal treatment significantly reduces the risk of local recurrence after conservative treatment of DCIS, as well the risk of contralateral carcinoma.
- The current management of DCIS does not vary across different subtypes and likely results in overtreatment of some patients.

■ LOBULAR NEOPLASIA

The term lobular neoplasia (LN) encompasses classic (C) LCIS and ALH. Lobular neoplasia has no specific clinical, radiologic, or macroscopic correlates and constitutes an incidental finding in about 8% to 10% of breast biopsies

obtained for calcifications, mass, or architectural distortion. The mean age at diagnosis of LN is 50 years, and the incidence of LN tends to spontaneously decrease in postmenopausal women due to physiologic reduction of estrogen and progesterone levels.

C-LCIS and ALH share similar deletion/functional inactivation of chromosome 16q and have comparable cytomorphology, but differ with regard to extent. According to the most commonly used definition, C-LCIS requires distension of at least 50% of the acini of a lobule, and less developed lesions are categorized as ALH (33). Nonetheless, no definite consensus exists regarding the degree of acinar distension, minimum number of acini, and total number of involved lobules required for the diagnosis of C-LCIS, with consequent limited interobserver and even intraobserver reproducibility.

The deletion/functional mutation of CDH1 (E-cadherin) gene, located at chromosome 16q22.1, is an early event in the progression of LN and translates into loss of membranous immunoreactivity for E-cadherin (34), which characterizes ALH, LCIS, and invasive lobular carcinoma. Immunoperoxidase stain for E-cadherin is a useful tool in the evaluation of solid carcinoma in situ with ambiguous morphology. Despite substantial molecular evidence, however, some pathologists still opt not to use E-cadherin to differentiate between ductal carcinoma and LN.

CDH1 gene germline mutations have been identified in patients with hereditary diffuse gastric carcinoma. The disease is autosomal dominant with high, but variable penetrance, which is greater in women than men. Although most patients present with gastric carcinoma, some affected individuals can first develop lobular carcinoma.

CDH1 germline mutation should be considered in patients with family history of invasive lobular carcinoma and/or diffuse-type gastric carcinoma and in women who

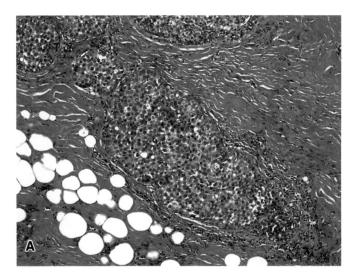
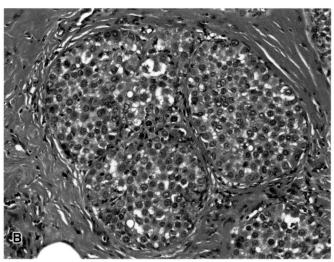

FIGURE 2.34 Lobular carcinoma in situ. (A) Monotonous and dyshesive nonpolarized cells with low-grade nuclear atypia expand all acini of a lobule. (B) Scattered cells show intracytoplasmic vacuoles. Small nucleoli are also noted.

are younger than 40 years at presentation of either disease (35).

Lobular Carcinoma In Situ, Classic Type

Lobules involved by C-LCIS are distended by a monotonous proliferation of small and dyshesive cells that fill most of the acini, obliterating the acinar lumen (Figure 2.34). The cells have a "fried egg" morphology and display a central round to ovoid nucleus, surrounded by a narrow rim of pale to lightly eosinophilic cytoplasm. The nuclei are small and uniform and show low-grade atypia. As described by Haagensen et al (36), C-LCIS can consist of two cell types: type A cells are small and have a scant cytoplasm, small nuclei with homogeneous chromatin, and no nucleolus; type B cells are slightly larger and have a more conspicuous cytoplasm, nuclei with paler and more open chromatin, and visible nucleoli. Types A and B cells often occur together in the same breast and can coexist in the same lobule.

Mucin-filled intracytoplasmic vacuoles are common in C-LCIS, although not specific for it, and often appear as intracytoplasmic targetoid inclusions that displace the nucleus to one side, with formation of signet ring cells. Rarely, focal signet ring cell morphology is secondary to intracytoplasmic mucin accumulation. This alteration is only focal in C-LN, and lobular carcinoma with widespread intracytoplasmic accumulation is to be regarded as a special variant of LCIS (S-LCIS) (see paragraph on S-LCIS).

C-LCIS is a lobulocentric lesion, but it can extend along the basement membrane of extralobular ducts, undermining the native luminal epithelium. This growth pattern, akin to that commonly seen in Paget's disease of the nipple, is referred to as pagetoid spread. A residual layer of attenuated ductal cells separates C-LCIS cells from the lumen of the involved duct (Figure 2.35). Pagetoid spread of C-LN is very common, but DCIS, especially DCIS with intermediate to high nuclear grade, can sometimes show a similar growth pattern.

Myoepithelial nuclei with crescentic nuclei and dense chromatin are sprinkled among LN cells, and LN often involves foci of myoepithelial hyperplasia, such as collagenous spherulosis.

LN is often difficult to appreciate in the context of postmenopausal breast atrophy and can amount to only one or two layers of neoplastic cells involving sclerotic extralobular ducts, whereas lobules are reduced in number and acini become sclerotic. Similarly, involvement of irradiated breast tissue by LN can be very subtle. Together

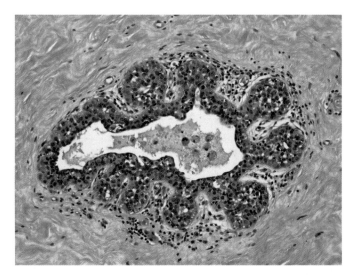

FIGURE 2.35 Lobular neoplasia with pagetoid involvement of a duct (pagetoid growth). Monotonous and dyshesive nonpolarized cells with low-grade nuclear atypia undermine the native epithelium of a duct seen in cross section. The residual native epithelium shows mark attenuation.

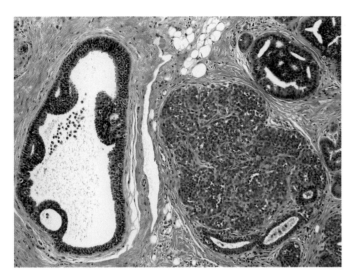

FIGURE 2.36 Atypical lobular hyperplasia (ALH). Monotonous and dyshesive nonpolarized cells with low-grade nuclear atypia cause minimal expansion of most of the acini of a lobule. In this case, ALH is adjacent to ADH.

with ALH, C-LCIS is strongly ER-positive, usually PR-positive, and HER2-negative.

Atypical Lobular Hyperplasia

ALH refers to a neoplastic proliferation cytologically similar to C-LCIS, but less developed. According to Page's definition, ALH involves fewer than 50% of the acini of a lobule, and causes only slight acinar distension (33) (Figure 2.36).

Differential Diagnosis of LN (C-LCIS and ALH)

DCIS With Low Nuclear Grade

Solid LG-DCIS closely mimics C-LCIS and vice versa. The C-LCIS cells are dyshesive, whereas the cells of solid LG-DCIS are polygonal, with linear cell borders, and arranged in a mosaic pattern. Cell polarity with formation of microacini supports ductal differentiation (Figure 2.37). Additional features useful in the differential diagnosis are summarized in Table 2.3. In ambiguous cases, lack of membranous immunoreactivity for E-cadherin and diffuse intracytoplasmic positivity for p120, the E-cadherin intra-cytoplasmic ligand, support lobular differentiation. Some authors, however, have reported rare cases of positive aberrant E-cadherin immunoreactivity in lobular carcinoma (37,38) (see also Chapter 10 on immunohistochemistry).

Myoepithelial Hyperplasia

Myoepithelial hyperplasia is often found in the context of a sclerosing lesion or postradiation and/or chemotherapy. Hyperplastic myoepithelial cells are usually prominent, have round to spindled shape, and conspicuous clear cytoplasm. The nucleus is small, can be round to spindled,

is centrally located, and shows no evident nucleolus. Focal indistinct cytoplasmic vacuoles can be observed, which can rarely indent the nucleus. Hyperplastic myoepithelium mimics C-LN, undermining the native luminal epithelium of ducts and acini; however, lobules involved by myoepithelial hyperplasia are not expanded, and the hyperplastic myoepithelium lacks cytologic atypia. Furthermore, hyperplastic myoepithelial cells do not display the well-formed intracytoplasmic targetoid inclusions and true signet ring cell morphology common in C-LN. Of note, small crescent-shaped myoepithelial nuclei are typically found sprinkled across C-LN, but they are not appreciable in the context of myoepithelial hyperplasia, as all cells are myoepithelial. Myoepithelial

■ **TABLE 2.3** Classic LCIS versus LG-DCIS

	LCIS	DCIS
Cell dyshesion	Present	Absent
Involvement of ducts	Frequent (pagetoid spread)	Present (cribriform, solid, micropapillary, etc); pagetoid growth is extremely rare
Involvement of lobules	Typical, expansive growth	Possible, "lobular cancerization"
Admixed myoepithelium	Common	Absent
Necrosis	Absent	Common
Mitoses	Absent	Common
Calcifications	Rare and incidental, minute	Frequent, often lamellar
Cell morphology	Round to ovoid, nonpolarized	Columnar and polarized
Cytoplasm	Scant	Usually fairly abundant
Nuclear pleomorphism	Absent	Absent
Nucleoli	Rare	Rare, inconspicuous
Adjacent invasive carcinoma	Possible	Possible

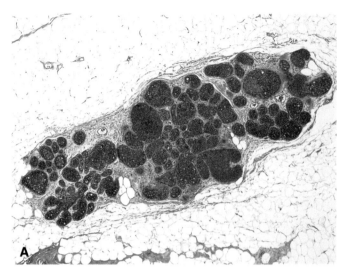
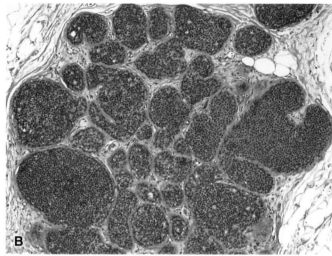

FIGURE 2.37 Ductal carcinoma in situ simulating LCIS. (A) A monotonous solid proliferation of cells with low-grade nuclear atypia uniformly distends the acini of a lobule. (B) The neoplastic cells form focal microacini, supporting ductal differentiation.

hyperplasia is often associated with an increased deposition of basement membrane material, which tends to surround individual myoepithelial cells, whereas it typically encircles multicellular aggregates of C-LN cells. Immunoperoxidase stains for myoepithelial markers, such as calponin and p63, are helpful to resolve difficult cases (Figures 2.38 and 2.39).

Secretory (Pregnancy-Like) Changes

Secretory (pregnancy-like) changes are a focal idiopathic alteration of the acinar epithelium that occurs outside of pregnancy or lactation. The acini of affected lobules are lined by a single layer of cuboidal to columnar cells with pale, vacuolated, and fragile cytoplasm. Nuclei are slightly enlarged with a small nucleolus, or are small and round with dense chromatin. Binucleation and hobnail nuclei are common. Frothy secretions are present within the enlarged

acini and can contain lamellar calcifications. In contrast to C-LCIS, cells with secretory changes are cohesive and do not fill the acinar lumen (Figure 2.27).

Poor Tissue Preservation

Artifactual cell dyshesion secondary to poor tissue preservation closely mimics LN, but the distorted acini show no cell proliferation or distension. On closer examination, poorly preserved cells lack nuclear and cytoplasmic detail and have frayed, indistinct cytoplasm. Suboptimal tissue preservation is usually not confined to only one lobule, but it also involves adjacent ducts. A definitive diagnosis sometimes cannot be rendered on poorly preserved material. Immunoperoxidase stains can sometimes be helpful, but only positive immunoreactivity can be interpreted with confidence, and any lack of staining should be regarded as noncontributory, as it could be due to antigen degradation.

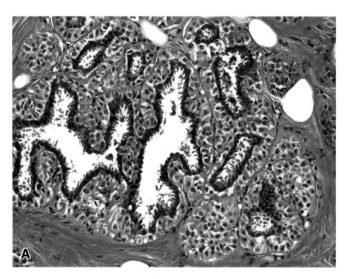
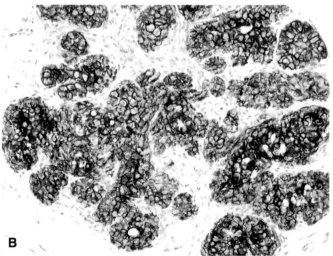

FIGURE 2.38 Myoepithelial hyperplasia. (A) Round to ovoid hyperplastic myoepithelial cells with abundant clear cytoplasm mimic C-LN. (B) Positive membranous immunoreactivity for E-cadherin in a characteristic dot-like linear pattern supports the diagnosis of myoepithelial cells hyperplasia.

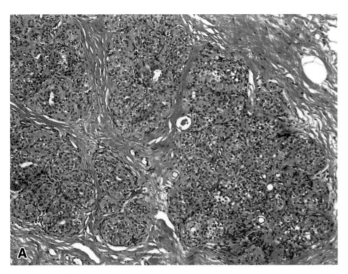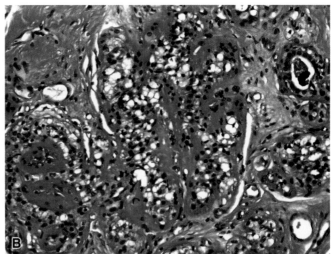

FIGURE 2.39 Postradiation myoepithelial hyperplasia. (A and B) Postradiation myoepithelial hyperplasia is characterized by pale and vacuolated cells admixed with abundant basement membrane-like material.

Clear Cell Change

Clear cell change is usually focal and limited to one or two lobules. The cells are polarized and have abundant clear cytoplasm. Nuclei are small and punctiform and are located at one pole of the cell or in the center. In contrast to C-LN, clear cells are cohesive and have a polygonal outline, with a sharp cell border (Figure 2.26).

Clear Cell DCIS

The cells of clear cell DCIS are polarized and have abundant clear cytoplasm. Nuclei are enlarged and hyperchromatic. In contrast to C-LN, clear cell DCIS consists of cohesive cells with more columnar shape, polygonal outline, with sharp cell borders (Figure 2.40).

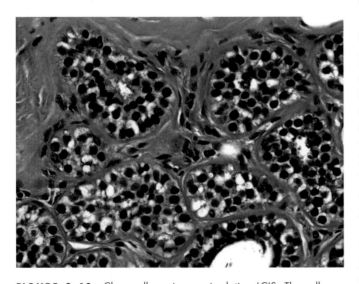

FIGURE 2.40 Clear cell carcinoma simulating LCIS. The cells are polarized and have abundant clear cytoplasm. Nuclei are enlarged and hyperchromatic. In contrast to LN, clear cells are cohesive and have a polygonal outline with sharp cell border.

Lobular Neoplasia Involving a Sclerosing Lesion Mimics Invasive Carcinoma

C-LN frequently involves sclerosing lesions in a pattern that can closely simulate invasive carcinoma. In these cases, comparative evaluation of the adjacent breast parenchyma is critical, in particular evaluation of adjacent sclerosing lesions uninvolved by LN. Sclerosing adenosis shows a characteristic lobulocentric swirling pattern, and radial scar has a concentric zonal arrangement. Sclerosed glands and tubules involved by C-LN are surrounded by a thick eosinophilic and refractive basement membrane, which is most helpful to rule out stromal invasion. Myoepithelial cells are often attenuated and sometimes cannot be reliably identified on routine sections, but immunoperoxidase stains for myoepithelial markers (calponin and p63) will help to resolve difficult cases (see also chapters on immunohistochemistry and adenosis).

Special LCIS

E-cadherin immunohistochemistry greatly facilitates categorization of morphologically ambiguous neoplastic in situ epithelial proliferations into ductal or lobular carcinoma. The widespread use of E-cadherin has revealed that some solid carcinomas in situ with uncertain morphology, uniformly categorized in the past as DCIS, actually have lobular differentiation. Classification of these special (S) variants of LCIS has not yet been standardized, and different terminology has been used by different authors. Some pathologists indiscriminately use the term pleomorphic (P)-LCIS for all forms of S-LCIS. Until more precise information on the biology of these lesions is available, it is preferable to distinguish the different variants of S-LCIS, as they can vary greatly in cytomorphology and nuclear pleomorphism.

Generally speaking, S-LCIS variants have solid growth and consist of round to ovoid neoplastic cells that fill

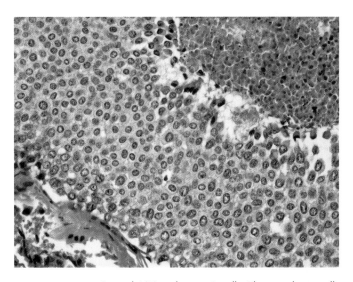

FIGURE 2.41 Special LCIS with type A cells. The neoplastic cells show low-grade nuclear atypia, but the growth pattern is that of massive acinar expansion with central necrosis.

entirely the lumen of ducts and lobules. Marked to massive acinar expansion, central necrosis and associated calcifications are characteristic and closely mimic DCIS. Just like C-LCIS, S-LCIS usually displays dyshesive growth but shows a much wider spectrum of nuclear atypia, ranging from low grade and indistinguishable from C-LCIS, to moderate or severe. Mitoses are numerous, and apoptosis frequent. Molecular data indicate that S-LCIS is genetically related to C-LCIS, although it shows a more complex pattern of genetic alterations. In particular, apocrine P-LCIS displays more genetic alterations than C-LCIS and nonapocrine P-LCIS (39). Apocrine P-LCIS is also more often negative for ER and PR and positive for HER2 (39). Despite substantial genetic evidence supporting lobular differentiation in these lesions, no uniform consensus exists on their classification, and some pathologists continue to regard them as DCIS.

S-LCIS variants are associated with stromal invasion in about 50% to 70% of cases, and invasive carcinoma is most often of lobular type (40,41). Associated

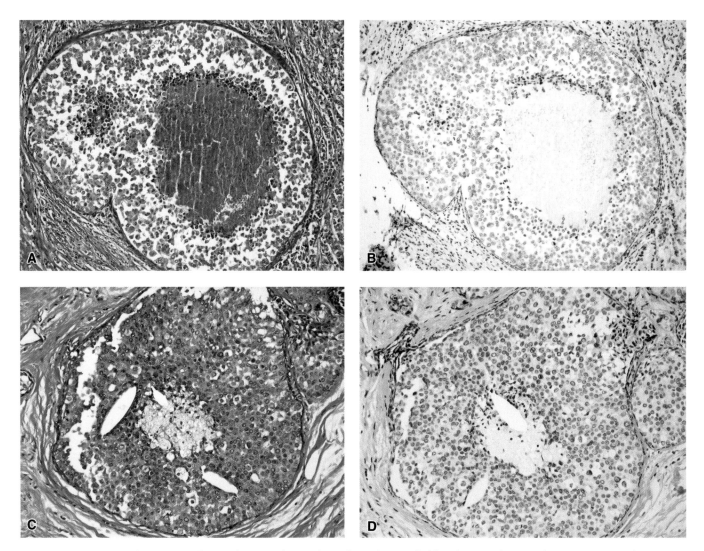

FIGURE 2.42 Special LCIS. (A and C) Dyshesive and nonpolarized neoplastic cells fill and massively expand an acinus. Central necrosis is present. (B and D) Lack of membranous immunoreactivity for E-cadherin supports lobular differentiation.

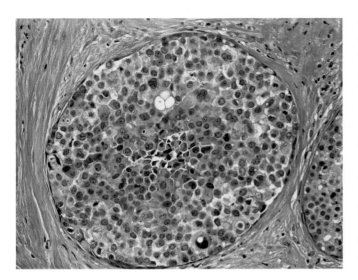

FIGURE 2.43 Pleomorphic LCIS. The neoplastic cells are markedly enlarged and dyshesive and show round to ovoid shape. Few cells display intracytoplasmic vacuoles. Nuclear atypia is marked with few binucleate cells, and nucleoli are prominent. Central necrosis is evident.

microinvasion is also very common and can be very subtle (see chapter on microinvasion). In contrast to C-LCIS, S-LCIS does not represent an incidental finding and is usually detected mammographically because of associated calcifications and/or a mass lesion (39–42).

Special LCIS Composed of Haagensen's Type A and/or Type B Cells

Massive acinar distension, with 50 or more cells across the diameter of each expanded acinus, is the hallmark of these S-LCIS. Necrosis is often present in the center of the solid proliferation. The tumor cells are round to ovoid and dyshesive, especially in the area immediately adjacent

to the central necrotic focus (Figure 2.40). Scattered apoptosis is also common, and mitotic figures are easily encountered. Nuclei range in size from ×1.5 to ×2.5 the size of a red blood cell and are indistinguishable from Haagensen's type A and/or B cells (Figure 2.41). Rare cells with larger and more atypical nuclei are sometimes present. Intracytoplasmic vacuoles and focal signet ring cell morphology are common.

Involved lobules are markedly expanded and clustered together and can form a discrete nodular area. These lesions are usually surrounded by C-LCIS and seamlessly merge with it.

Dr. Rosen (43) refers to these lesions as florid LCIS, whereas Dr. Tavassoli uses the term LCIS with comedone-crosis (40) (Figure 2.42).

Pleomorphic LCIS

P-LCIS is composed of round to ovoid neoplastic cells with abundant cytoplasm, enlarged nuclei, and prominent nucleoli (Figure 2.43). The nucleus is often located off to the cell center, with resulting plasmacytoid appearance (41). Intracytoplasmic light blue to gray mucin can be abundant and indent the nucleus, and some P-LCIS consist entirely of signet ring cells (Figure 2.44). Some cells have pale, foamy, and abundant cytoplasm, which mimics the appearance of foamy histiocytes. P-LCIS with apocrine cytology has also been described (39) and consists of large cells with abundant densely eosinophilic cytoplasm (Figure 2.45). In most cases, P-LCIS shows massive acinar distension, but the proliferation can, sometimes be more subtle and show pagetoid growth with only minimal acinar expansion (Figure 2.46). Large pleomorphic nuclei (about 3 to 4 times the size of a small lymphocyte) with irregular nuclear membrane and coarse chromatin are the

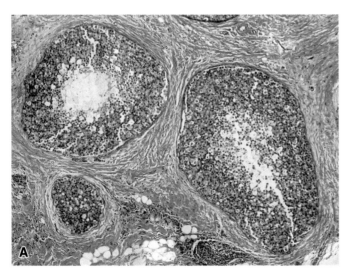

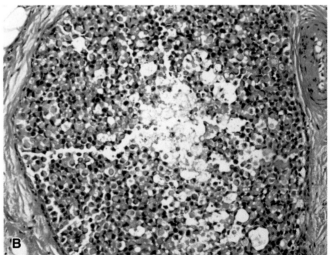

FIGURE 2.44 Pleomorphic LCIS composed of signet ring cells. The neoplastic cells uniformly show signet ring cell morphology, secondary to accumulation of intracytoplasmic mucin.

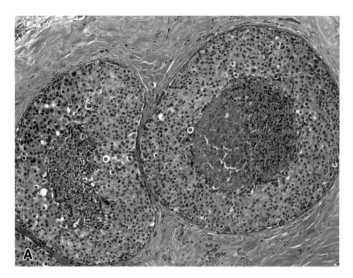
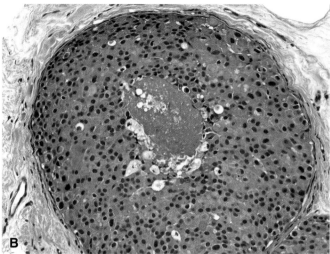

FIGURE 2.45 Apocrine LCIS. (A and B) The neoplastic cells are markedly enlarged and dyshesive and have abundant eosinophilic cytoplasm, consistent with apocrine differentiation.

hallmark of P-LCIS (39,41). Nucleoli are prominent, often irregular, and can be multiple. Binucleate cells are also common, especially in apocrine P-LCIS. P-LCIS is usually surrounded by C-LCIS and appears to merge seamlessly with it.

In one study evaluating molecular alterations of P-LCIS without associated invasion, investigators found that C-LCIS and P-LCIS are genetically related, but the latter displays a more complex pattern of changes. In particular, apocrine P-LCIS carries more chromosomal alterations than C-LCIS and nonapocrine P-LCIS. In the same study, investigators observed that P-LCIS presents at a median age of 55 years (vs median age of 50 years for C-LCIS), raising the possibility of late progression from C-LCIS. In contrast to C-LCIS and to other variants of S-LCIS, P-LCIS included, apocrine P-LCIS is frequently negative for ER/PR and positive for HER2 (39).

Differential Diagnosis of S-LCIS

Ductal Carcinoma In Situ

In all its possible cytomorphologic variants, S-LCIS with central necrosis very closely resembles DCIS. The differential diagnosis of S-LCIS composed of Haagensen's type A and/or type B cells includes LG-DCIS, whereas P-LCIS and apocrine P-LCIS resemble solid DCIS with intermediate to high nuclear grade, including apocrine DCIS. Lack of cell cohesion, round to ovoid cytomorphology, and presence of intracytoplasmic lumina all favor lobular over ductal differentiation. In contrast to DCIS, S-LCIS is often surrounded by C-LCIS and merges seamlessly with it. Lack of membranous immunoreactivity for E-cadherin supports lobular differentiation in problematic cases.

All S-LCIS variants were classified and managed as DCIS in the past, and this information always needs to

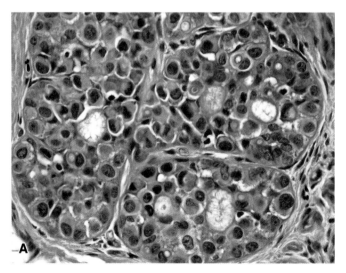
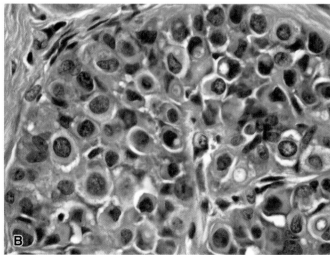

FIGURE 2.46 Pleomorphic LCIS with minimal acinar expansion. (A) The neoplastic cells are enlarged and dyshesive and grow admixed with residual myoepithelial cells, but massive acinar distension is not present. (B) Note large cell size and marked nuclear atypia.

be related and discussed with the treating clinicians, especially in the rare cases of S-LCIS without associated invasive carcinoma.

In some cases, DCIS with intermediate to high nuclear grade is present adjacent to carcinoma in situ morphologically similar to P-LCIS, and transition between the two can be observed, including gradual, patchy, and incomplete loss of E-cadherin immunoreactivity. No molecular data are available at present that can help determine if these cases represent true P-LCIS or DCIS undergoing loss of E-cadherin. In particular, close proximity of apocrine DCIS and P-LCIS/apocrine P-LCIS can be observed.

Classic LCIS

Special LCIS composed of Haagenesen's type A and/or type B cells (florid LCIS/LCIS with comedonecrosis) can raise the differential diagnosis of C-LCIS. Massive acinar expansion, necrosis, and associated calcifications are not characteristic of C-LCIS. Some of the morphologic features useful in the differential diagnosis between C-LCIS and S-LCIS are summarized in Table 2.4.

Management of Lobular Lesions

Women with ALH have a 4- to 5-fold higher risk of developing invasive breast carcinoma (44), and the risk is 8- to 10- fold higher in patients with C-LCIS (1). For risk stratification and patient management, it is therefore preferable to render a specific diagnosis of ALH or C-LCIS rather than use the more generic term of classic LN. In a recent study, Page et al reported that invasive carcinoma in patients with prior diagnosis of ALH is about 3 times more likely to involve the same breast as the index lesion (45), suggesting that ALH constitutes a possible precursor of carcinoma in addition to a generalized high-risk lesion. According to a recent systematic review of the published literature, the cumulative average risk of invasive breast carcinoma in patients with classic LN is 8.7% (range, 0–33), and it is similar in the ipsilateral (4.7%; range, 0–25) and contralateral breast (4.2%; range, 0–16). In the same analysis, about half (52%) of breast carcinoma in patients with classic LN occurred more than 10 years after the index lesion, and about a third showed lobular morphology (range, 0%–67%). On the basis of these findings, the authors concluded that classic LN should be regarded both as a risk factor and a nonobligate precursor of breast carcinoma. As a risk factor, classic LN is associated with similar low risk of invasive breast carcinoma in both breasts. As a nonobligate precursor of invasive carcinoma, classic LN is characterized by a long delay between the index lesion and subsequent invasive carcinoma, which has lobular histology in most cases (46).

■ **Table 2.4** Lobular carcinoma in situ

	Classic	Special
Cell dyshesion	Present	Present
Cell shape	Round	Round to ovoid[a]
Nuclear atypia	Low	Low to severe
Cytoplasm	Scant	Scant to abundant
Intracytoplasmic vacuoles	Present	Present
Intracytoplasmic mucin	Rare and only focal	Common, can be focal or present in most cells
Nucleoli	Rare	Common, prominent
Necrosis	Absent	Present
Mitoses	Absent	Present
Calcifications	Incidental	Common
E-cadherin	Negative	Negative
ER	100% positive	[b]Nonapocrine P-LCIS 100% positive [b]Apocrine P-LCIS 20%–25% positive
HER2[b]	100% negative	[b]Nonapocrine P-LCIS 100% negative [b]Apocrine P-LCIS 30% positive

[a]Plasmacytoid morphology is common.
[b]Based on findings reported by Chen et al (39).

Even if classic LN likely represents a precursor lesion, the margin status of classic LN (C-LCIS or ALH) is not reported, and no reexcision is performed for classic LN which is close or at a margin.

Conflicting data exist on whether LCIS increases the risk of local recurrence in patients with invasive carcinoma (47–49) or DCIS managed with breast conservation (50). Similarly, there is no consensus on the need to excise classic LN found in a core needle biopsy with good radiologic-pathologic correlation. The reported rate of upgrade in excision specimens after diagnosis of classic LN at core biopsy ranges from 4% to 28%, but most series are retrospective and selection bias likely overestimates the actual risk (51–54).

The management of S-LCIS is also controversial, as these lesions were classified and treated as DCIS in the past, and no information is available on the natural history of the disease. Only limited guidelines are available at present (9). Surgical excision of S-LCIS in a core biopsy is mandated. Most experts advocate reporting the presence of S-LCIS with necrosis, mitoses, nuclear pleomorphism, and/or predominant signet ring cell morphology near a margin to prompt reexcision, although no consensus exists on this matter. At the periphery of the lesion, S-LCIS frequently transitions into C-LCIS, and margin status of the latter is not reported.

In the past, S-LCIS misdiagnosed as DCIS and managed with breast-conserving surgery was treated with adjuvant radiotherapy. Some clinicians continue this practice for S-LCIS without invasion, whereas others object to treating a lobular lesion with radiotherapy. Unfortunately, S-LCIS without associated invasion is very rare, which precludes the design of randomized prospective trials.

Key Points

Lobular Neoplasia

- Lobular neoplasia consists of atypical lobular hyperplasia (ALH) and classic-lobular carcinoma in situ (C-LCIS).
- ALH and C-LCIS are cytologically indistinguishable and differ only in extent (C-LCIS > ALH).
- Classic LN has no specific clinical, radiologic, or macroscopic findings.
- Classic LN cells are nonpolarized, with a central nucleus and scant cytoplasm ("fried egg" morphology).
- Mitoses and necrosis are not characteristic of classic LN.
- C-LCIS carries an ×8 to ×10 risk of invasive carcinoma; the risk associated with ALH is ×4 to ×5.
- ALH and C-LCIS are also indolent nonobligate precursors of invasive carcinoma.

Special LCIS

- The term S-LCIS indicates solid carcinoma in situ with ambiguous morphology that lack membranous immunoreactivity for E-cadherin.
- Central necrosis with coarse calcifications is common.

- Cells are dyshesive and not polarized.
- Mitoses are frequent.
- Associated stromal (micro) invasion is common (about 50%–60% of cases).
- S-LCIS is usually surrounded by C-LCIS and merges with it.
- S-LCIS can be roughly subdivided into 2 types based on cytomorphology:

  (a) S-LCIS composed of Haagensen's type A cells and/or type B cells, alone or in combination shows massive acinar distention (>50 cells across the diameter of an acinus), necrosis and associated calcifications. Other terms include florid LCIS or LCIS with comedonecrosis. Binucleate cells are common.

  (b) S-LCIS composed of large cells with abundant cytoplasm, intracytoplasmic vacuoles, and large (×≥4 size of lymphocytes) pleomorphic (×2-×3 size variation) nuclei is also referred to as P-LCIS. Binucleate cells are common. Apocrine P-LCIS has abundant eosinophilic cytoplasm or consists predominantly of signet ring cells with abundant intracytoplasmic mucin.

- S-LCIS is usually ER- and PR-positive and HER2-negative, but apocrine P-LCIS can be ER/PR-negative and HER2-positive in about a third of cases.
- S-LCIS presents clinically as mammographic calcifications, a mass lesion, or architectural distortion.
- Management of S-LCIS is controversial:

  (a) S-LCIS in a core biopsy always need to be excised.

  (b) Reexcision of S-LCIS with massive acinar distension/necrosis/mitoses/nuclear pleomorphism and/or signet ring morphology near a margin is recommended.

  (c) Adjuvant radiotherapy in cases of S-LCIS without invasion managed with breast conservation is subject of debate.

■ REFERENCES

1. Page DL, Dupont WD, Rogers LW, Rados MS. Atypical hyperplastic lesions of the female breast. A long-term follow-up study. *Cancer.* 1985; 55:2698–2708.
2. Tavassoli FA, Norris HJ. A comparison of the results of long-term follow-up for atypical intraductal hyperplasia and intraductal hyperplasia of the breast. *Cancer.* 1990;65:518–529.

3. Rosai J. Borderline epithelial lesions of the breast. *Am J Surg Pathol*. 1991;15:209–221.

4. Schnitt SJ, Connolly JL, Tavassoli FA, et al. Interobserver reproducibility in the diagnosis of ductal proliferative breast lesions using standardized criteria. *Am J Surg Pathol*. 1992;16:1133–1143.

5. Page DL, Rogers LW. Combined histologic and cytologic criteria for the diagnosis of mammary atypical ductal hyperplasia. *Hum Pathol*. 1992;23:1095–1097.

6. Dupont WD, Page DL. Breast cancer risk associated with proliferative disease, age at first birth, and a family history of breast cancer. *Am J Epidemiol*. 1987;125:769–779.

7. Carter CL, Corle DK, Micozzi MS, Schatzkin A, Taylor PR. A prospective study of the development of breast cancer in 16,692 women with benign breast disease. *Am J Epidemiol*. 1988;128:467–477.

8. Collins LC, Achacoso NA, Nekhlyudov L, et al. Clinical and pathologic features of ductal carcinoma in situ associated with the presence of flat epithelial atypia: an analysis of 543 patients. *Mod Pathol*. 2007;20:1149–1155.

9. Tavassoli FA, Devilee P, eds. *World Health Organization Classification of Tumours. Pathology and Genetics. Tumours of the Breast and Female Genital Organs*. Lyon: IARC Press; 2003.

10. Abdel-Fatah TM, Powe DG, Hodi Z, Lee AH, Reis-Filho JS, Ellis IO. High frequency of coexistence of columnar cell lesions, lobular neoplasia, and low grade ductal carcinoma in situ with invasive tubular carcinoma and invasive lobular carcinoma. *Am J Surg Pathol*. 2007;31:417–426.

11. Abdel-Fatah TM, Powe DG, Hodi Z, Reis-Filho JS, Lee AH, Ellis IO. Morphologic and molecular evolutionary pathways of low nuclear grade invasive breast cancers and their putative precursor lesions: further evidence to support the concept of low nuclear grade breast neoplasia family. *Am J Surg Pathol*. 2008;32:513–523.

12. Aulmann S, Elsawaf Z, Penzel R, Schirmacher P, Sinn HP. Invasive tubular carcinoma of the breast frequently is clonally related to flat epithelial atypia and low-grade ductal carcinoma in situ. *Am J Surg Pathol*. 2009;33:1646–1653.

13. Sgroi D, Koerner FC. Involvement of collagenous spherulosis by lobular carcinoma in situ. Potential confusion with cribriform ductal carcinoma in situ. *Am J Surg Pathol*. 1995;19:1366–1370.

14. Page DL, Dixon JM, Anderson TJ, Lee D, Stewart HJ. Invasive cribriform carcinoma of the breast. *Histopathology*. 1983;7:525–536.

15. Farshid G, Moinfar F, Meredith DJ, Peiterse S, Tavassoli FA. Spindle cell ductal carcinoma in situ. An unusual variant of ductal intra-epithelial neoplasia that simulates ductal hyperplasia or a myoepithelial proliferation. *Virchows Arch*. 2001;439:70–77.

16. Leal C, Henrique R, Monteiro P, et al. Apocrine ductal carcinoma in situ of the breast: histologic classification and expression of biologic markers. *Hum Pathol*. 2001;32:487–493.

17. Jones C, Damiani S, Wells D, Chaggar R, Lakhani SR, Eusebi V. Molecular cytogenetic comparison of apocrine hyperplasia and apocrine carcinoma of the breast. *Am J Pathol*. 2001;158:207–214.

18. Livasy CA, Perou CM, Karaca G, et al. Identification of a basal-like subtype of breast ductal carcinoma in situ. *Hum Pathol*. 2007;38:197–204.

19. Bryan BB, Schnitt SJ, Collins LC. Ductal carcinoma in situ with basal-like phenotype: a possible precursor to invasive basal-like breast cancer. *Mod Pathol*. 2006;19:617–621.

20. Guerry P, Erlandson RA, Rosen PP. Cystic hypersecretory hyperplasia and cystic hypersecretory duct carcinoma of the breast. Pathology, therapy, and follow-up of 39 patients. *Cancer*. 1988;61:1611–1620.

21. Rosen PP, Scott M. Cystic hypersecretory duct carcinoma of the breast. *Am J Surg Pathol*. 1984;8:31–41.

22. Shin SJ, Rosen PP. Carcinoma arising from preexisting pregnancy-like and cystic hypersecretory hyperplasia lesions of the breast: a clinicopathologic study of 9 patients. *Am J Surg Pathol*. 2004;28:789–793.

23. Shin SJ, Rosen PP. Pregnancy-like (pseudolactational) hyperplasia: a primary diagnosis in mammographically detected lesions of the breast and its relationship to cystic hypersecretory hyperplasia. *Am J Surg Pathol*. 2000;24:1670–1674.

24. Van Zee KJ, Liberman L, Samli B, et al. Long term follow-up of women with ductal carcinoma in situ treated with breast-conserving surgery: the effect of age. *Cancer*. 1999;86:1757–1767.

25. Rudloff U, Jacks LM, Goldberg JI, et al. Nomogram for predicting the risk of local recurrence after breast-conserving surgery for ductal carcinoma in situ. *J Clin Oncol*. 2010;28:3762–3769.

26. Fisher B, Dignam J, Wolmark N, et al. Lumpectomy and radiation therapy for the treatment of intraductal breast cancer: findings from National Surgical Adjuvant Breast and Bowel Project B-17. *J Clin Oncol*. 1998;16:441–452.

27. Bijker N, Meijnen P, Peterse JL, et al. Breast-conserving treatment with or without radiotherapy in ductal carcinoma-in-situ: ten-year results of European Organisation for Research and Treatment of Cancer randomized phase III trial 10853—a study by the EORTC Breast Cancer Cooperative Group and EORTC Radiotherapy Group. *J Clin Oncol*. 2006;24:3381–3387.

28. Wong JS, Kaelin CM, Troyan SL, et al. Prospective study of wide excision alone for ductal carcinoma in situ of the breast. *J Clin Oncol.* 2006;24:1031–1036.

29. Rudloff U, Brogi E, Reiner AS, et al. The influence of margin width and volume of disease near margin on benefit of radiation therapy for women with DCIS treated with breast-conserving therapy. *Ann Surg.* 2010;251:583–591.

30. Fisher B, Dignam J, Wolmark N, et al. Tamoxifen in treatment of intraductal breast cancer: National Surgical Adjuvant Breast and Bowel Project B-24 randomised controlled trial. *Lancet.* 1999;353:1993–2000.

31. Moore KH, Sweeney KJ, Wilson ME, et al. Outcomes for women with ductal carcinoma-in-situ and a positive sentinel node: a multi-institutional audit. *Ann Surg Oncol.* 2007;14:2911–2917.

32. Shapiro-Wright HM, Julian TB. Sentinel lymph node biopsy and management of the axilla in ductal carcinoma in situ. *J Natl Cancer Inst Monogr.* 2010;2010:145–149.

33. Page DL. *Diagnostic Histopathology of the Breast.* New York: Churchill Livingstone; 1987.

34. Vos CB, Cleton-Jansen AM, Berx G, et al. E-cadherin inactivation in lobular carcinoma in situ of the breast: an early event in tumorigenesis. *Br J Cancer.* 1997;76:1131–1133.

35. Fitzgerald RC, Hardwick R, Huntsman D, et al. Hereditary diffuse gastric cancer: updated consensus guidelines for clinical management and directions for future research. *J Med Genet.* 2010;47:436–444.

36. Haagensen CD, Lane N, Lattes R, Bodian C. Lobular neoplasia (so-called lobular carcinoma in situ) of the breast. *Cancer.* 1978;42:737–769.

37. Harigopal M, Shin SJ, Murray MP, Tickoo SK, Brogi E, Rosen PP. Aberrant E-cadherin staining patterns in invasive mammary carcinoma. *World J Surg Oncol.* 2005;3:73.

38. Da Silva L, Parry S, Reid L, et al. Aberrant expression of E-cadherin in lobular carcinomas of the breast. *Am J Surg Pathol.* 2008;32:773–783.

39. Chen YY, Hwang ES, Roy R, et al. Genetic and phenotypic characteristics of pleomorphic lobular carcinoma in situ of the breast. *Am J Surg Pathol.* 2009;33:1683–1694.

40. Fadare O, Dadmanesh F, Alvarado-Cabrero I, et al. Lobular intraepithelial neoplasia [lobular carcinoma in situ] with comedo-type necrosis: a clinicopathologic study of 18 cases. *Am J Surg Pathol.* 2006;30:1445–1453.

41. Sneige N, Wang J, Baker BA, Krishnamurthy S, Middleton LP. Clinical, histopathologic, and biologic features of pleomorphic lobular (ductal-lobular) carcinoma in situ of the breast: a report of 24 cases. *Mod Pathol.* 2002;15:1044–1050.

42. Sapino A, Frigerio A, Peterse JL, Arisio R, Coluccia C, Bussolati G. Mammographically detected in situ lobular carcinomas of the breast. *Virchows Arch.* 2000;436:421–430.

43. Rosen PP. *Rosen's Breast Pathology.* 3rd ed. Philadelphia: Lippincott, Williams & Wilkins; 2008.

44. Page DL, Dupont WD. Anatomic markers of human premalignancy and risk of breast cancer. *Cancer.* 1990;66:1326–1335.

45. Page DL Schuyler PA, Dupont WD, Jensen RA, Plummer WD, Simpson JF. Atypical lobular hyperplasia as a unilateral predictor of breast cancer risk: a retrospective cohort study. *Lancet.* 2003;361:125–129.

46. Ansquer Y, Delaney S, Santulli P, Salomon L, Carbonne B, Salmon R. Risk of invasive breast cancer after lobular intra-epithelial neoplasia: review of the literature. *Eur J Surg Oncol.* 2010;36:604–609.

47. Abner AL, Connolly JL, Recht A, et al. The relation between the presence and extent of lobular carcinoma in situ and the risk of local recurrence for patients with infiltrating carcinoma of the breast treated with conservative surgery and radiation therapy. *Cancer.* 2000;88:1072–1077.

48. Sasson AR, Fowble B, Hanlon AL, et al. Lobular carcinoma in situ increases the risk of local recurrence in selected patients with stages I and II breast carcinoma treated with conservative surgery and radiation. *Cancer.* 2001;91:1862–1869.

49. Ben-David MA, Kleer CG, Paramagul C, Griffith KA, Pierce LJ. Is lobular carcinoma in situ as a component of breast carcinoma a risk factor for local failure after breast-conserving therapy? Results of a matched pair analysis. *Cancer.* 2006;106:28–34.

50. Rudloff U, Brogi E, Brockway JP, et al. Concurrent lobular neoplasia increases the risk of ipsilateral breast cancer recurrence in patients with ductal carcinoma in situ treated with breast-conserving therapy. *Cancer.* 2009;115:1203–1214.

51. Subhawong AP, Subhawong TK, Khouri N, Tsangaris T, Nassar H. Incidental minimal atypical lobular hyperplasia on core needle biopsy: correlation with findings on follow-up excision. *Am J Surg Pathol.* 2010;34:822–828.

52. Shin SJ, Rosen PP. Excisional biopsy should be performed if lobular carcinoma in situ is seen on needle core biopsy. *Arch Pathol Lab Med.* 2002;126:697–701.

53. Elsheikh TM, Silverman JF. Follow-up surgical excision is indicated when breast core needle biopsies show atypical lobular hyperplasia or lobular

carcinoma in situ: a correlative study of 33 patients with review of the literature. *Am J Surg Pathol.* 2005;29:534–543.

54. Cangiarella J, Guth A, Axelrod D, et al. Is surgical excision necessary for the management of atypical lobular hyperplasia and lobular carcinoma in situ diagnosed on core needle biopsy? A report of 38 cases and review of the literature. *Arch Pathol Lab Med.* 2008;132:979–983.

3

Papillary Lesions of the Breast

CANSU KARAKAS

ERIKA RESETKOVA

AYSEGUL A. SAHIN

■ BENIGN PAPILLARY LESIONS OF THE BREAST

Intraductal Papilloma

Clinical Presentation

Intraductal papilloma is typically a solitary lesion located centrally in the breast within the major or lactiferous ducts; hence, it has been often referred to as a central papilloma. This tumor occurs most frequently in the fifth or sixth decade of life and often manifests with a serous or serosanguineous nipple discharge (1,2). Although frequently not palpable, it may be detected as a subareolar mass (central solitary papilloma), or it may be detected in one of the breast quadrants. Intraductal papilloma typically is not seen on mammogram because of its small size and intraductal location. However, mammographic findings may include a round- to oval-shaped nodule or a solitary dense mass (3,4). Microcalcifications suggest a long-standing lesion (5).

Ultrasonography may be useful in determining the cystic or solid nature of a papillary lesion (1). Galactography is a safe and simple technique for imaging the affected duct system in cases of nipple discharge. Intraductal papilloma may appear as an intraductal filling defect or obstruction of the flow of contrast material (4,6). Magnetic resonance imaging (MRI) is a relatively new imaging tool, useful especially in younger women with denser breast tissue. Intraductal papilloma may present with varying appearance on MRI, ranging from occult lesion to "small intraluminal mass" or irregular, rapidly enhancing lesion (7). Mammary ductoscopy is a useful endoscopic technique that is direct and accurate in characterizing intraductal lesions (8).

Although any of these imaging techniques may be helpful in establishing the diagnosis of a papillary lesion, neither mammographic nor sonographic features are sensitive and specific enough to allow accurate differentiation between benign and malignant papillary lesions. Both can appear as an architectural distortion, a mass, or solid, round, and clustered suspect calcifications (3,4,6).

Pathologic Features

Intraductal papilloma is characterized by branching fibrovascular cores that protrude into the ductal lumina (Figure 3.1). The fibrovascular cores are composed of fibrous branches with centrally located vessels lined by endothelial cells and a fairly uniform myoepithelial cell layer at the base of the core with the epithelial cell layer facing the lumen (1,9) (Figure 3.2). The myoepithelial cells are usually round to cuboidal and often have clear cytoplasm (Figures 3.3–3.5). The epithelial cells are cuboidal to columnar and sometimes demonstrate varying degrees of hyperchromasia. Epithelial hyperplasia may lead to more complex structures exhibiting fusion of papillary fronds and formation of irregular secondary lumina (1,5,9,10) (Figures 3.6–3.7).

Often, a portion of the epithelium can be replaced by apocrine metaplasia and less often by squamous metaplasia (Figures 3.8–3.13). Squamous metaplasia is a result of a reparative process usually related to prior infarction. Clear cell, mucinous, and sebaceous metaplasia could be present, but those are less frequent (1,10,11).

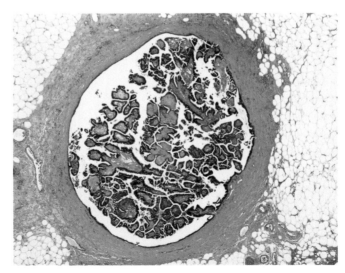

FIGURE 3.1 An intraductal papilloma. Low-power magnification of intraductal papilloma completely filling the entire duct.

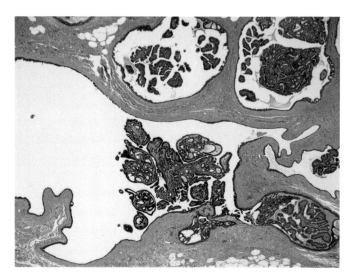

FIGURE 3.2   An intraductal papilloma, partially involving duct.

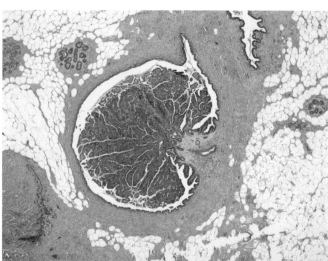

FIGURE 3.3   An intraducal papilloma. The arborescent proliferation of the epithelium resulting in fusion of the papillary fronds.

When there is extensive sclerosis in the intraductal papilloma, the lesion is defined as *sclerosing papilloma* (Figures 3.14–3.18). Sometimes, distorted tubules entrapped in the sclerotic areas mimic an invasion (Figure 3.19). Benign cytologic features, lack of desmoplastic reaction, and preservation of the myoepithelial cell layer surrounding small glands facilitate the correct diagnosis (5,10,11). Papillomas are frequently associated with adjacent sclerosing adenosis (Figures 3.20–3.22). Papillary torsion may cause hemorrhagic infarction (Figure 3.8). In most cases, the specific cause for the infarction is unclear. Needling procedures may lead to infarction and hemorrhage (1,10,11).

Cytologic Features

Cytologic diagnosis of intraductal papilloma can be made either by examining the serous or bloody nipple secretions or by fine-needle aspiration of a palpable lesion (12–15). Benign papillary lesions usually yield cellular aspirate that contains clusters of ductal cells, often exhibiting papillary configuration (Figure 3.23). The ductal cells within groups are tightly packed, but groups can occasionally appear crowded and may show varying degrees of cytologic atypia ranging from mild to moderate in the form of variability of nuclear sizes and presence of nuclear hyperchromasia (Figures 3.24–3.25). Myoepithelial cells

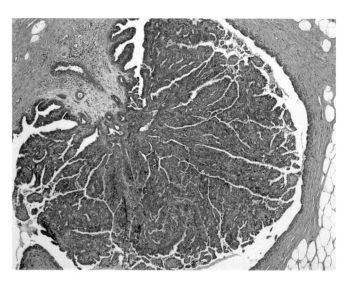

FIGURE 3.4   An intraductal papilloma. On a higher magnification, the attachment point of the papillary proliferation from the duct wall is apparent.

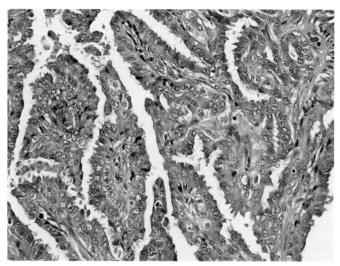

FIGURE 3.5   High-power view of an intraductal papilloma illustrated in Figures 3.3 and 3.4 showing that the papillary fronds consist of fibrovascular cores covered by an inner myoepithelial cell layer and outer epithelial cell layer.

CHAPTER 3 • Papillary Lesions of the Breast

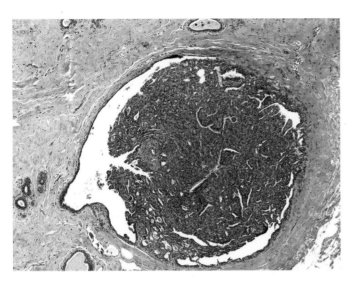

FIGURE 3.6 A papilloma with usual ductal epithelial hyperplasia. This lesion displays more complex architecture with the presence of ductal epithelial hyperplasia that fills the spaces between fibrovascular stalks causing fusion of papillary fronds and forming a solid area in the central portion of the papilloma with irregular fenestrations at the periphery.

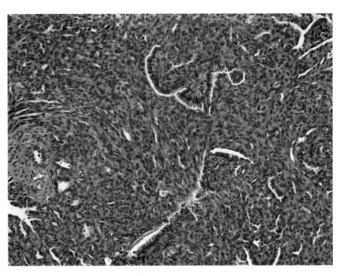

FIGURE 3.7 A papilloma with usual ductal epithelial hyperplasia. At higher magnification, the epithelial proliferation in papilloma in Figure 3.6 exhibits the architectural and cytologic features consistent with usual ductal hyperplasia. The streaming of ovoid-shaped cells, the presence of cellular overlapping, and a heterogeneous pattern indicates two-cell-types and is consistent with benign epithelial proliferation.

and naked nuclei are present in benign papillary lesions (Figure 3.26), and apocrine metaplastic cells (Figure 3.27), foamy macrophages (Figure 3.28), and squamous metaplastic cells are frequently noted in the proteinaceous background. More pronounced atypia and necrosis may sometimes be seen in the presence of infarction and do not necessary signify malignant nature of the lesion. In such cases, an additional sampling either by core needle biopsy (CNB) or excisional biopsy should be recommended

by the pathologist to rule out a more worrisome lesion (12,16,17).

Differential Diagnosis

Although most intraductal papillomas share specific histopathologic features, there are several difficulties regarding their diagnosis and classification. The criteria for differentiating benign intraductal papilloma from papillary ductal carcinoma in situ (DCIS) were first defined by Kraus and Neubecker (18) 48 years ago and are still in use today. The most important histologic feature distinguishing benign

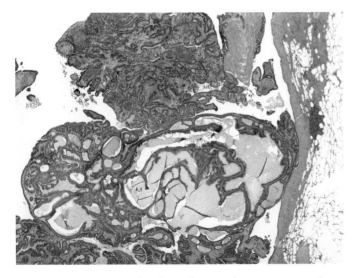

FIGURE 3.8 An intraductal papilloma with apocrine metaplasia. The foci of apocrine metaplasia are frequent in benign papillomas. In this case, the papillary proliferation forms a cystic nodule that protrudes into the cyst lumen and is surrounded by a fibrous capsule. Apocrine epithelium is evident in the midportion of the papillary lesion.

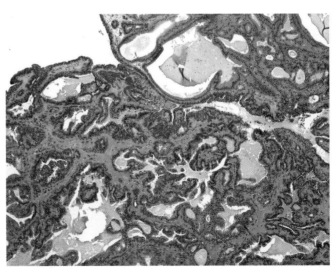

FIGURE 3.9 On higher magnification, an intraductal papilloma from Figure 3.8, usual duct hyperplasia (bottom portion), is admixed with metaplastic apocrine cells (top portion).

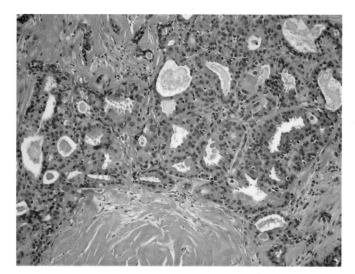

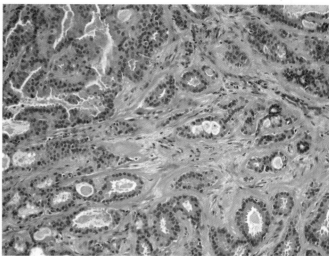

FIGURE 3.10 Apocrine metaplasia is characterized by enlarged epithelial cells with abundant granular, eosinophilic cytoplasm that frequently shows apical snouting. The nuclei are round, of variable size, and generally have vesicular chromatin and prominent nucleoli. The myoepithelial cell layer is less distinct in areas of apocrine metaplasia. The presence of apocrine metaplasia within the papillary lesion favors benignity.

FIGURE 3.11 Some areas within the center of the intraductal lesion show increased stromal sclerosis. A high-power magnification illustrating an irregular, entrapped glandular epithelium within sclerotic stroma. This may mimic invasion especially in small core biopsy sample.

intraductal papilloma from atypical papilloma or malignant counterparts (papillary intraductal carcinoma) is the epithelium. In benign papilloma, the epithelial layer is supported by myoepithelial cells, which are ordinarily visible on hematoxylin and eosin stain in most lesions. The continuous, basally oriented myoepithelial cell layer is discohesive or completely absent within papillary carcinoma (1,19).

In certain cases, demonstrating the myoepithelial cells at the base of the epithelium requires immunohistochemical analysis. Cytoplasmic expression in myoepithelial cells can be demonstrated by many markers, including S-100, CK14,

34βE12, CD10, smooth muscle actin, calponin, CK5/6, and heavy chain myosin. Several of the above markers can cross-react with stromal myofibroblasts or vascular structures and are difficult to interpret. The nuclear marker p63 is more specific for myoepithelial cells, and it exhibits no cross-reactivity for stromal cells, but sometimes, it can also be expressed in the nuclei of overlying epithelial cells in a papillary lesion. However, p63-positive epithelial cells can be readily distinguished from myoepithelium by their position in the fibrovascular cores (Figures 3.29–3.30). In clinical practice, it is prudent to use a panel composed of several cytoplasmic and nuclear myoepithelial markers because variable staining of myoepithelium and stromal elements may occur with some but not all markers in benign intraductal papillomas (1).

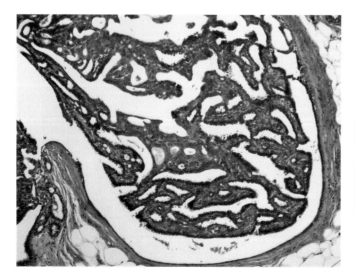

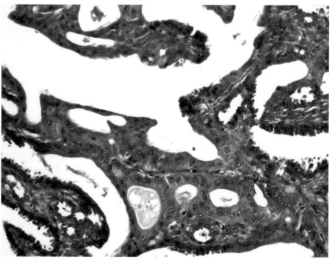

FIGURE 3.12 Another example of low magnification illustrating apocrine metaplasia in intraductal papilloma.

FIGURE 3.13 Another example of high magnification of apocrine metaplasia in intraductal papilloma.

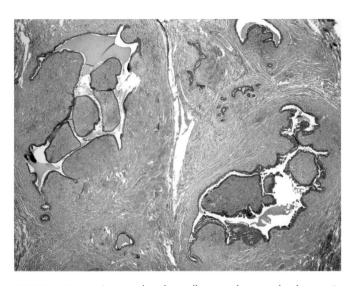

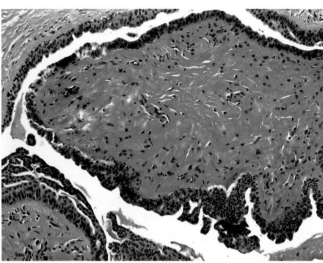

FIGURE 3.14 An intraductal papilloma with stromal sclerosis. In some cases, sclerosis may be diffuse, thus transforming the involved duct into a completely hyalinized nodule.

FIGURE 3.15 At a higher magnification, the papillary stalk has a dense, hypocellular, collagenized stroma lined with epithelial and myo-epithelial cell layer.

Certain degree of epithelial proliferation could be observed either focally or diffusely in many benign intraductal papillomas. When hyperplastic epithelium extensively and/or completely fills the duct lumen, it can obscure the papillary nature of the lesion and may mimic malignancy, especially in small samples, such as in CNB. Solid areas of hyperplastic cells with nuclear overlapping, admixture of cell types, streaming, and fenestrated areas favor benign epithelial proliferation (1,11). Moreover, myoepithelial cells are evenly distributed throughout the base of the epithelium in benign intraductal papillomas. In addition to myoepithelial cell markers, high-molecular-weight cytokeratin and basement membrane markers are useful in distinguishing papillary lesions, which are suggestive of atypia, involvement by carcinoma, or presence of peripheral invasion (11). The role of these markers will

be further discussed in the section of papillary carcinoma. A papilloma with prominent stromal sclerosis may simulate an invasive carcinoma but may also mimic fibroadenoma. In infarcted papillomas, fibrosis at the periphery of the lesion can mimic an invasive process (10). The presence of clusters of squamous metaplastic cells surrounded by fibrous tissue can also be interpreted as invasive carcinoma. Benign cytologic features, lack of desmoplastic reaction, and presence of myoepithelial cells around the entrapped tubules and glandular structures facilitate benign diagnosis (1).

Management

Central papilloma when not associated with epithelial atypia is considered a benign lesion. In a large

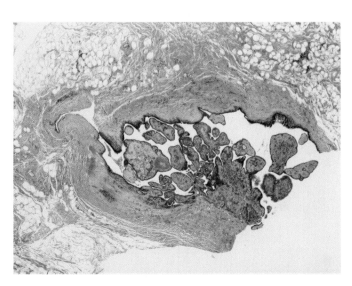

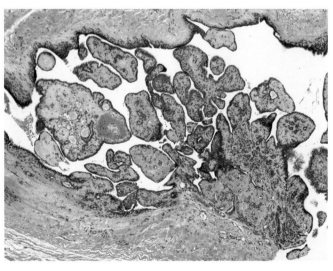

FIGURE 3.16 Sclerosing papilloma, low magnification.

FIGURE 3.17 Sclerosing papilloma, higher magnification of the lesion in Figure 3.16. Stromal sclerosis is present throughout this papilloma.

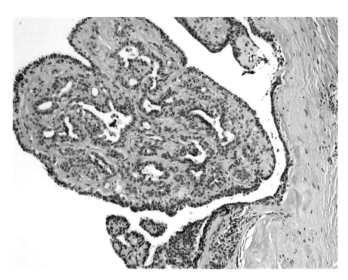

FIGURE 3.18 A high-power magnification of the papilloma from Figure 3.16 shows small, irregular, distorted ductal glands entrapped within one sclerotic nodule.

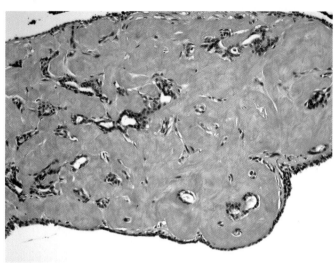

FIGURE 3.19 Sometimes distorted tubules entrapped in the sclerotic areas may mimic an invasion. However, in benign intraductal papillomas with sclerosis, myoepithelial cells are visible around at least some of these entrapped glands.

retrospective study that included 372 solitary papillomas after a mean follow-up period of 16 years, patients with a solitary papilloma lacking epithelial atypia had a slight increased chance for subsequent development of breast cancer, which is similar to the risk in patients with proliferative fibrocystic disease without atypia (20). In the past, papilloma was regarded as a precancerous lesion, and surgical excision was indicated for the diagnosis and treatment of these lesions. Recently, ultrasound-guided and stereotactic CNBs have been increasingly replacing surgical excision in the diagnosis of both clinically occult and palpable breast lesions (21–23). However, the optimal diagnostic modality and management of benign papillary lesions still remain highly controversial.

Large series reveal that the percentage of papillary lesions detected by CNB ranges from 0.7% to 4% (21,24–27). Sampling error could be a problem in the correct classification of papillary lesions on CNB, particularly if only a small portion of the lesion is sampled (27). Distinguishing a benign from a malignant lesion may be difficult on the limited, fragmented material obtained by CNB. Areas of atypia or carcinoma may be totally missed in the limited sample (22). Several published studies have suggested that excision of a larger volume of tissue, as with directional vacuum-assisted biopsy, may improve the accuracy of core biopsy evaluation (28,29). Another problem associated with CNB sampling is displacement due to needling procedures. Benign epithelial cells can be

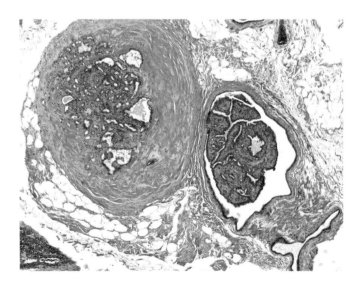

FIGURE 3.20 An intraductal papilloma with adjacent sclerosing adenosis. Intraductal papillomas are frequently associated with other benign epithelial proliferations and fibrocystic changes.

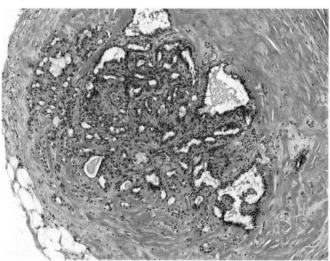

FIGURE 3.21 Sclerosing adenosis is characterized by a lobulated proliferation of closely packed ductules. The central portion of the lesion is more cellular, in the periphery of the lesion, the sclerosis dominates.

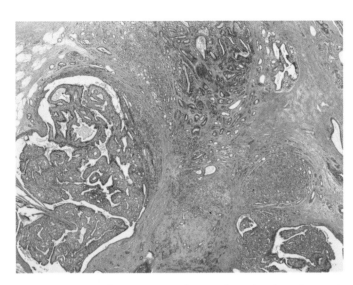

FIGURE 3.22 A low-power magnification of intraductal papilloma with adjacent foci of sclerosing adenosis. In this case, numerous small tubules are proliferating around and parallel to the intraductal papilloma.

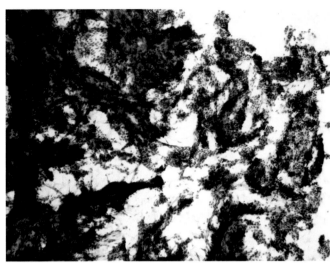

FIGURE 3.23 Cytology of an intraductal papilloma. Highly cellular aspirate is composed of sheets of ductal epithelium arranged in papillary configuration with central fibrovascular stalks.

displaced within the biopsy site, along the needle tract, and travel through lymphatic channels to axillary lymph nodes, which may simulate an invasive carcinoma (30, 31). A history of a recent needling procedure, presence of prior biopsy site changes, and/or granulation tissue and hemorrhage surrounding the epithelial cell clusters favor mechanical transport (32,33).

In certain cases, it is difficult to distinguish a benign papillary lesion with sclerosis and entrapment of epithelial elements from invasive carcinoma based on morphologic evaluation (22). The presence of a myoepithelial cell layer and lack of cytologic atypia help to distinguish benign lesions from carcinoma (21). Benign papillary

lesions of the breast are more likely to be marked by sclerosis, stromal hyalinization, or fibrocystic changes after CNB than atypical papillomas or papillary carcinomas (21).

The reported frequency of finding a more worrisome lesion on subsequent excision (such as atypical ductal hyperplasia [ADH] or carcinoma) after a diagnosis of benign papilloma on CNB ranges from 0% to 25% (26,28,29,34–36). As a consequence of frequent upgrade, some investigators recommend surgical excision for all papillary lesions diagnosed on CNB (9,22,24,25,34,37–41). Some authors have suggested that stereotactic or ultrasound-guided CNB may be reliable in differentiating most

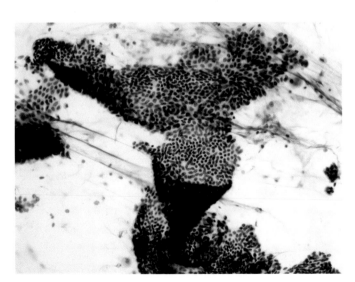

FIGURE 3.24 Cytology of an intraductal papilloma. On a higher magnification, sheets of ductal epithelium are arranged in papillary configuration. Myoepithelial cells and macrophages are noted in a background. Small fragment of apocrine metaplastic cells is present in the upper left portion.

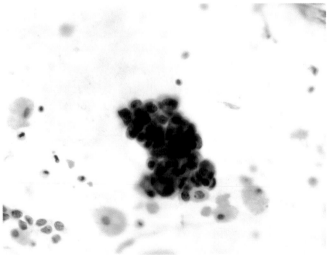

FIGURE 3.25 Cytology of an intraductal papilloma. Papillary cluster of benign ductal cells is well demonstrated, although the chromatin detail is difficult to visualize, and the group appears crowded and shows some variability of nuclear size and nuclear hyperchromasia. Macrophages are noticeable in a background.

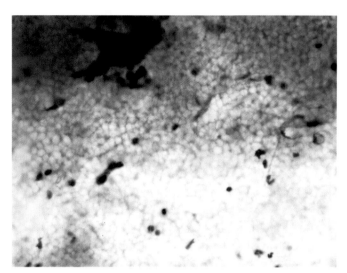

FIGURE 3.26 Cytology of an intraductal papilloma. Papillary cluster of benign ductal cells in a proteinaceous background with scattered naked nuclei present in a background.

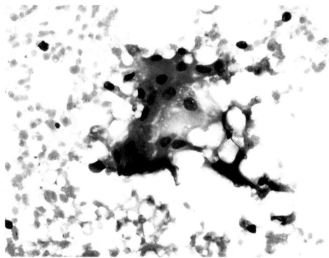

FIGURE 3.27 Cytology of an intraductal papilloma. Apocrine meta-plastic cells are frequently noted in intraductal papilloma and are better illustrated in Diff quick stained smears and are a very helpful feature in distinguishing this benign entity from papillary carcinoma.

benign and malignant papillary lesions, especially when the results correlate with clinical and imaging findings. The patients may be monitored clinically without undergoing surgical excision, and surgical excision is recommended for those patients with discrepancy of radiologic and pathologic findings or if the tissue obtained on CNB shows atypia or is considered inadequate for definitive diagnosis (21,26–28,36,42–44).

Multiple Intraductal Papillomas

Clinical Presentation

Papillomatosis, which is defined as peripheral/multiple intraductal papillomas, is characterized by papillary proliferations within multiple terminal ductal lobular units or in the distal branches of the duct system. Papillomatosis

has been defined by several authors as at least 5 microscopic foci separated by uninvolved mammary tissue within a localized segment of breast tissue (2,45,46). Multiple intraductal papillomas are more likely to occur bilaterally. The incidence of multiple papillomas is less than 10% that of solitary papilloma (47). Patients with multiple papillomas tend to be younger than patients with a solitary/central papilloma; cases of multiple papillomas appear most often in the fourth or fifth decade of life. Nipple discharge occurs rarely, only when the lesion is extensive and extends to the subareolar region. Most lesions are clinically occult. When abundant, nodular masses or, rarely, calcifications may be seen on mammography (9).

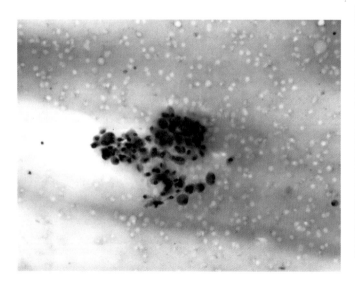

FIGURE 3.28 Cytology of an intraductal papilloma. Foamy macrophages in a proteinaceous background.

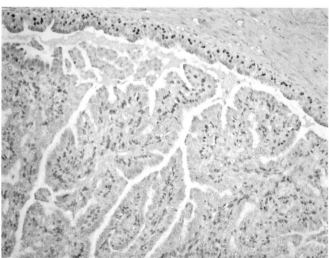

FIGURE 3.29 p63 immunostain demonstrates myoepithelial cells within the papillae and at the periphery of the duct in a benign intraductal papilloma.

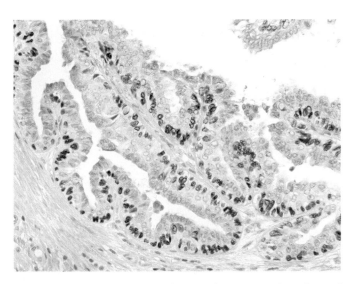

FIGURE 3.30 A higher magnification of p63 immunohistochemical staining from Figure 3.29 demonstrating labeling of myoepithelial cells at the base of each frond.

Pathologic Features

The morphologic and cytologic features of multiple intraductal papillomas are similar to those of solitary/central intraductal papilloma. Proliferation or protrusions with multiple points of attachment are more common findings in papillomatosis (9).

Management

The slightly higher risk of developing breast cancer has been reported in patients with multiple intraductal papillomas than in those with a solitary/central intraductal papilloma (11,20,48–50). In 1977, Carter (51) found that 6 of 64 patients with a benign intraductal papilloma developed carcinoma after 5 to 17 years of clinical monitoring. The incidence was higher in patients with multiple papillomas and was further elevated by coexisting proliferative fibrocystic disease (51). A retrospective study by Ali-Fehmi et al in 2003, which included 28 patients with various coexisting atypical and malignant lesions, showed that patients with multiple papillomas were more likely to have an atypical or malignant epithelial lesion than those with a solitary/central papilloma. Although atypical lesions (ADH or lobular neoplasia) were observed frequently in sections of the breast outside the field of papillomas, DCIS and invasive carcinomas almost always arose within the area of papillomatosis or atypical multiple papillomas. These pathologic findings suggest that papillomatosis might be characterized by progressive growth and histologic alteration into increasingly aggressive lesions (48). A more recent, larger study in the Mayo Clinic series, which included 372 patients, reported that the risk of developing cancer was 3 to 7 times greater in patients with papillomatosis than in those with a solitary/central papilloma and that multiple

papillomas with atypia carried even higher relative risk (20).

The findings of these studies, besides the known increased risk of cancer, suggest that patients with multiple papillomas should be carefully followed. In view of the significant frequency of bilaterality, diagnostic radiographic imaging of contralateral breast tissue may be appropriate. Open biopsy should be considered to exclude in situ or invasive carcinoma if the lesion is mammographically silent or the patient is premenopausal (20,48).

Juvenile Papillomatosis

Clinical Presentation

Juvenile papillomatosis (JP) of the breast (Swiss cheese disease) is a proliferative epithelial lesion of the breast that occurs almost exclusively in young adult women. There are only 8 JP male cases reported in the literature (52). Clinically, JP is detected as a solitary, firm, unilateral mass, often in the upper outer quadrant of the breast that clinically suggests a fibroadenoma (53,54). Mammography is not routinely performed in the diagnosis of JP because of the young age of the patients. If performed, it shows changes similar to those observed in a fibroadenoma or a cyst (55). The sonographic appearance of JP is an ill-defined and nonhomogeneus, hypoechoic mass with multiple cysts (56,57). The MRI shows several internal cysts best observed on T2-weighted sequence (58). A high proportion of patients with JP have a family history of breast cancer, and increased frequency of concurrent and subsequent carcinoma has been described in a few case reports (53,55). Up to 10% to 15% of patients with JP also have breast carcinoma (54,59). The types of breast carcinoma that have been encountered include intraductal carcinoma, infiltrating lobular carcinoma, lobular carcinoma in situ (LCIS), infiltrating ductal carcinoma, and secretory carcinoma. Patients with this lesion often have a family history of breast carcinoma, although the long-term risk for the development of carcinoma in patients with JP remains unknown (59,60).

Pathologic Features

The histopathologic criteria for the diagnosis of this lesion were defined by Rosen et al (53) and are as follows: (1) duct papillomatosis with or without epithelial atypia, (2) cysts and apocrine cysts with papillary apocrine hyperplasia, (3) sclerosing adenosis, and (4) duct stasis and duct ectasia. Cysts and ductal hyperplasia are common features. In most cases, the ductal proliferative changes consist of usual ductal hyperplasia, which is often florid and may show foci of necrosis. Atypical ductal hyperplasia may be also seen. Sometimes, ductal hyperplasia is accompanied by sclerosis that may mimic a radial scar pattern. The epithelium of the cysts or duct hyperplasia frequently exhibits apocrine metaplasia, which may either be flat or papillary (53,59). None

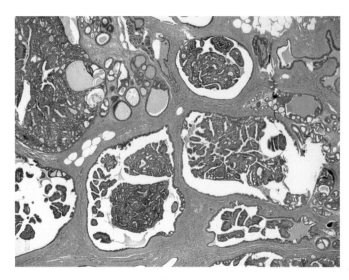

FIGURE 3.31 Papillomas with atypical epithelial proliferation. A low-power magnification shows multiple peripheral ducts with various patterns of papillary proliferation at different stages of the development.

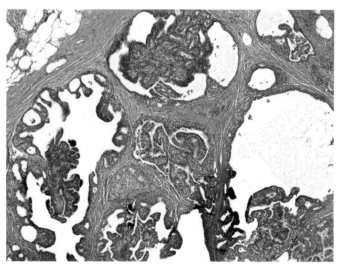

FIGURE 3.32 Papillomas with foci of atypical epithelial proliferation. On a higher magnification of Figure 3.31, there are small foci of monomorphic epithelial cells with a cribriform pattern that are associated with microcalcifications.

of these histologic features are unique to this lesion, and the diagnosis of JP should be made by correlation of age with the clinical features and pathologic parameters (53).

Cytologic Features

Cytologic findings of JP are nonspecific and could be similar to fibrocystic changes. Typical lesions may feature cellular smears with numerous papillary epithelial fragments, some of which may exhibit moderate to severe atypia. Cystic background with naked nuclei and fragments of apocrine epithelium are also noted. Clinical correlation and further sampling are typically necessary to rule out involvement by carcinoma in these cases.

Management

Although JP is a rarely encountered lesion, the reported findings suggest that it is a marker for increased risk of breast cancer in patients and their families. Consequently, wide local excision is necessary followed by long-term clinical follow-up and monitoring family members. Inadequate excision may invariably lead to local recurrence. Follow-up examination should be scheduled annually or more frequently for patients who have multifocal, bilateral, or recurrent JP and if there are other risk factors such as a positive family history for breast carcinoma. Mammography is useful to follow up the patients, especially those older than 35 years. Ultrasonography is a simple technique alternative to mammography (54,61).

Atypical Papilloma

Clinical Presentation

Atypical papilloma is defined as a papilloma with foci of atypical epithelial proliferation that has combined

architectural and cytologic criteria for the diagnosis of ADH but insufficient for diagnosis of DCIS (19). Patients with atypical papilloma are usually older than patients with benign intraductal papilloma (21,43). Although imaging studies are not reliable in distinguishing benign, atypical, and malignant papillary lesions, the atypical lesion is almost always observed as a well-defined mass with or without associated calcifications (28).

Pathologic Features

Page et al (50) uses the term *atypical papilloma* to define papillomas that contain epithelial proliferation with atypia

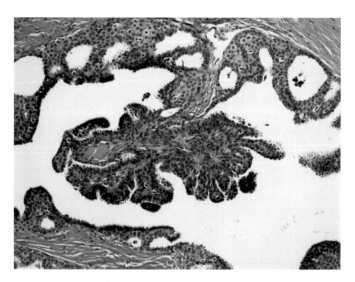

FIGURE 3.33 Papillomas with foci of atypical epithelial proliferation. A high-power view of Figure 3.31 illustrates that the atypical epithelial cells are uniform with low nuclear grade forming fenestrated proliferation with rigid structures.

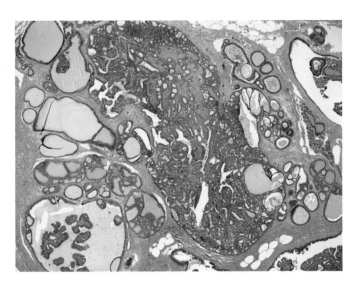

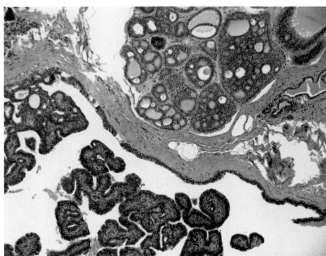

FIGURE 3.34 Papillomatosis associated with concurrent low-grade DCIS. Papillomas are often associated with other proliferative fibrocystic changes, but atypical lesions may be also present. Atypical epithelial proliferation is noted to involve only 4 ducts in the left lower portion of the figure.

FIGURE 3.35 Papillomatosis associated with concurrent low-grade DCIS. The DCIS component is in the upper portion of the figure.

measuring less than 3 mm in size. Tavassoli (2) suggested using the term *atypical papilloma* if less than one third of the lesion shows atypical epithelial changes. The size or proportion criteria are valid only for low-grade lesions; for high-grade lesions or if necrosis is present, the diagnosis of carcinoma in papilloma is made regardless of extent of atypia (5,10). Atypical papilloma may exhibit different types of atypical proliferation, but features of underlying benign papilloma are always notable in the rest of the lesion (5,19). The most common architectural patterns of atypical epithelial proliferation are cribriform, solid, and/or

micropapillary (50,62) (Figures 3.31–3.37). Myoepithelial cells are diminished or absent in the foci of ADH or DCIS but remain clearly visible in areas of residual benign papilloma and around the periphery (19). Moreover, several studies have demonstrated that the epithelial cells in atypical foci lack immunoreactivity to CK5/6 and 34βE12 in 80% to 100% of lesions, whereas 88% to 100% of benign intraductal proliferations display strong mosaic distribution of immunoreactivity with these markers (63–66) (Figures 3.38–3.39). In addition to ductal lesions, lobular neoplasis can involve papillomas (Figures 3.40–3.42). Immunohistochemical staining for E-cadherin can be very helpful to delineate lobular neoplasia cells (Figure 3.43).

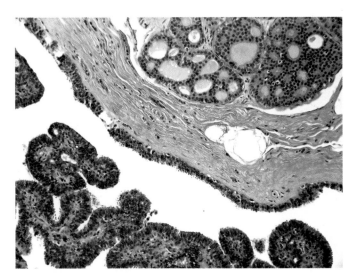

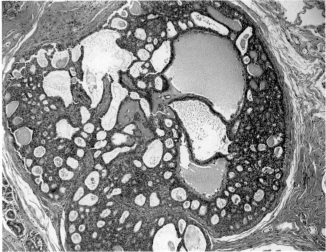

FIGURE 3.36 Papillomatosis associated with concurrent low-grade DCIS. On a high-power magnification of Figure 3.34, the DCIS shows a classic cribriform growth pattern with an atypical monotonous cell population forming round lumens and rigid epithelial bridges, which is distinctly different from that of the epithelial cells present in benign intraductal papilloma.

FIGURE 3.37 Papilloma involved by low-grade DCIS. More than half of this papilloma are involved by atypical epithelial proliferation with low nuclear grade, which shows the architectural and cytologic features of DCIS. An area of atypical cells with round monotonous non-overlapping nuclei is organized around cribriform spaces. An area reminiscent of a benign papilloma is also noted.

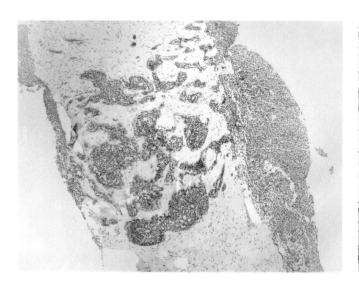

FIGURE 3.38 Cytokeratin 5/6. Nuclear reactivity is absent in atypical epithelial proliferation within the papillary lesion.

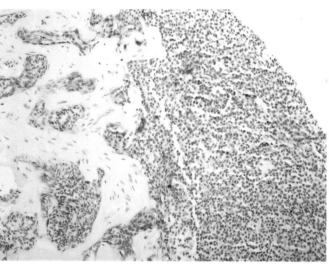

FIGURE 3.39 Cytokeratin 5/6. A higher-power magnification of Figure 3.37 showing scattered immunoreactivity within myoepithelial cells within small entrapped glands but not in the epithelium.

Cytologic Features

Cytology is not extremely helpful in the definitive classification of papillary lesions. Aspirates from atypical papillomas may show predominately benign cytologic features similar to those described in the chapter on benign intraductal papilloma, but rare epithelial groups may exhibit monotony or cellular or architectural atypia (Figure 3.44). When focal atypia is noted in aspirates, additional sampling should be recommended for definitive diagnosis and classification.

Management

At present, clinical trials studying the clinical significance of atypical papilloma are limited. Page et al reported that

the risk of subsequent breast cancer for women with atypical papilloma was 4 times greater than that of patients with papilloma without atypia. Moreover, the increased relative risk of subsequent breast cancer in atypical papilloma appeared to be linked also to the presence of ADH in the surrounding breast tissue. Most of the subsequent invasive cancers developed in the ipsilateral breast and near the site of the atypical papilloma. However, the number of patients in the study was limited (50). In another retrospective study that included 119 central papillomas, MacGrogan et al reported a similar finding: the increased risk of invasive carcinoma was related to the presence of ADH in the surrounding breast tissue. On the other

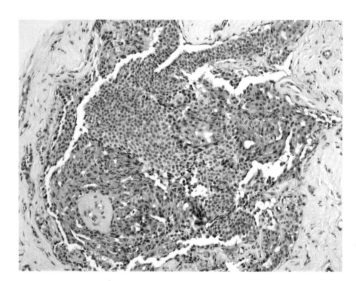

FIGURE 3.40 Lobular neoplasia involving an intraductal papilloma. An intraductal papilloma is involved by the monotonous, discohesive cells in the middle portion; the residual portion of the benign papilloma is present in the lower part of the figure.

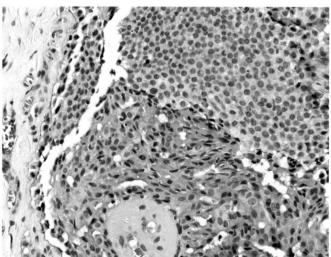

FIGURE 3.41 Lobular neoplasia involving an intraductal papilloma. The higher magnification of Figure 3.40 showing contrast of morphologic features of lobular neoplasia with small, loosely cohesive, uniform epithelial proliferation to the rest of the papillary lesion, which shows usual ductal hyperplasia with an admixture of epithelial and myoepithelial cells.

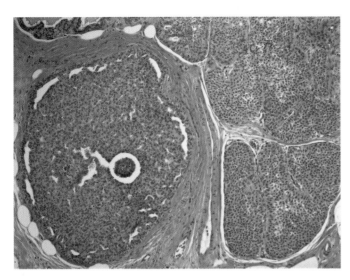

FIGURE 3.42 Another example of an intraductal papilloma with adjacent LCIS.

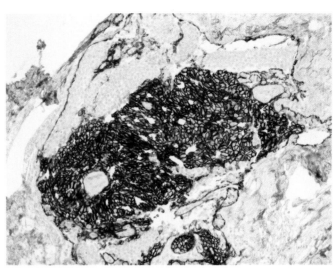

FIGURE 3.43 E-cadherin immunostaining demonstrates strong positivity in the cells of usual ductal hyperplasia, whereas lobular neoplasia shows a complete loss of an E-cadherin expression.

hand, no statistically significant difference was observed in relation to recurrence for the various categories of papilloma in this study. Recurrence appeared to be associated with the presence of proliferative lesions (ADH, epithelial hyperplasia, lobular neoplasia) in the surrounding breast tissue (62). In the study by Lewis et al (20), the authors found that the risk of developing subsequent breast cancer in atypical papillomas is similar to that of patients with ADH elsewhere in the breast (4- to 5-fold). These authors also emphasized that the breast cancer risk is significantly higher among patients with multiple papillomas with atypia.

The above-mentioned studies indicate that papilloma with atypia is a marker of increased risk of developing cancer rather than a precursor lesion. Most authorities in the field recommend excision and radiologic follow-up for a papillary lesion with atypia to exclude in situ or invasive carcinoma (21,28,29,35,42). The surrounding breast tissue should be carefully evaluated to exclude the presence of ADH and DCIS at the periphery of the lesion (10,19).

■ MALIGNANCIES INVOLVING PAPILLARY LESIONS

Papilloma Involved by DCIS

Clinical Presentation

Although there is limited information from clinicopathologic studies about papilloma involved by DCIS, the clinical and radiologic features of this lesion are similar to those of atypical papillomas. On mammography, the lesion usually appears as a circumscribed or irregular mass with or without associated calcifications (27).

Pathologic Features

Although there are no agreed criteria for the definition of papilloma with DCIS, some authors use this designation when the papilloma exhibits any area of epithelial atypia with uniform histology and single-cell–type cytology consistent with low-grade DCIS that is greater than 3 mm in size (50) (Figures 3.37,3.45–3.47). Tavassoli (2) classifies a lesion as an "intraductal carcinoma arising in papilloma" when the atypical epithelial proliferation occupies at least one third but less than 90% of the underlying papillary lesion. In these lesions, the DCIS foci are most often low to intermediate grade with a solid, cribriform, and/or micropapillary pattern (1). Even when the DCIS

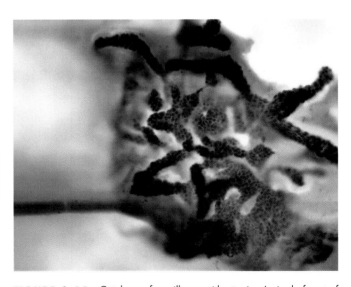

FIGURE 3.44 Cytology of papilloma with atypia. A single focus of ductal epithelium with monotony and architectural atypia was noted in a background of an otherwise benign papillary lesion. Excision showed intraductal papilloma with focal atypia. Careful screening of all cytology smears is warranted for such atypical foci.

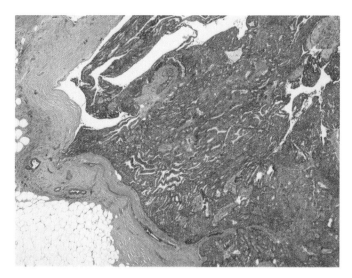

FIGURE 3.45 An atypical papillary lesion with adjacent focus of invasive ductal carcinoma. A low-power view illustrating a circumscribed, cystic dilated nodule surrounded by a thick, fibrous capsule in which complex, branching, hypercellular atypical papillary proliferation protrudes to the duct lumen. Small, irregular, suspicious ductal structures are dispersed in the fibrous wall of the papillary lesion.

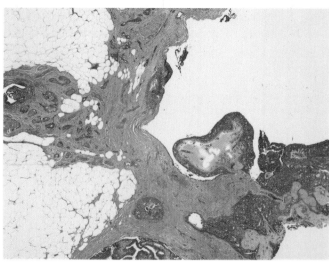

FIGURE 3.46 An atypical papillary lesion with adjacent focus of invasive ductal carcinoma. In another area of the same lesion as in Figure 3.45, many more irregular, atypical ductal glands and clusters invading the stroma extend to the left portion of the papillary lesion around the benign ductal gland.

extensively involves the underlying papilloma, preexisting benign papilloma remains evident at least in part of the lesion (19). Myoepithelial cells are diminished or absent in the DCIS foci but can be seen in areas of residual benign papilloma and around the periphery of the involved duct (19). A combination of myoepithelial cell markers and high-molecular-weight cytokeratins such as CK5/6 and 34βE12 may be useful in the differentiation of atypical papilloma, papilloma with DCIS, from benign papilloma. The high-molecular weight cytokeratins are reactive with myoepithelial and epithelial cells in usual ductal hyperplasia within benign papilloma but show decreased or absent

reactivity in atypical epithelium of ADH or intraductal carcinoma involving papillary lesion (64,66). Some authors have shown that CD44s and cyclin D1 are useful in differentiating benign from malignant papillary lesions, but these markers are currently not used in routine practice (67–69).

Cytologic Features

Aspirates from papillomas involved by DCIS may show benign cytologic features similar to those described in the

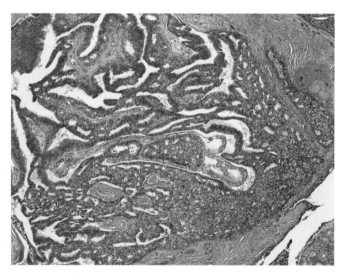

FIGURE 3.47 An atypical papillary lesion with adjacent focus of invasive ductal carcinoma. On a high-power magnification, a portion of the papillary lesion appears more monotonous and more cellular than the rest of the papillary proliferation.

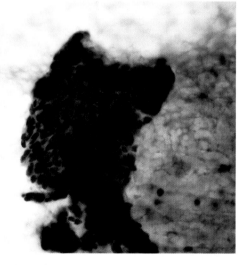

FIGURE 3.48 Cytology of papilloma involved by DCIS. Rare atypical groups of ductal epithelium present are typically noted in the otherwise benign papillary lesion. This group may be considered worrisome for involvement of papilloma by DCIS because of the crowding of cells and nuclear hyperchromasia. Subsequent excision showed papilloma focally involved by DCIS with intermediate nuclear grade.

chapter on benign intraductal papilloma, but several epithelial groups exhibit monotony or architectural or cellular atypia similar to those of atypical papilloma (Figures 3.48–3.49). When atypia is noted within aspirates, additional sampling is usually recommended for definitive diagnosis and classification.

Management

Although the clinical importance and prognostic differences between atypical papilloma and papilloma involved by DCIS are not well defined, these 2 lesions appear to exhibit the same clinical behavior based on limited report. One retrospective study demonstrated that neither the extent nor the quantity of epithelial atypia in papilloma had prognostic significance or influenced the outcome of the patient. The same study revealed that in most lesions, epithelial atypia comprised 20% to 60% of the papillary lesion. As in atypical papilloma, the presence of epithelial hyperplasia, ADH, or lobular neoplasia in the surrounding breast tissue is a significant factor in recurrence (62). The recommended management of these lesions is complete excision with a rim of uninvolved breast tissue and follow-up monitoring (11,62). The surrounding breast tissue should be carefully evaluated to exclude ADH or DCIS (19). Although these lesions have an excellent prognosis, they should be carefully considered before being diagnosed as "papilloma with DCIS" because this diagnosis may lead to unnecessary overtreatment of the ipsilateral breast (70).

■ MALIGNANT PAPILLARY LESIONS OF THE BREAST

Papillary DCIS

Clinical Presentation

Papillary DCIS is a variant of DCIS composed of papillary epithelial tufts or fronds projecting into the lumen (1,2). The mean patient age at diagnosis is between 50 and 59 years, quite similar to the mean age of women with invasive carcinoma (1). There are no significant differences in the age distribution of subtypes of intraductal carcinoma (1). Like the other types of intraductal carcinoma, papillary DCIS is not palpable in most patients (71). Mammography is the most sensitive procedure in detecting papillary DCIS, which usually appears as a density or asymmetric soft tissue changes with or without calcifications (1,71). Papillary DCIS is commonly associated with linear, granular, or mixed types of calcifications (1). The lesion may not be detected by sonography. When detected, it usually present as a hypoechoic mass or multiple small lesions (71). Magnetic resonance imaging is an effective method for detecting papillary DCIS that lack calcifications or is not visible by the other imaging methods (1).

Pathologic Features

Papillary DCIS has a papillary growth pattern characterized by fibrovascular cores lined by neoplastic epithelium. There is no evidence of preexisting papilloma (Figures 3.50–3.52). The epithelium is usually composed of a single-cell–type population with uniform monotonous appearance. The nuclei of the epithelial cells are mostly low to intermediate nuclear grade (1,2,19). The epithelium may consist of one

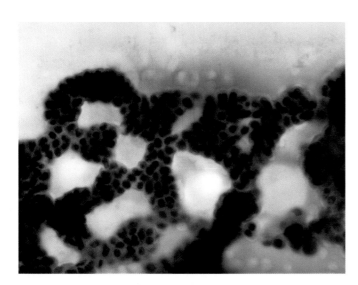

FIGURE 3.49 Cytology of papilloma involved by DCIS. Rare atypical groups of ductal epithelium present within the otherwise benign papillary lesion. This group shows monotony, open spaces mimicking cribriforming, but cells are cytologically bland. Excision showed papilloma focally involved by low-grade DCIS.

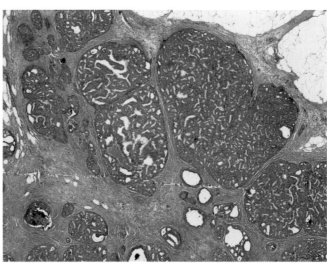

FIGURE 3.50 Multiple papillary DCIS. A low-power magnification view illustrating multiple papillary lesions involved by malignant papillary proliferation in various sizes.

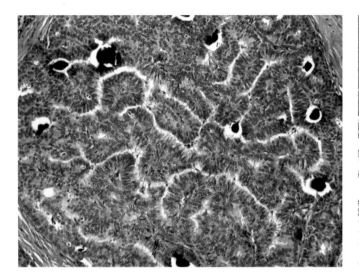

FIGURE 3.51 At high-power magnification of Figure 3.50, the papillae are lined by a single population of elongated, stratified columnar cells. No discernible myoepithelial cells are identified beneath the epithelial cells. There is no evidence of residual benign papilloma. Microcalcifications are noted within the lesion.

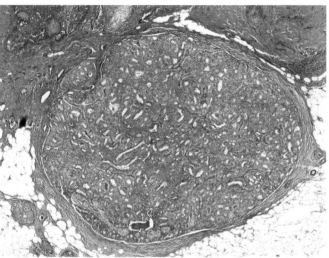

FIGURE 3.52 Medium-power view of Figure 3.50 illustrating complex branching papillary processes with delicate fibrovascular cores not supported by myoepithelial cell layer. Microinvasion is present at the periphery of the lesion (left upper portion).

to several layers of columnar cells with varying degrees of stratification or may show a more significant proliferation of uniform cells in a solid, cribriform, or micropapillary growth pattern. The myoepithelial cell layer is absent in fibrovascular cores within the lesion but is present at the periphery of the lesion, a feature that implicates in situ process (19). In several instances, small foci of invasive carcinoma can be demonstrated at the periphery of lesion (Figures 3.52–3.54).

Cytologic Features

Aspirates of papillary carcinomas are highly cellular and may have a bloody background with hemosiderin-containing macrophages. The presence of single papillae

and 3-dimensional papillary clusters are distinctive features. Cells may be dispersed and fibrovascular cores denuded. The tumor cells have a monotonous appearance and are distinctly columnar in appearance and may appear in small rows or palisades (Figure 3.55). Immunohistochemistry may be necessary before definitive diagnosis is made (Figure 3.56). The degree of anisonucleosis and nuclear membrane abnormality varies and may not be significant. Occasionally, necrotic debris can be seen in the background.

Management

Prognosis and management of papillary DCIS are similar to that of other types of DCIS. Careful mammographic and pathologic evaluation is essential to assess each patient's

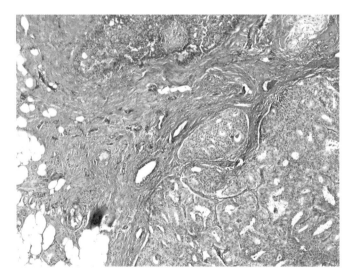

FIGURE 3.53 On a higher magnification of Figure 3.52, in the left portion of the papillary lesion, there is a small cluster of invasive tumor cells arising adjacent to the papillary lesion.

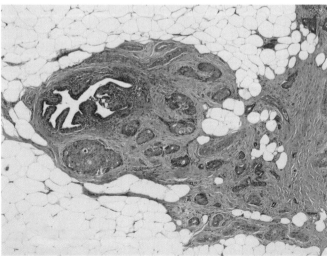

FIGURE 3.54 Adjacent invasive carcinoma. Low-power magnification shows invasive carcinoma of ductal type, NOS, arising in a periphery of papillary carcinoma.

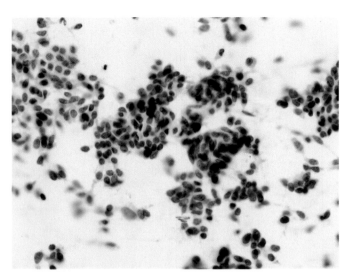

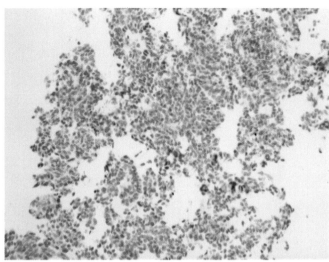

FIGURE 3.55 Cytology of papillary carcinoma. Discohesive papillary structures composed of monotonous atypical cells with high nuclear-to-cytoplasmic ratio are noted in a background of elongated spindle cells. No myoepithelial cells are visible in the groups, and no naked nuclei are noted in a background.

FIGURE 3.56 Cytology of papillary carcinoma. p63 immunostaining can be performed on cytology smears. p63 is negative in tumor cells with staining present only in rare naked nuclei in a background.

candidacy for breast-conserving treatment. Although excision followed by radiation therapy has significantly reduced the recurrence rate, some small, low-grade lesions appear to be adequately treated with excision alone. On the other hand, extensive lesions involving large areas of the breast may require mastectomy (1). The most important factor in the risk assessment of recurrence is based on the presence of a residual tumor. Moreover, retrospective studies showed that high nuclear grade, larger lesion size, necrosis, and involved margins of excision are the factors predictive of local recurrence after breast-conserving treatment for DCIS (1).

Encapsulated (Intracystic) Papillary Carcinoma

Clinical Presentation

Encapsulated (intracystic) papillary carcinoma is a rare entity that accounts for 1% to 2% of all breast carcinomas. It has distinct pathologic features and overall favorable prognosis. It usually occurs in older patients (60 years and older) and arises centrally in the breast (19). Clinically, encapsulated (intracystic) papillary carcinoma frequently appears as a mass in the retroareolar region. The neoplastic papillary proliferation grows within a cystically dilated duct and tends to bleed into the cystic space, which causes bloody nipple discharge in at least one third of patients (10). The average lesion is 2 to 3 cm in size, but in rare cases, it can be as large as 10 cm in diameter (10). On mammography, it often appears as an ill-defined, lobulated mass lesion that less likely contains calcifications than DCIS (71). When the lesion is well circumscribed, it is difficult to differentiate it from benign lesions, such as fibroadenoma and cyst, or malignant lesions, such as medullary carcinoma, mucinous carcinoma, or phyllodes

tumor by mammography (71). On sonography, irregular borders and microlobulation suggest malignancy. The lesion often appears as a solid, hypoechoic mass with a cystic component that demonstrates distal enhancement (72). When there is spontaneous hemorrhage within the tumor or bleeding related to biopsy, a fluid-fluid level or internal echoes may be detected (71,73). In its early stage, intracystic papillary carcinoma could be clinically indistinguishable from a cyst, a fibroadenoma, or a papilloma (74).

Pathologic Features

Encapsulated (intracystic) papillary carcinoma of the breast has traditionally been considered as a variant of DCIS (75). However, it is still controversial whether these lesions should be considered in situ carcinomas or invasive carcinomas.

Hill and Yeh (76) first proposed the term *encapsulated* papillary carcinoma to describe intracystic papillary carcinomas that are surrounded by a thick fibrous capsule but have no detectable myoepithelial cell layer at the border by hematoxylin and eosin stain or immunohistochemical analysis. On microscopy, this lesion consists of a single expanded duct that is completely filled by a neoplastic epithelium with papillary features and surrounded by a fibrous capsule that gives the tumor an encysted appearance (19) (Figures 3.57–3.60). The neoplastic epithelial proliferation may exhibit various architectural patterns, including cribriform, papillary, micropapillary, trabecular, or solid (5,10). The cytology of the neoplastic epithelium is usually low to intermediate nuclear grade, but higher-grade and more prominent necrosis could be present (Figure 3.61). Associated DCIS may be present in the surrounding breast tissue at the tumor periphery (75,77,78). Encapsulated (intracystic) papillary carcinoma may be associated with stromal invasion.

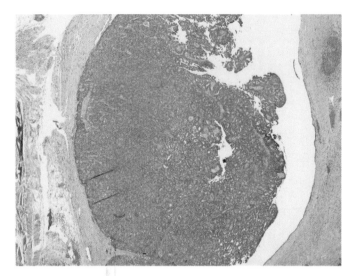

FIGURE 3.57 Encapsulated papillary carcinoma with solid growth pattern. Low-power magnification showing well-circumscribed dilated duct filled with a solid nodular proliferation of monotonous neoplastic cells surrounded by a thickened fibrous wall.

Interestingly, when invasion is present, it is usually invasive ductal carcinoma, not otherwise specified (NOS) (19). Rare variants such as secretory carcinoma, carcinoma with endometrium-like morphology, and tall cell variant of thyroid papillary carcinoma have been described arising within these tumors (79,80).

A distinctive feature of encapsulated (intracystic) papillary carcinoma is the complete or partial absence of myoepithelial cells not only within the intraductal neoplastic proliferation as in papillary DCIS but also at tumor periphery (10,19). Hill and Yeh evaluated the presence of myoepithelial cells by using a panel of sensitive myoepithelial markers including calponin, smooth muscle myosin heavy chain, and p63. Of 9 cases diagnosed as encapsulated

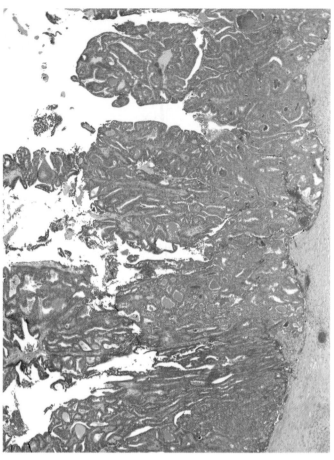

FIGURE 3.58 Encapsulated papillary carcinoma. Another area of the same lesion as in Figure 3.57 showing slender, finger-like papillae, which display sheet-like cellular proliferation and open cystic-like structures.

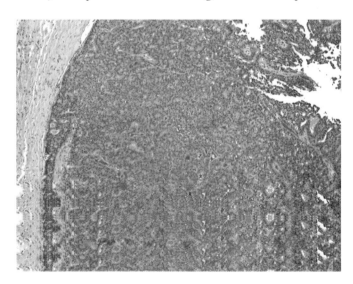

FIGURE 3.59 Encapsulated papillary carcinoma. At medium magnification, the cellular proliferation from Figure 3.57 shows solid architectural pattern. Discrete papillae are not appearent, and the underlying papillary structure is represented by a network of fibrovascular cores among the solid, cellular proliferation.

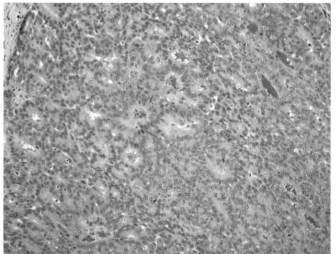

FIGURE 3.60 Encapsulated papillary carcinoma. On high magnification, the neoplastic cells within the nodule are composed of a uniform population of ovoid- to spindle-shaped epithelial cells growing in a solid architectural pattern. The cells are organized around the fibrovascular cores, and they show neuroendocrine appearance and rosette-like pattern.

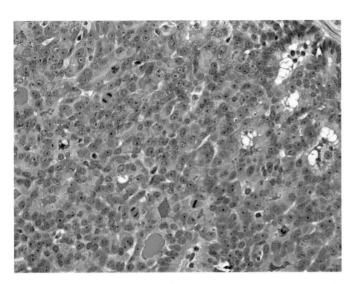

FIGURE 3.61 Encapsulated papillary carcinoma. In some areas, cells exhibit high nuclear grade and mitotic figures can be easily identified.

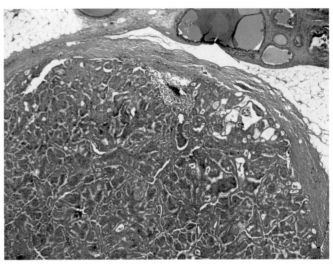

FIGURE 3.62 Another example of encapsulated papillary carcinoma. The lesion forms a well-demarcated, cystic nodule, which is characterized by a complex arborescent growth pattern, surrounded by a thick fibrous capsule.

(intracystic) papillary carcinoma in their series, a myoepithelial cell layer was identified only in 4 cases by one or more of the above-mentioned myoepithelial markers. Size and nuclear grade did not correlate with presence or absence of myoepithelial cells (76) (Figures 3.62–3.64). In another study, Collins et al (77) reported results on immunohistochemical studies using a panel of 5 markers in 22 encapsulated (intracystic) papillary carcinomas. All of the lesions showed absence of a myoepithelial cell layer at the periphery of tumors, whereas a myoepithelial cell layer was detected around the foci of the DCIS present near the encapsulated (intracystic) papillary carcinoma. The authors suggested that these lesions might represent a spectrum of progression between in situ and invasive papillary carcinomas and that the term *encapsulated papillary*

carcinoma is preferred for circumscribed nodules of papillary carcinoma surrounded by a fibrous capsule in which a peripheral myoepithelial layer is not demonstrable (76) (Figures 3.62–3.64). On the other hand, Esposito et al (81) studied basement membrane immunostainings, including type IV collagen and laminin, to evaluate possible invasion at the periphery of these lesions. They demonstrated moderate to intense collagen type IV expression in all encapsulated (intracystic) papillary carcinomas. In contrast, all invasive ductal carcinomas showed diminished or absent expression of basement membrane proteins (81). Although not routinely used, these markers may be helpful in evaluating early invasion in clinically suspicious cases of encapsulated (intracystic) carcinoma.

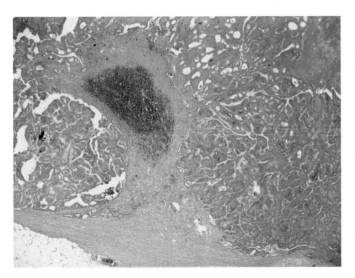

FIGURE 3.63 Encapsulated papillary carcinoma. In another area, biopsy site–related changes are seen adjacent to the complex, branching papillary process. Fibroblastic proliferation, with abundant hemorrhage, hemosiderophages, and lymphoplasmacytic infiltrate, is helpful in recognizing these changes as biopsy related.

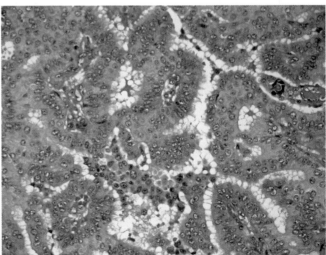

FIGURE 3.64 At a high-power magnification of Figure 3.62, the papillae are covered by a single-cell, uniform, stratified population of columnar epithelial cells with intermediate nuclear grade. No myoepithelial cells are noted.

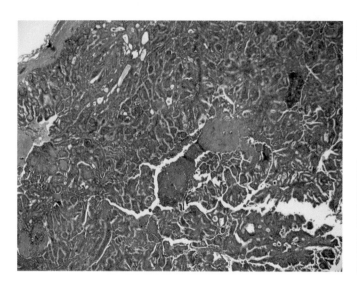

FIGURE 3.65 Encapsulated papillary carcinoma. At low-power magnification, the neoplastic papillary proliferation grows within a cystically dilated duct in a cribriform pattern and is surrounded by a fibrous capsule.

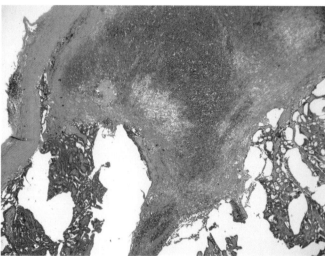

FIGURE 3.66 Encapsulated papillary carcinoma. In another area, infarction and hemorrhage are evident in a part of the lesion. Encysted papillary carcinomas tend to bleed into the cavity, which may cause bloody nipple discharge.

Cytologic Features

Aspirates have similar cytomorphologic features to papillary DCIS.

Differential Diagnosis

The differentiation of encapsulated (intracystic) papillary carcinoma from benign intraductal papilloma may be complicated by the presence of a dimorphic type of neoplastic cell population in some cases. *Dimorphic papillary carcinoma* is a term that has been used to refer to papillary carcinomas that have 2 types of neoplastic cells, with a second population of cells showing pale cytoplasm. These cells could grow in solid or cribriform nests beneath a superficial layer of malignant columnar epithelial cells. This second cell type can be misinterpreted as myoepithelial cells. The nuclear features are similar in both populations, but immunohistochemical staining confirms their epithelial origin (1,10). In some cases, encapsulated (intracystic) papillary carcinoma, especially with low nuclear grade, may also be confused with benign intraductal papilloma exhibiting florid ductal epithelial hyperplasia (78). In these cases, a single-cell type surrounding thin papillary fronds at the tumor periphery by immunohistochemical analysis facilitates the diagnosis.

Complex sclerosing papilloma can mimic encapsulated (intracystic) papillary carcinoma. Entrapped and distorted tubules in a dense collagenized stroma favor sclerosing papilloma. Immunohistochemical stains are helpful to exclude sclerosing papilloma since they highlight the myoepithelial cell layer surrounding small glands within the sclerotic stroma (78). Metastatic thyroid carcinoma or metastatic ovarian carcinoma may mimic intracystic papillary carcinoma, but this is relatively rare and clinical history should lead to correct diagnosis and utilization of appropriate

immunostainings (78). Encapsulated (intracystic) papillary carcinoma associated with an invasion should be distinguished from the papillary variant of invasive carcinoma. The invasive carcinoma associated with encapsulated (intracystic) papillary carcinoma is usually nonpapillary type and most often is invasive ductal carcinoma, NOS (82).

Displaced malignant epithelial cells in the stroma of the fibrotic wall of the lesion or within the needle tract after needling procedures, such as fine-needle aspiration biopsy or CNB, may cause the erroneous diagnosis of invasive carcinoma in certain cases (Figures 3.65–3.67). Despite the presence of a supporting fibrovascular core, loose,

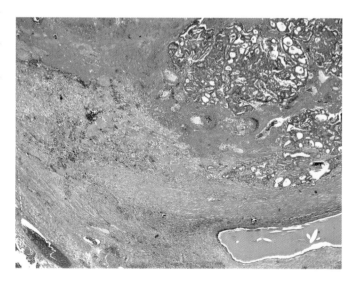

FIGURE 3.67 Encapsulated papillary carcinoma. The same lesion as in Figure 3.65. On low-power view, biopsy site–related reaction due to CNB is noted. The duct wall of the papilloma has been disrupted. It is prudent to avoid an interpretation of invasion around these areas.

exophytic papillary clusters may break off the lesion and mimic true invasion. Immnunohistochemical stains are not helpful in such cases and recommendation is that the diagnosis of invasion should be considered only if the foci of invasion are noted away from any area that exhibits hemorrhage, fibrosis, granulation tissue, or scarring, which may be due to prior needling or surgical procedure (30,32,33).

Management

The prognosis of patients with encapsulated (intracystic) papillary carcinoma is good (1,10,19). However, encapsulated (intracystic) papillary carcinoma carries a less favorable prognosis than other intraductal carcinomas (78). Rare cases with metastases have been reported in the literature (78,83,84). The presence of metastases favors the concept that this lesion may be a low-grade invasive carcinoma with expansile growth pattern (19).

Some studies have demonstrated that the presence of DCIS in the breast tissue adjacent to an intracystic papillary carcinoma is associated with an increased risk of recurrence (75). MacGrogan and Tavassoli (62) reported similar findings, and, based on their study, the presence of atypia when confined to the papillary lesion only did not influence increased risk of recurrence of either benign or malignant papillary lesions. When invasive carcinoma is associated with encapsulated (intracystic) papillary carcinoma, it is most prudent to separately report the size of the true invasive component to avoid possible overstaging and/or overtreatment based on the size of the entire lesion (10,19). Pathologists should avoid categorizing these lesions as "invasive" papillary carcinomas, and these lesions are adequately managed with local therapy only (10,19,78).

Solid Papillary Carcinoma

Clinical Presentation

Solid papillary carcinoma is a distinctive breast tumor first described as such by Maluf and Koerner (85). It is considered to be a variant of DCIS that is characterized by circumscribed, solid cellular proliferation presenting as single or multiple nodules (Figure 3.68). This tumor usually occurs in older patients and infrequently presents as a mass lesion, but the lesion could measure a few centimeters in diameter. On mammography, it is an ill-defined and lobulated mass with or without single or multiple calcifications (71). The lesion when small may not be detected by sonography. When detectable, it usually presents as a hypoechoic mass with distal enhancement due to transmission of the ultrasound waves through the abundant mucinous material (71).

Pathologic Features

Solid papillary carcinoma is an uncommon tumor typically forming well-circumscribed nodules composed of solid

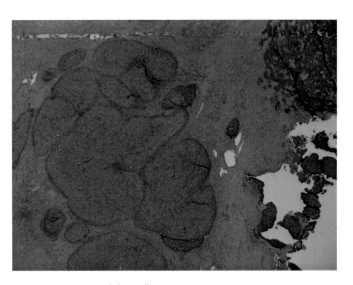

FIGURE 3.68 Solid papillary carcinoma.

epithelial cell proliferation separated by thin fibrotic septa. The neoplastic cells are usually ovoid or spindle shaped and with a low to intermediate nuclear grade, an eosinophilic cytoplasm, and a streaming pattern that may resemble florid hyperplasia at low magnification (85,86). The cells are organized around the fibrovascular cores with their nuclei polarized on the basal side, and they may exhibit a rosette-like pattern and neuroendocrine differentiation with granular eosinophilic cytoplasm and immunoreactivity for neuroendocrine markers (85) (Figures 3.68 and 3.70). Extracellular and intracellular mucin production is a common feature, and therefore, solid papillary carcinoma is thought to be a precursor of colloid (mucinous) carcinoma, with which it is frequently associated. In a large study, Nassar et al (86) analyzed 58 solid papillary carcinomas. In 30% of the cases, the invasion had a neuroendocrine-like pattern. All of the tumors were positive for estrogen and progesterone receptors and negative for HER-2 protein overexpression by immunohistochemical analysis (86). Otsuki et al (87) published a report on 15 cases of solid papillary carcinoma associated with an invasive component. The histologic types of the invasive cancers were mucinous carcinoma in 5 cases and neuroendocrine carcinoma in 10 cases. These authors suggested that solid papillary carcinoma may be a precursor of neuroendocrine carcinoma and mucinous carcinoma (87). Uncommon variants of solid papillary carcinoma include glycogen-rich clear cell tumors, spindle cell tumors, and carcinoma with mucoepidermoid features (1).

It is still controversial whether solid papillary carcinoma is a purely in situ lesion or a low-grade invasive carcinoma with pushing borders. In several reports, the authors who studied the presence of myoepithelial cells by sensitive myoepithelial markers in these lesions showed that most solid papillary carcinomas completely lack myoepithelial cells (85,88,89). However, the behavior of these tumors is indolent, especially when there is no associated invasive component identified.

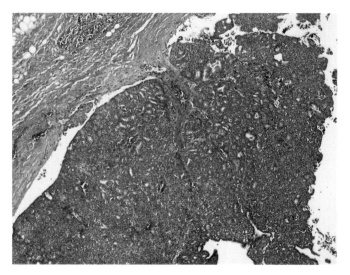

FIGURE 3.69 Solid papillary carcinoma.

Cytologic Findings

Smears are typically cellular with cell groups consisting of moderate to large discohesive epithelial clusters, nests, and many single isolated cells in a background showing plasmacytoid appearance. Several groups of short spindle cells could be noted. No naked nuclei of myoepithelial cell origin are typically noted in a background (Figure 3.71) (90,91).

Differential Diagnosis

Although solid papillary carcinoma shows distinct histologic features, it is sometimes difficult to distinguish it from some benign and malignant entities. The lesion can mimic florid hyperplasia due to cellular streaming and spindle and ovoid cellular morphology. The monotonous population, significant mitotic activity, hyalinized fibrovascular cores, and peripheral palisading of cells favor the diagnosis of solid papillary carcinoma (85). In cases of solid papillary carcinoma associated with mucinous carcinoma, it is important not to mistake solid papillary carcinoma with mucin extravasation for an invasive component. Irregular, angulated cell clusters and loose myxoid stroma are helpful in distinguishing these lesions (85). The uncommon encapsulated (intracystic) papillary carcinoma could show some similarities to solid papillary carcinoma. The cells of encapsulated (intracystic) papillary carcinoma are cuboidal to columnar in shape, and they more often show intermediate- to high-nuclear-grade features, whereas cells of solid papillary carcinoma have spindle and/or plasmocytoid morphology and are low to intermediate nuclear grade (78). There is no neuroendocrine-like pattern and no association with colloid carcinoma in encapsulated (intracystic) papillary carcinoma. Solid papillary carcinoma can be confused with low-grade DCIS in small foci. The fibrovascular cores and intracellular and extracellular mucin production usually

favor solid papillary carcinoma. The monotonous plasmacytoid cells of solid papillary carcinoma may mimic an LCIS, although the cells are not discohesive and the pattern of solid papillary carcinoma is different from that of LCIS (86). The solid variant of adenoid cystic carcinoma may rarely resemble solid papillary carcinoma, but the cells of adenoid cystic carcinoma have prominent basaloid features, hyperchromatic nuclei, inconspicuous nucleoli, and scant cytoplasm, and the lesion has infiltrative pattern whereas solid papillary carcinoma is circumscribed (92).

Management

Solid papillary carcinoma of the breast is a low-grade malignant neoplasm in elderly patients and shows an indolent behavior. Even when associated with invasive carcinoma, the prognosis is favorable compared with that of other variants of invasive carcinomas of comparable size (85,86). Low-grade cytologic features, estrogen receptor positivity, and association with mucinous carcinomas are favorable features. Lymph node and distant metastases are rare and limited to cases with associated invasive components (85,86). The recent reports seem to support that conservative approach with locoregional excision is satisfactory in the management of cases of solid papillary carcinomas (86).

Invasive Papillary Carcinoma

Clinical Presentation

Some authors prefer the term *invasive papillary carcinoma* to refer to a rare entity accounting for less than 2% of breast-invasive cancers (93,94). It occurs mostly in elderly people of African American origin (93). The mean

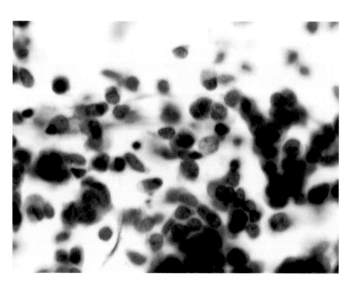

FIGURE 3.70 Another example of solid papillary carcinoma with more pronounced histiocytoid/plasmacytoid features.

age of the patients ranges from 63 to 71 years. Nearly 50% of papillary carcinomas occur in the central part of the breast and often manifest themselves with nipple discharge. The average size of the tumor is 2 to 3 cm (93). On mammography, invasive papillary carcinoma often appears as a rounded or lobulated lesion. Although it is difficult to differentiate papillary carcinoma from benign lesions by imaging, the irregular contours of the lesion and the detection of any suspect axillary lymph node on mammography or sonography would suggest a malignant nature (71).

Pathologic and Cytologic Features

The most important diagnostic feature of invasive papillary carcinoma is that the invasive component is composed of papillary structures surrounding thin fibrovascular cores lined by a neoplastic cell population invading the stroma of the breast parenchyma (Figures 3.72–3.73). Carcinoma cells usually extend into ducts at the periphery of papillary carcinoma. The nuclei of tumor cells are hyperchromatic and usually intermediate nuclear grade with a high ratio of nucleus to cytoplasm. Mitotic figures are variably present and are seen more often with increasing grade of cytologic atypia. The cytoplasm is amphophilic, but apocrine changes can be seen in a number of lesions; furthermore, the tumor cells may exhibit "apical snouts" at the luminal surface. In some cases, the stroma show prominent mucin extravasation. Microcalcifications are seen often in papillary carcinomas in the glandular component and in the stroma. Many cases have adjacent DCIS, usually the papillary or cribriform type. Pure papillary carcinoma is rare and is usually seen admixed with another type of carcinomas, often with invasive ductal carcinoma (93).

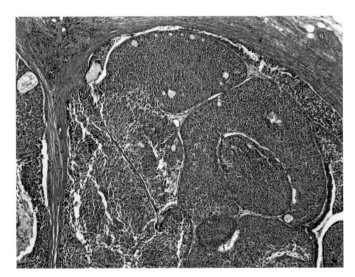

FIGURE 3.71 Cytology of solid papillary carcinoma. A high-power magnification of imprint cytologic findings showing moderate to large cell nests with many isolated cells showing plasmacytoid appearance. Short spindle cells are seen in a background.

Differential Diagnosis

Benign papillary lesions must be considered in the differential diagnosis. The distinction between a benign papilloma and an invasive papillary carcinoma is determined by the cytologic and histologic features of the lesion and architectural pattern. The epithelial cells in invasive papillary carcinoma grow disorganized, with uneven stratification and loss of polarity. The nuclei are hyperchromatic, and the nucleus-to-cytoplasm ratio is increased. The number of mitotic figures varies but are more frequent in papillary carcinomas and more numerous in lesions with more severe cytologic atypia. The presence of benign apocrine changes is associated with intraductal papilloma but is rarely seen in papillary carcinoma. Myoepithelial cells, which are distributed at the base of the epithelium in benign intraductal papilloma, tend to be discontinuous or completely absent in the carcinoma. Demonstrating the distribution of myoepithelial cells at the base of the epithelium by using immunohistochemical studies is helpful in recognizing these lesions. Invasive micropapillary carcinoma is a rare entity that is morphologically different from invasive papillary carcinoma, with clear spaces surrounding tumor clusters that lack true fibrovascular cores (1).

Management

Clinical behavior and prognosis of invasive papillary carcinoma are not well studied due to their rarity. Fisher et al (93) reported the presence of lymph node metastases in 32% of the 22 patients. Only 2 (9%) of 22 patients had 4 or more lymph nodes with metastasis. Overall, 5-year disease-free survival was in the range of 90%, similar to mucinous carcinoma. Furthermore, of the 3 patients who had a recurrence, only 1 died of disease. The results of this study indicated that invasive papillary carcinoma represents a histologic type of breast carcinoma with favorable prognosis (93).

Invasive Micropapillary Carcinoma

Clinical Presentation

Invasive micropapillary carcinoma is a rare, clinically aggressive variant of invasive carcinoma, first described by Tavassoli and Sıriaunkgul in 1993. After being recognized as a distinctive entity in the breast, multiple studies reported the same pattern in other organs, including the urinary bladder, the lung, and major salivary glands (95–98). The incidence of invasive micropapillary carcinoma varies from 0.9% (99), when occurring in its pure form, to 7% (100), when mixed with other types of breast carcinoma. The mean ages at presentation for patients with invasive micropapillary carcinoma range from 25 to 92 years, similar to that of patients with invasive ductal carcinoma, NOS (100–105). Two cases have been described in male patients (102,104). The most common

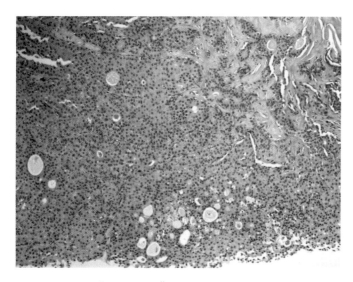

FIGURE 3.72 Invasive papillary carcinoma.

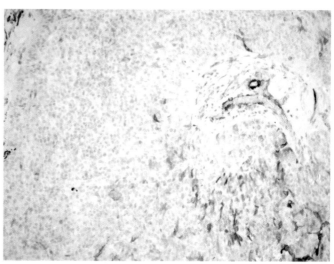

FIGURE 3.73 Invasive papillary carcinoma. Smooth muscle myosin heavy chain immunostain demonstrates an absence of myoepithelial cells within the papillary lesion. Vascular smooth muscle cells and pericytes within the fibrovascular stroma are positive.

clinical finding is a palpable mass. On mammography, it usually appears as a high-density, irregular mass with spiculated margins, with or without associated calcifications. The sonographic finding is frequently a solid hypoechoic, irregular, or multilobulated mass with posterior acoustic shadowing or normal sound transmission (99,106).

Pathologic and Cytologic Features

The invasive micropapillary pattern is characterized by small micropapillary clusters and tubuloalveolar structures of tumor cells that lack true fibrovascular cores. The tumor cells often occupy clear, empty spaces, and these frequently resemble lymphatic channels (Figures 3.74–3.77). The nonvascular nature of these spaces can be demonstrated by negative immunostaining for endothelial markers (100,104,107). The clear, empty spaces are thought to be an artifact of fixation because they are not seen on frozen tissue sections (100). The tumor cells have abundant finely granular eosinophilic cytoplasm and intermediate- to high-grade nuclei with a high nucleus-to-cytoplasmic ratio (103,104). In some tumors, intracytoplasmic vacuoles displaced the nucleus eccentrically, causing a signet ring–like appearance. Mitotic activity is variable. The stroma is typically spongy with little or no desmoplastic reaction in the surrounding breast tissue (108). Psammoma bodies have been found in association

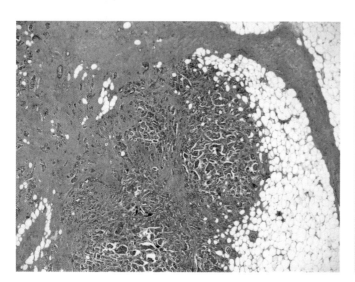

FIGURE 3.74 Invasive micropapillary carcinoma. A low-magnification of a portion of the tumor shows micropapillary architectural pattern, showing the neoplastic cell clusters floating in a spongy stroma. There are focal microcalcifications in association with the tumor.

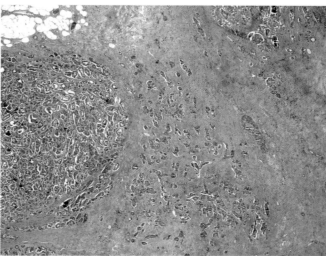

FIGURE 3.75 Invasive micropapillary carcinoma with retraction artifact leaving spaces between the epithelial groups and the surrounding stroma. Clusters of neoplastic cells are devoid of fibrovascular cores and appear to be floating in clear spaces.

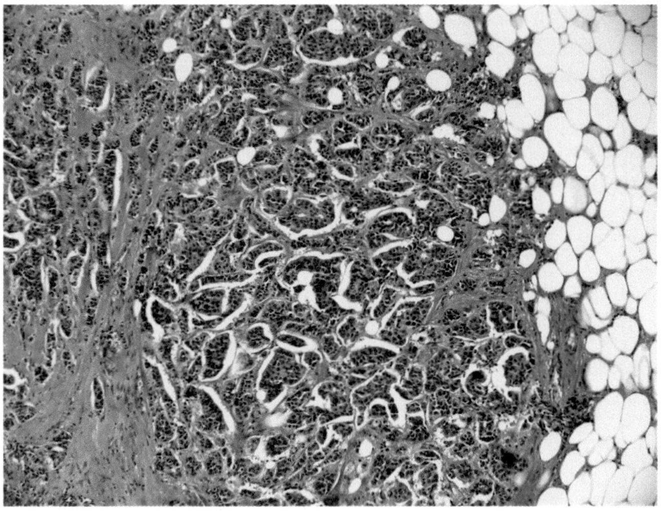

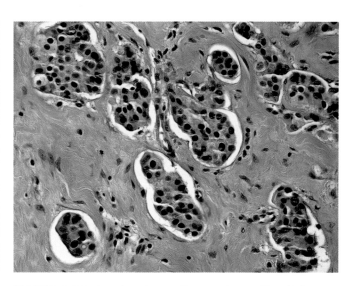

FIGURE 3.76 Invasive micropapillary carcinoma. On a medium-power view, the cell clusters are surrounded by empty lacunar spaces.

FIGURE 3.77 Invasive micropapillary carcinoma. On a high-power view, the neoplastic cells have abundant slightly granular cytoplasm exhibiting intermediate to high nuclear grade.

with this tumor in 47% to 62% of cases. Some authors have suggested that the lack of fibrovascular cores and subsequent ischemic cell degeneration might cause the formation of concentric calcifications (109). An intraductal component is present in more than half of cases, and it is often micropapillary, cribriform, or papillary type with intermediate to high nuclear grade. Necrosis is frequently observed (100,105,109). A characteristic feature of invasive micropapillary carcinoma is a prominent tendency toward lymphovascular spread. The authors of 2 studies have found that regardless of the extent, tumors with any amount of micropapillary differentiation are associated with a significant lymphotrophism (100,102).

Studies have revealed that the characteristic feature of this tumor is related to the inversion of polarization of the neoplastic cells. The stroma-facing (basal) surface of the cells acquires apical secretory properties, and cells are covered with microvilli directed toward the surrounding stroma (108). Moreover, MUC1 glycoprotein, normally expressed in the apical membrane of many secretory organs, shows an inverted membrane cytoplasmic reactivity in these tumors (104,107,110).

A pure invasive micropapillary carcinoma is unusual. Most cases are mixed with invasive ductal carcinoma, NOS, or less often, one of its variants, including tubular, papillary, or mucinous carcinoma, or less frequently invasive lobular carcinoma (100,101,104). In such cases, an abrupt transition is observed between the invasive micropapillary pattern and the other component of the tumor. Moreover, the foci of the micropapillary carcinoma are usually observed at the periphery of the tumor rather than at the center (102). Another unique characteristic of this lesion is its high percentage of estrogen receptor and progesterone receptor positivity, interestingly combined with

a high positivity for HER-2 oncoprotein (100,103,111). Multiple studies have reported that these tumors express p53 protein at a high level compared with invasive ductal carcinoma, NOS (109). An overexpression of N-cadherin was shown recently by Nagi et al (112). Thor et al (113) demonstrated loss of the short arm of chromosome 8 in all of the invasive micropapillary carcinomas. Middleton et al (109) reported loss of heterozygosity in locus 17p13.1 in 4 of 5 cases of invasive micropapillary carcinoma, with 80% concordance between molecular and immunohistochemical analyses. All these studies show the aggressive nature of this tumor.

Differential Diagnosis

Other rare breast tumors should be considered in the differential diagnosis. Invasive papillary carcinoma is histologically different from invasive micropapillary carcinoma. It exhibits complex papillary structures within a cystically dilated duct lined by low-nuclear-grade neoplastic cells and lacking the clear spaces surrounding tumor clusters seen in invasive micropapillary carcinoma (100,102). In some cases, invasive micropapillary carcinoma may resemble colloid carcinoma, with the neoplastic cell clusters floating in a small amount of mucin. Clusters of cells in invasive micropapillary carcinoma are typically smaller, with well-defined reversed cellular polarity or tubule formation. Larger extracellular mucin pools are also a feature of colloid carcinoma (100,102).

Extensive lymphatic invasion at the periphery of invasive ductal carcinoma may mimic invasive micropapillary carcinoma. It should be kept in mind that many spaces within the invasive micropapillary carcinoma are not lined by true endothelial cells, and this appearance is most likely related to a shrinkage artifact due to fixation (100). Retraction artifact may also mimic invasive micropapillary carcinoma, but retraction artifact occurs usually in association with dense collagenous stroma, whereas invasive micropapillary carcinoma exhibits a loose, typically spongy stroma (102). Metastatic tumors should also be considered in the differential diagnosis, especially ovarian serous papillary adenocarcinoma and the less common micropapillary variant of transitional cell carcinoma of the bladder. The clinicopathologic correlation and the presence of DCIS can help to distinguish invasive micropapillary carcinoma from the metastatic tumors (95).

Management

Most studies have reported a poor outcome for patients with invasive micropapillary carcinoma compared with patients with a conventional invasive carcinoma arising in the same organ site. In one study, the rate of skin and chest wall recurrence was reported as 90% after a mean follow-up interval of 24 months (109). Similarly, Pettinato et al (104) reported that 71% of patients experienced local relapse after a mean follow-up period of 24 months. In one retrospective study, Nassar et al (102) reported that 46% of patients died from breast cancer with invasive micropapillary carcinoma after a mean follow-up duration of 35.8 months. Death of disease was not correlated with the extent of micropapillary carcinoma. It was, however, correlated with size of lymph node involvement and the number of lymph nodes involved. Skin invasion were significantly higher in the group of patients who died of breast cancer. When the outcomes of patients with invasive micropapillary carcinoma and those of patients with invasive ductal carcinoma, NOS, were compared, the former group exhibited worse overall disease behavior. However, the survival of patients with invasive micropapillary carcinoma did not differ from those with invasive ductal carcinoma, NOS, of similar nodal status (102).

All these results suggest that invasive micropapillary carcinoma of the breast is a distinct and aggressive variant of breast cancer, with marked lymphotropism, frequent axillary lymph node and skin involvement, frequent local recurrence, and distant metastasis. This aggressive behavior seems independent of patient age, tumor size, location, histologic grade, or extent of the micropapillary growth pattern. These adverse morphologic features are supported by prognostic markers such as HER-2 neu and p53, high proliferation index, aneuploidy, and down-regulation of adhesion molecules. The recognition of a micropapillary growth pattern in carcinoma of the breast, even if it is a small component relative to the more

ordinary carcinoma, is important because of its association with extensive lymphovascular invasion and aggressive tumor behavior (100,104). Aggressive neoadjuvant chemotherapy before surgery should be evaluated in these patients (104). Further studies are necessary to clarify the mechanism of lymphotropism of this unique pattern of invasive carcinoma (100).

■ CONCLUSION

Papillary lesions of the breast are commonly encountered in routine surgical pathology practice and consist of a heterogeneous group of lesions that include a wide spectrum in their morphologic appearance, malignant potential, and clinical behavior. The evaluation of papillary lesions remains one of the most problematic areas in breast pathology. In this chapter, we review the clinicopathologic features, histology, differential diagnosis, and biological behavior of the papillary lesions, and we discuss various diagnostic difficulties to accurately diagnose and manage these lesions. We also define the importance of immunohistochemistry in evaluating these lesions. In current pathology practice, there are several difficulties regarding diagnosis and the subsequent management of papillary lesions encountered on the CNB specimens. Epithelial displacement by needling procedures is not infrequently encountered because of the increasing popularity of these procedures, and the pathologist should be aware of this possibility. In this review, the difficulties of cytology in the diagnosis and classification of papillary lesions have also been addressed.

Finally, in evaluations of the breast papillary lesions, radiologic, clinical, and histopathologic correlation is essential. The limitations of fine-needle aspiration and CNB should be kept in mind. Discordant imaging and histopathologic findings should always prompt a repeat biopsy.

■ KEY POINTS

- Papillary lesions encompass the spectrum of lesions ranging from benign to frankly malignant entities.
- Intraductal papilloma, sclerosing papilloma, and papillomatosis, a benign spectrum of lesions characterized by fronds with broad to blunt configuration, different amounts of stroma, and epithelium composed of 2 layers and 2 types of cells (epithelial and myoepithelial).
- Superimposed epithelial proliferations in intraductal papilloma, such as apocrine metaplasia, squamous

metaplasia, usual ductal hyperplasia, ADH, lobular neoplasia, and DCIS, can involve intraductal papilloma, and the extent and type of epithelial proliferation are hallmarks of classification of papillomas as "atypical" or involved by lobular neoplasia or DCIS.

- Papillary carcinoma is malignant in situ lesion and is composed of numerous fronds with preponderance of the epithelium over the stroma. A proliferative population is composed solely of neoplastic epithelial cells.

- Variants of papillary carcinoma such as an encapsulated (intracystic) papillary carcinoma, solid papillary carcinoma, and invasive papillary and micropapillary carcinoma are rare variants of ductal carcinoma.

■ REFERENCES

1. Rosen P. *Rosen's Breast Pathology.* Philadelphia: Lippincott, Williams & Wilkins; 2008.

2. Tavassoli FA. *Pathology of the Breast.* Stamford, Conn: Appleton & Lange; 1999.

3. Cardenosa G, Eklund GW. Benign papillary neoplasms of the breast: mammographic findings. *Radiology.* 1991;181:751–755.

4. Woods ER, Helvie MA, Ikeda DM, et al. Solitary breast papilloma: comparison of mammographic, galactographic, and pathologic findings. *AJR Am J Roentgenol.* 1992;159:487–491.

5. Ibarra JA. Papillary lesions of the breast. *Breast J.* 2006;12:237–251.

6. Lam WW, Chu WC, Tang AP, et al. Role of radiologic features in the management of papillary lesions of the breast. *AJR Am J Roentgenol.* 2006;186:1322–1327.

7. Daniel BL, Gardner RW, Birdwell RL, et al. Magnetic resonance imaging of intraductal papilloma of the breast. *Magn Reson Imaging.* 2003;21:887–892.

8. Makita M, Akiyama F, Gomi N, et al. Endoscopic and histologic findings of intraductal lesions presenting with nipple discharge. *Breast J.* 2006;12:S210–S217.

9. Tseng HS, Chen YL, Chen ST, et al. The management of papillary lesion of the breast by core needle biopsy. *Eur J Surg Oncol.* 2009;35:21–24.

10. Mulligan AM, O'Malley FP. Papillary lesions of the breast: a review. *Adv Anat Pathol.* 2007;14:108–119.

11. Ueng SH, Mezzetti T, Tavassoli FA. Papillary neoplasms of the breast: a review. *Arch Pathol Lab Med.* 2009;133:893–907.

12. Lieske B, Ravichandran D, Wright D. Role of fine-needle aspiration cytology and core needle biopsy in the preoperative diagnosis of screen-detected breast carcinoma. *Br J Cancer.* 2006;95:62–66.

13. Gomez-Aracil V, Mayayo E, Azua J, Arraza A. Papillary neoplasms of the breast: clues in fine needle cytology. *Cytopathology.* 2002;13:22–30.

14. Simsir A, Waissman J, Thorner K, Cangiarella J. Mammary lesions diagnosed as "papillary" by aspiration cytology: 70 cases with follow-up. *Cancer.* 2003;99:156–165.

15. Saad RS, Kanbour-Shakir A, Syed A, Kanbour A. Sclerosing papillary lesion of the breast: a diagnostic pitfall for malignancy in fine needle aspiration biopsy. *Diagn Cytopathol.* 2006;34:114–118.

16. Michael CW, Buschmann B. Can true papillary neoplasms of breast and their mimickers be accurately classified by cytology? *Cancer.* 2002;96:92–100.

17. Massod S, Loya A, Khalbuss W. Is core needle biopsy superior to fine needle aspiration biopsy in the diagnosis of papillary breast lesions? *Diagn Cytopathol.* 2003;28:329–334.

18. Kraus FT, Neubecker RD. The differential diagnosis of papillary tumors of the breast. *Cancer.* 1962;15:444–455.

19. Collins LC, Schnitt SJ. Papillary lesions of the breast: selected diagnostic and management issues. *Histopathology.* 2008;52:20–29.

20. Lewis JT, Hartmann LC, Vierkant RA, et al. An analysis of breast cancer risk in women with single, multiple, and atypical papilloma. *Am J Surg Pathol.* 2006;30:665–672.

21. Ivan D, Selinko V, Sahin AA, et al. Accuracy of core needle biopsy diagnosis in assessing papillary breast lesions: histologic predictors of malignancy. *Mod Pathol.* 2004;17:165–171.

22. Jacobs TW, Connolly JL, Schnitt SJ. Nonmalignant lesions in breast core needle biopsies: to excise or not to excise? *Am J Surg Pathol.* 2002;26:1095–1110.

23. Liberman L. Percutaneous image-guided core breast biopsy. *Radiol Clin North Am.* 2002;40:483–500, vi.

24. Gendler LS, Feldman SM, Balassanian R, et al. Association of breast cancer with papillary lesions identified at percutaneous image-guided breast biopsy. *Am J Surg.* 2004;188:365–370.

25. Puglisi F, Zuiani C, Bazzocchi M, et al. Role of mammography, ultrasound and large core biopsy in the diagnostic evaluation of papillary breast lesions. *Oncology.* 2003;65:311–315.

26. Renshaw AA, Derhagopian RP, Tizol-Blanco DM, Gould EW. Papillomas and atypical papillomas in breast core needle biopsy specimens: risk of carcinoma in subsequent excision. *Am J Clin Pathol.* 2004;122:217–221.

27. Rosen EL, Bentley RC, Baker JA, Soo MS. Imaging-guided core needle biopsy of papillary lesions of the breast. *AJR Am J Roentgenol.* 2002;179:1185–1192.

28. Liberman L, Bracero N, Vuolo MA, et al. Percutaneous large-core biopsy of papillary breast lesions. *AJR Am J Roentgenol.* 1999;172:331–337.

29. Mercado CL, Hamele-Bena D, Singer C, et al. Papillary lesions of the breast: evaluation with stereotactic directional vacuum-assisted biopsy. *Radiology.* 2001;221:650–655.

30. Bleiweiss IJ, Nagi CS, Jaffer S. Axillary sentinel lymph nodes can be falsely positive due to iatrogenic displacement and transport of benign epithelial cells in patients with breast carcinoma. *J Clin Oncol.* 2006;24:2013–2018.

31. Carter BA, Jensen RA, Simpson JF, Page DL. Benign transport of breast epithelium into axillary lymph nodes after biopsy. *Am J Clin Pathol.* 2000;113:259–265.

32. Nagi C, Bleiweiss I, Jaffer S. Epithelial displacement in breast lesions: a papillary phenomenon. *Arch Pathol Lab Med.* 2005;129:1465–1469.

33. Youngson BJ, Cranor M, Rosen PP. Epithelial displacement in surgical breast specimens following needling procedures. *Am J Surg Pathol.* 1994;18:896–903.

34. Mercado CL, Hamele-Bena D, Oken SM, et al. Papillary lesions of the breast at percutaneous core-needle biopsy. *Radiology.* 2006;238:801–808.

35. Philpotts LE, Shaheen NA, Jain KS, et al. Uncommon high-risk lesions of the breast diagnosed at stereotactic core-needle biopsy: clinical importance. *Radiology.* 2000;216:831–837.

36. Sydnor MK, Wilson JD, Hijaz TA, et al. Underestimation of the presence of breast carcinoma in papillary lesions initially diagnosed at core-needle biopsy. *Radiology.* 2007;242:58–62.

37. Cheng TY, Chen CM, Lee MY, et al. Risk factors associated with conversion from nonmalignant to malignant diagnosis after surgical excision of breast papillary lesions. *Ann Surg Oncol.* 2009;16:3375–3379.

38. Liberman L, Tornos C, Huzjan R, et al. Is surgical excision warranted after benign, concordant diagnosis of papilloma at percutaneous breast biopsy? *AJR Am J Roentgenol.* 2006;186:1328–1334.

39. Rizzo M, Lund MJ, Oprea G, et al. Surgical follow-up and clinical presentation of 142 breast papillary lesions diagnosed by ultrasound-guided core-needle biopsy. *Ann Surg Oncol.* 2008;15:1040–1047.

40. Skandarajah AR, Field L, Yuen Larn Mou A, et al. Benign papilloma on core biopsy requires surgical excision. *Ann Surg Oncol.* 2008;15:2272–2277.

41. Valdes EK, Tartter PI, Genelus-Dominique E, et al. Significance of papillary lesions at percutaneous breast biopsy. *Ann Surg Oncol.* 2006;13:480–482.

42. Agoff SN, Lawton TJ. Papillary lesions of the breast with and without atypical ductal hyperplasia: can we accurately predict benign behavior from core needle biopsy? *Am J Clin Pathol.* 2004;122:440–443.

43. Ashkenazi I, Ferrer K, Sekosan M, et al. Papillary lesions of the breast discovered on percutaneous large core and vacuum-assisted biopsies: reliability of clinical and pathological parameters in identifying benign lesions. *Am J Surg.* 2007;194:183–188.

44. Bennett LE, Ghate SV, Bentley R, Baker JA. Is surgical excision of core biopsy proven benign papillomas of the breast necessary? *Acad Radiol.* 2010;17:553–557.

45. Papotti M, Gugliotta P, Ghiringhello B, Bussolati G. Association of breast carcinoma and multiple intraductal papillomas: an histological and immunohistochemical investigation. *Histopathology.* 1984;8:963–975.

46. Sapino A, Botta G, Cassoni P, et al. Multiple papillomas of the breast: morphologic findings and clinical evolution. *Anat Pathol.* 1996;1:205–218.

47. Azzopardi JG, Ahmed A, Millis RR. Problems in breast pathology. *Major Probl Pathol.* 1979;11:i-xvi, 1–466.

48. Ali-Fehmi R, Carolin K, Wallis T, Visscher DW. Clinicopathologic analysis of breast lesions associated with multiple papillomas. *Hum Pathol.* 2003;34:234–239.

49. Ohuchi N, Abe R, Kasai M. Possible cancerous change of intraductal papillomas of the breast. A 3-D reconstruction study of 25 cases. *Cancer.* 1984;54:605–611.

50. Page DL, Salhany KE, Jensen RA, Dupont WD. Subsequent breast carcinoma risk after biopsy with atypia in a breast papilloma. *Cancer.* 1996;78:258–266.

51. Carter D. Intraductal papillary tumors of the breast: a study of 78 cases. *Cancer.* 1977;39:1689–1692.

52. Pacilli M, Sebire NJ, Thambapillai E, Pierro A. Juvenile papillomatosis of the breast in a male infant with Noonan syndrome, cafe au lait spots, and family history of breast carcinoma. *Pediatr Blood Cancer.* 2005;45:991–993.

53. Rosen PP, Cantrell B, Mullen DL, DePalo A. Juvenile papillomatosis (Swiss cheese disease) of the breast. *Am J Surg Pathol.* 1980;4:3–12.

54. Rosen PP, Holmes G, Lesser ML, et al. Juvenile papillomatosis and breast carcinoma. *Cancer.* 1985;55:1345–1352.

55. Taffurelli M, Santini D, Martinelli, G et al. Juvenile papillomatosis of the breast. A multidisciplinary study. *Pathol Annu.* 1991;26(pt 1):25–35.

56. Hidalgo F, Llano JM, Marhuenda A. Juvenile papillomatosis of the breast (Swiss cheese disease). *AJR Am J Roentgenol.* 1997;169:912.

57. Kersschot EA, Hermans ME, Pauwels C, et al. Juvenile papillomatosis of the breast: sonographic appearance. *Radiology* 1988;169:631–633.

58. Mussurakis S, Carleton PJ, Turnbull LW. Case report: MR imaging of juvenile papillomatosis of the breast. *Br J Radiol.* 1996;69:867–870.

59. Rosen PP, Kimmel M. Juvenile papillomatosis of the breast. A follow-up study of 41 patients having biopsies before 1979. *Am J Clin Pathol.* 1990;93:599–603.

60. Bazzocchi F, Santini D, Martinelli G, et al. Juvenile papillomatosis (epitheliosis) of the breast. A clinical and pathologic study of 13 cases. *Am J Clin Pathol.* 1986;86:745–748.

61. Rosen PP, Lyngholm B, Kinne DW, Beattie EJ, Jr. Juvenile papillomatosis of the breast and family history of breast carcinoma. *Cancer.* 1982;49:2591–2595.

62. MacGrogan G, Tavassoli FA. Central atypical papillomas of the breast: a clinicopathological study of 119 cases. *Virchows Arch.* 2003;443:609–617.

63. Lacroix-Triki M, Mery E, Voigt JJ, et al. Value of cytokeratin 5/6 immunostaining using D5/16 B4 antibody in the spectrum of proliferative intraepithelial lesions of the breast. A comparative study with 34betaE12 antibody. *Virchows Arch.* 2003;442:548–554.

64. Otterbach F, Bankfalvi A, Bergner S, et al. Cytokeratin 5/6 immunohistochemistry assists the differential diagnosis of atypical proliferations of the breast. *Histopathology.* 2000;37:232–240.

65. Rabban JT, Koerner FC, Lerwill MF. Solid papillary ductal carcinoma in situ versus usual ductal hyperplasia in the breast: a potentially difficult distinction resolved by cytokeratin 5/6. *Hum Pathol.* 2006;37:787–793.

66. Tse GM, Tan PH, Moriya T. The role of immunohistochemistry in the differential diagnosis of papillary lesions of the breast. *J Clin Pathol.* 2009;62:407–413.

67. Saddik M, Lai R. CD44s as a surrogate marker for distinguishing intraductal papilloma from papillary carcinoma of the breast. *J Clin Pathol.* 1999;52:862–864.

68. Saddik M, Lai R, Medeiros LJ, et al. Differential expression of cyclin D1 in breast papillary carcinomas and benign papillomas: an immunohistochemical study. *Arch Pathol Lab Med.* 1999;123:152–156.

69. Tse GM, Tan PH, Ma TK, et al. CD44s is useful in the differentiation of benign and malignant papillary lesions of the breast. *J Clin Pathol.* 2005;58:1185–1188.

70. Raju U, Vertes D. Breast papillomas with atypical ductal hyperplasia: a clinicopathologic study. *Hum Pathol.* 1996;27:1231–1238.

71. Lam WW, Tang AP, Tse G, Chu WC. Radiology-Pathology conference: papillary carcinoma of the breast. *Clin Imaging.* 2005;29:396–400.

72. McCulloch GL, Evans AJ, Yeoman L, et al. Radiological features of papillary carcinoma of the breast. *Clin Radiol.* 1997;52:865–868.

73. Muttarak M, Lerttumnongtum P, Chaiwun B, Peh WC. Spectrum of papillary lesions of the breast: clinical, imaging, and pathologic correlation. *AJR Am J Roentgenol.* 2008;191:700–707.

74. Knelson MH, el Yousef SJ, Goldberg RE, Ballance W. Intracystic papillary carcinoma of the breast: mammographic, sonographic, and MR appearance with pathologic correlation. *J Comput Assist Tomogr.* 1987;11:1074–1076.

75. Carter D, Orr SL, Merino MJ. Intracystic papillary carcinoma of the breast. After mastectomy, radiotherapy or excisional biopsy alone. *Cancer.* 1983;52:14–19.

76. Hill CB, Yeh IT. Myoepithelial cell staining patterns of papillary breast lesions: from intraductal papillomas to invasive papillary carcinomas. *Am J Clin Pathol.* 2005;123:36–44.

77. Collins LC, Carlo VP, Hwang H, et al. Intracystic papillary carcinomas of the breast: a reevaluation using a panel of myoepithelial cell markers. *Am J Surg Pathol.* 2006;30:1002–1007.

78. Lefkowitz M, Lefkowitz W, Wargotz ES. Intraductal (intracystic) papillary carcinoma of the breast and its variants: a clinicopathological study of 77 cases. *Hum Pathol.* 1994;25:802–809.

79. Eusebi V, Damiani S, Ellis IO, et al. Breast tumor resembling the tall cell variant of papillary thyroid carcinoma: report of 5 cases. *Am J Surg Pathol.* 2003;27:1114–1118.

80. Fadare O, Rose TA, Tavassoli FA. Papillary intraductal carcinoma with extensive secretory endometrium-like subnuclear vacuolization. *Breast J.* 2005;11:470–471.

81. Esposito NN, Dabbs DJ, Bhargava R. Are encapsulated papillary carcinomas of the breast in situ or invasive? A basement membrane study of 27 cases. *Am J Clin Pathol.* 2009;131:228–242.

82. Leal C, Costa I, Fonseca D, et al. Intracystic (encysted) papillary carcinoma of the breast: a clinical, pathological, and immunohistochemical study. *Hum Pathol.* 1998;29:1097–1104.

83. Mulligan AM, O'Malley FP. Metastatic potential of encapsulated (intracystic) papillary carcinoma of the breast: a report of 2 cases with axillary lymph node micrometastases. *Int J Surg Pathol.* 2007;15:143–147.

84. Solorzano CC, Middleton LP, Hunt KK, et al. Treatment and outcome of patients with intracystic papillary carcinoma of the breast. *Am J Surg.* 2002;184:364–368.

85. Maluf HM, Koerner FC. Solid papillary carcinoma of the breast. A form of intraductal carcinoma with endocrine differentiation frequently associated with mucinous carcinoma. *Am J Surg Pathol.* 1995;19:1237–1244.

86. Nassar H, Qureshi H, Volkanadsay N, Visscher D. Clinicopathologic analysis of solid papillary carcinoma of the breast and associated invasive carcinomas. *Am J Surg Pathol.* 2006;30:501–507.

87. Otsuki Y, Yamada M, Shimizu S, et al. Solid-papillary carcinoma of the breast: clinicopathological study of 20 cases. *Pathol Int.* 2007;57:421–429.

88. Dickersin GR, Maluf HM, Koerner FC. Solid papillary carcinoma of breast: an ultrastructural study. *Ultrastruct Pathol.* 1997;21:153–161.

89. Nicolas MM, Wu Y, Middleton LP, Gilcrease MZ. Loss of myoepithelium is variable in solid papillary carcinoma of the breast. *Histopathology.* 2007;51:657–665.

90. Yamada M, Otsuki Y, Shimitzu S, Tanioka F, Ogawa H, Kobayashi H. Cytologistudy of 20 cases of solid papillary carcinoma if the breast. *Diagn Cytopathol.* 2007;35:417–422.

91. Kuroda N, Fujishima N, Inoue K, Chara M, Nizouro K, Lee GH. Solid papillary carcinoma of the breast: imprint cytological and histological findings. *Med Mol Morphol.* 2010;43:48–52.

92. Shin SJ, Rosen PP. Solid variant of mammary adenoid cystic carcinoma with basaloid features: a study of nine cases. *Am J Surg Pathol.* 2002;26:413–420.

93. Fisher ER, Palekar AS, Redmond C, et al. Pathologic findings from the National Surgical Adjuvant Breast Project (protocol no. 4). VI. Invasive papillary cancer. *Am J Clin Pathol.* 1980;73:313–322.

94. McDivitt RW, Holleb AI, Foote FW Jr. Prior breast disease in patients treated for papillary carcinoma. *Arch Pathol.* 1968;85:117–124.

95. Amin MB, Ro JY, el-Sharkawy T, et al. Micropapillary variant of transitional cell carcinoma of the urinary bladder. Histologic pattern resembling ovarian papillary serous carcinoma. *Am J Surg Pathol.* 1994;18:1224–1232.

96. Amin MB, Tamboli P, Merchant SH, et al. Micropapillary component in lung adenocarcinoma: a distinctive histologic feature with possible prognostic significance. *Am J Surg Pathol.* 2002;26:358–364.

97. Johansson SL, Borghede G, Holmang S. Micropapillary bladder carcinoma: a clinicopathological study of 20 cases. *J Urol.* 1999;161:1798–1802.

98. Nagao T, Gaffey TA, Visscher DW, et al. Invasive micropapillary salivary duct carcinoma: a distinct histologic variant with biologic significance. *Am J Surg Pathol.* 2004;28:319–326.

99. Gunhan-Bilgen I, Zekioglu O, Ustun EE, et al. Invasive micropapillary carcinoma of the breast: clinical, mammographic, and sonographic findings with histopathologic correlation. *AJR Am J Roentgenol.* 2002;179:927–931.

100. Walsh MM, Bleiweiss IJ. Invasive micropapillary carcinoma of the breast: eighty cases of an underrecognized entity. *Hum Pathol.* 2001;32:583–589.

101. Luna-More S, Casquero S, Perez-Mellado A, et al. Importance of estrogen receptors for the behavior of invasive micropapillary carcinoma of the breast. Review of 68 cases with follow-up of 54. *Pathol Res Pract.* 2000;196:35–39.

102. Nassar H, Wallis T, Andea A, et al. Clinicopathologic analysis of invasive micropapillary differentiation in breast carcinoma. *Mod Pathol.* 2001;14:836–841.

103. Paterakos M, Watkin WG, Edgerton SM, et al. Invasive micropapillary carcinoma of the breast: a prognostic study. *Hum Pathol.* 1999;30:1459–1463.

104. Pettinato G, Manivel CJ, Panico L, et al. Invasive micropapillary carcinoma of the breast: clinicopathologic study of 62 cases of a poorly recognized variant with highly aggressive behavior. *Am J Clin Pathol.* 2004;121:857–866.

105. Siriaunkgul S, Tavassoli FA. Invasive micropapillary carcinoma of the breast. *Mod Pathol.* 1993;6:660–662.

106. Adrada B, Arribas E, Gilcrease M, Yang WT. Invasive micropapillary carcinoma of the breast: mammographic, sonographic, and MRI features. *AJR Am J Roentgenol.* 2009;193:W58–63.

107. Nassar H, Pansare V, Zhang H, et al. Pathogenesis of invasive micropapillary carcinoma: role of MUC1 glycoprotein. *Mod Pathol.* 2004;17:1045–1050.

108. Luna-More S, Gonzalez B, Acedo C, et al. Invasive micropapillary carcinoma of the breast. A new special type of invasive mammary carcinoma. *Pathol Res Pract.* 1994;190:668–674.

109. Middleton LP, Tressera F, Sobel ME, et al. Infiltrating micropapillary carcinoma of the breast. *Mod Pathol.* 1999;12:499–504.

110. Li YS, Kaneko M, Sakamoto DG, et al. The reversed apical pattern of MUC1 expression is characteristics of invasive micropapillary carcinoma of the breast. *Breast Cancer.* 2006;13:58–63.

111. Luna-More S, de los Santos F, Breton JJ, Canadas MA. Estrogen and progesterone receptors, c-erbB-2,

p53, and Bcl-2 in thirty-three invasive micropapillary breast carcinomas. *Pathol Res Pract.* 1996;192: 27–32.

112. Nagi C, Guttman M, Jaffer S, et al. N-cadherin expression in breast cancer: correlation with an aggressive histologic variant--invasive micropapillary carcinoma. *Breast Cancer Res Treat.* 2005;94: 225–235.

113. Thor AD, Eng C, Devries S, et al. Invasive micropapillary carcinoma of the breast is associated with chromosome 8 abnormalities detected by comparative genomic hybridization. *Hum Pathol.* 2002;33:628–631.

4

Flat Epithelial Atypia

MELINDA F. LERWILL

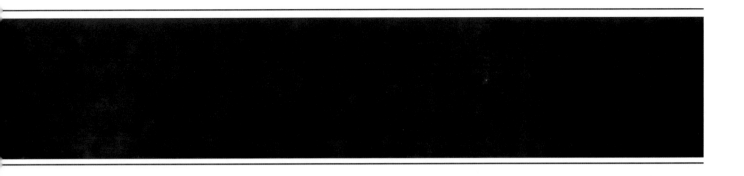

Flat epithelial atypia is an early form of ductal neoplasia that is characterized by the replacement of normal luminal cells by those demonstrating low-grade cytologic atypia. The atypical cells grow either as a single cell layer or as a pseudostratified cell layer along the walls of the involved glandular spaces. Because the atypical cells do not fill the glandular lumens, flat epithelial atypia is often not recognized as an abnormal, proliferative process. In fact, it is commonly mistaken for unremarkable breast tissue or fibrocystic changes. Such diagnostic problems stem, in large part, from the fact that flat epithelial atypia is primarily identified by its cytologic features rather than its architectural ones. The approach to its diagnosis therefore differs considerably from the architecture-based evaluation that many pathologists are accustomed to using for epithelial proliferations in the breast.

The recognition of low-grade cytologic atypia in the breast can be challenging because the definitional features run in opposition to conventional notions of atypia. Mammary low-grade ductal atypia is characterized by cellular uniformity, nuclear monomorphism, evenly distributed chromatin, smooth nuclear membranes, and inconspicuous nucleoli. The cells do not look overtly alarming, and they all look alike. In contrast, cellular atypia in most other organ systems is characterized by nuclear pleomorphism, unevenly distributed chromatin, irregular nuclear membranes, and enlarged nucleoli—cytologic heterogeneity rather than uniformity. Although the latter description of atypia is applicable to higher-grade lesions in the breast, the former set of characteristics defines the type of atypia seen in flat epithelial atypia.

The identification of low-grade cytologic atypia forms the crux of a diagnosis of flat epithelial atypia, but there are also accompanying changes in the terminal duct-lobular unit architecture, the stroma, and the myoepithelial cells that can provide important diagnostic clues. In this chapter, we will examine the histologic features of flat epithelial atypia and contrast them with those of benign and malignant entities in the differential diagnosis. We will also review the current clinical management of patients with flat epithelial atypia and discuss the terminological confusion surrounding this oft-renamed form of early ductal neoplasia.

■ PATHOLOGIC FEATURES

The histologic changes of flat epithelial atypia are most readily identified in the terminal duct-lobular units. Involved terminal duct-lobular units appear enlarged when compared with adjacent normal ones (Figure 4.1). The increase in the size of the lobules is due to dilatation of the terminal ductules and acini, which develops progressively as the atypical ductal cells increase in number along the glandular walls. The degree of dilatation and lobular enlargement is variable from case to case and lobule to lobule. In some examples, the glands can be markedly cystic (Figure 4.2) and even span a millimeter or more in diameter (Figure 4.3). Others show a more modest degree of dilatation, but an overall increase in lobule size is still readily appreciated (Figures 4.1 and 4.4–4.6). Lobules with early involvement by flat epithelial atypia show only a mild degree of lobular enlargement and minimal

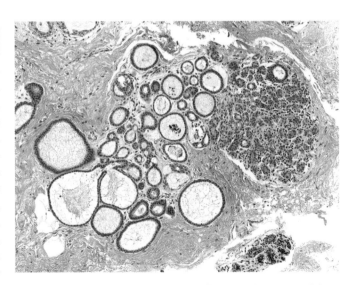

FIGURE 4.1 The lobule involved by flat epithelial atypia (left) is larger than the adjacent normal lobule (right).

89

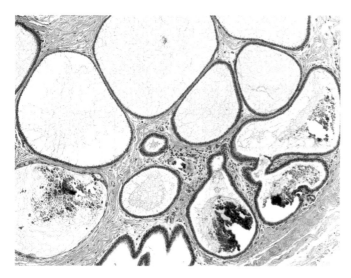

FIGURE 4.2 Cystic dilatation is common in flat epithelial atypia, as are intraluminal calcifications.

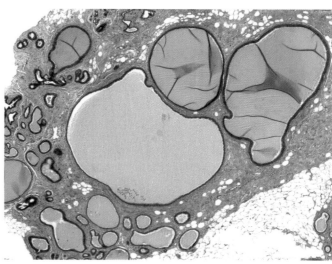

FIGURE 4.3 Marked cystic dilatation in flat epithelial atypia.

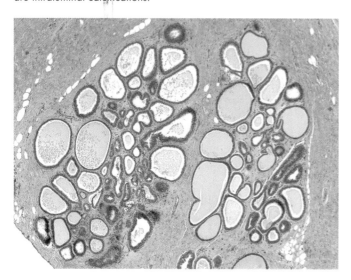

FIGURE 4.4 Both lobules are involved by flat epithelial atypia and exhibit a moderate degree of enlargement and cystic change.

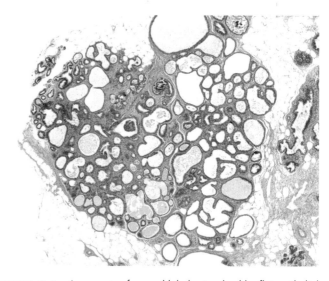

FIGURE 4.5 Aggregate of several lobules involved by flat epithelial atypia.

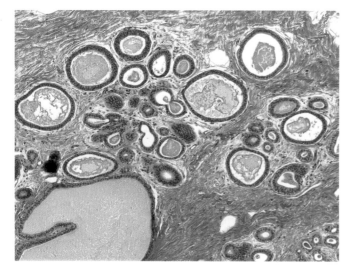

FIGURE 4.6 Less complex lobules involved by flat epithelial atypia. The degree of dilatation is most pronounced in the preterminal ductule (bottom left), which is the anatomic site of origin for flat epithelial atypia.

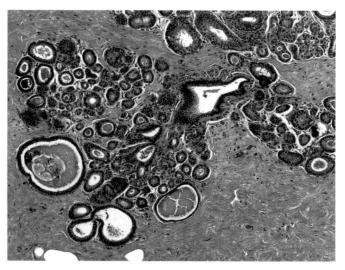

FIGURE 4.7 Early example of flat epithelial atypia. The atypical changes extend from the central ductule into several adjacent lobules. The involved lobules show only a mild degree of acinar distension.

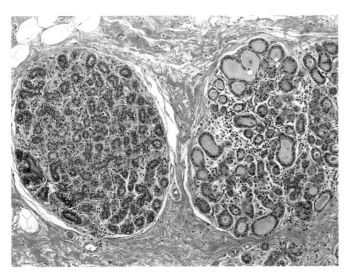

FIGURE 4.8 Early example of flat epithelial atypia (right) demonstrating mild lobular enlargement and glandular dilatation in comparison to normal lobule (left).

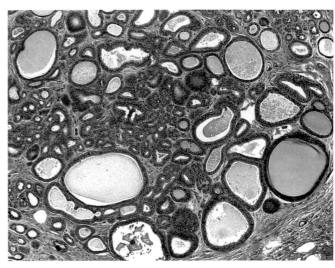

FIGURE 4.9 Well-developed example of flat epithelial atypia with thickened epithelium, cystic change, and diminished intralobular stroma.

glandular distension (Figures 4.7–4.8). As the acini within a lobule become dilated, the intralobular stroma decreases in amount (Figure 4.9). Occasionally, medium to large extralobular ducts are involved by flat epithelial atypia, and they demonstrate similar enlargement and dilatation depending on the degree of atypical proliferation (Figures 4.10–4.11).

The diagnostic hallmark of flat epithelial atypia is the presence of low-grade cytologic atypia (Table 4.1, Figures 4.12–4.28). The atypia is identical to that seen in both low-grade ductal carcinoma in situ (Figure 4.12) and atypical ductal hyperplasia. The atypical ductal cells have a monomorphic appearance and contain round or oval, mildly enlarged nuclei. The chromatin is typically fine, hyperchromatic, and evenly distributed. The nuclear membranes are smoothly contoured. The nucleoli are generally inconspicuous. Occasional examples may demonstrate slightly more granular chromatin and 1 or 2 small,

distinct nucleoli (Figure 4.22). Mitotic activity is absent to minimal.

The cytoplasm of the atypical cells is increased in comparison with normal luminal cells (Figures 4.19, 4.23, and 4.24). It tends to be pale eosinophilic or amphophilic in color and fine and nongranular in quality. Much of the cytoplasm is present in the apices of the cells, creating the typical tall columnar cell morphology of flat epithelial atypia. In some instances, however, the atypical cells are cuboidal in shape (Figures 4.25–4.26). The luminal border in flat epithelial atypia tends to be sharply defined, and apical cytoplasmic snouts are common (Figure 4.21). Intercellular borders are often more distinct than in benign epithelial proliferations.

The atypical ductal cells may grow as a single cell layer or in a pseudostratified manner (Figures 4.13–4.28). The nuclei maintain a basal location when only a single layer of

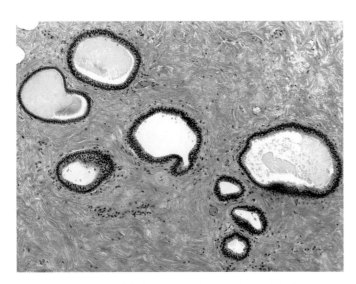

FIGURE 4.10 Extralobular ducts harboring flat epithelial atypia.

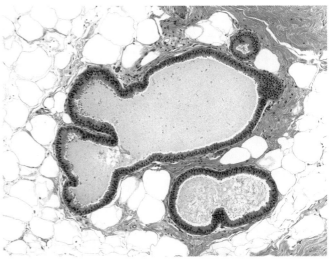

FIGURE 4.11 Extralobular ducts involved by flat epithelial atypia. Even on relatively low-power magnification, the epithelial layer appears abnormally thickened, crowded, and hyperchromatic.

■ **Table 4.1** Cytologic features of low-grade ductal atypia

Cell population	Monomorphic
Nuclear shape	Round or oval
Nuclear contours	Smooth
Chromatin	Homogeneous, fine, hyperchromatic
Nucleoli	Often inconspicuous
Nuclear pseudoinclusions	Absent
Cytoplasm, amount	Increased
Cytoplasm, staining quality	Eosinophilic or amphophilic, pallorous
Cell borders	Sometimes distinct

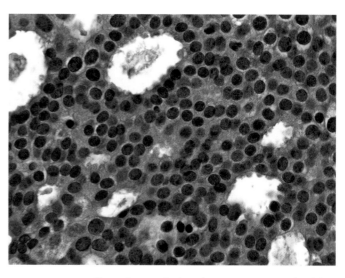

FIGURE 4.12 Classic low-grade ductal atypia in an example of ductal carcinoma in situ. The same type of cytologic atypia is seen in flat epithelial atypia.

cells is present. When the proliferation is pseudostratified, the nuclei come to occupy variable positions in the cells. This is sometimes described as a loss of polarity, since the nuclei are no longer basally located. The nuclei, however, do maintain polarity relative to the basal-apical axis of the cell. When the nuclei are oval in shape, one can appreciate that they are arranged with their long axes in parallel with the long axes of the cells (Figure 4.17). This maintenance of cellular polarity imparts a very orderly appearance to flat epithelial atypia, with evenly distributed nuclei organized in radial array around the luminal space.

Genuine stratification of the atypical ductal cells in the form of micropapillae, trabecular bars, Roman arches, cribriform spaces, or solid growth is, by definition, absent

in flat epithelial atypia. When these types of architectural atypia are superimposed upon an otherwise flat atypical proliferation, a diagnosis of either atypical ductal hyperplasia or ductal carcinoma in situ is warranted.

The myoepithelial cell layer is frequently attenuated in flat epithelial atypia (Figure 4.27), much as it is in many examples of ductal carcinoma in situ and atypical ductal hyperplasia. The degree of attenuation is variable, but in some examples, it may be so extreme that the myoepithelial cells appear to be altogether absent on routine sections, although a few remaining ones can usually be identified by immunohistochemistry. The loss of myoepithelial cells tends to be most evident in affected terminal duct-lobular

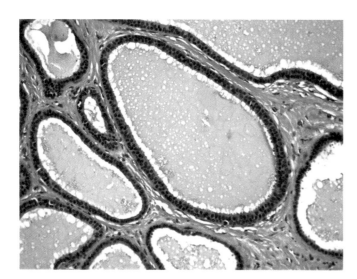

FIGURE 4.13 Monomorphic, hyperchromatic nuclei indicate the presence of low-grade ductal atypia.

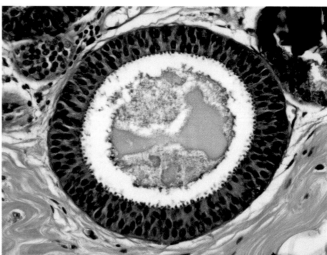

FIGURE 4.14 Strikingly uniform population of cells with hyperchromatic nuclei. As the atypical cells increase in number, they pseudostratify, resulting in a band-like thickening of the epithelial layer with cellular crowding.

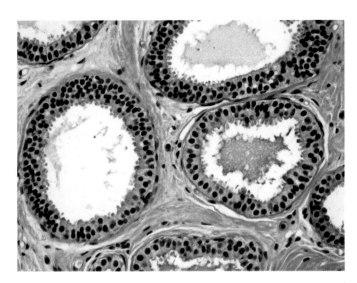

FIGURE 4.15 Example of flat epithelial atypia with round, hyperchromatic nuclei and distinctive amphophilic cytoplasm.

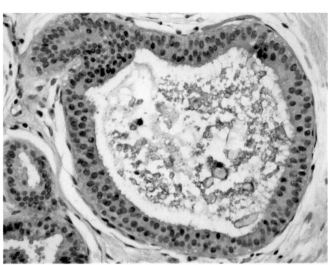

FIGURE 4.16 Nuclear uniformity and pseudostratification in flat epithelial atypia.

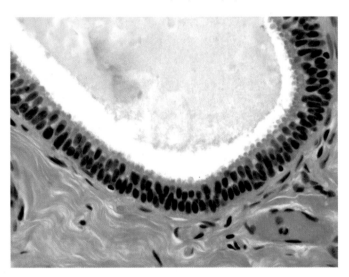

FIGURE 4.17 Orderly distribution of cells in flat epithelial atypia with maintenance of cellular polarity around the luminal space.

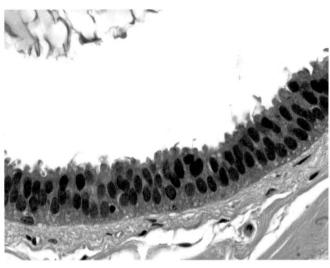

FIGURE 4.18 Classic low-grade cytologic atypia in flat epithelial atypia.

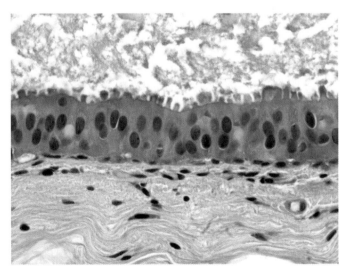

FIGURE 4.19 Ductal cells demonstrating low-grade nuclear atypia usually have increased amounts of pale cytoplasm, which tends to accumulate at the apical poles.

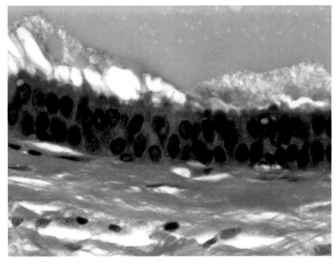

FIGURE 4.20 Uniform pseudostratification of the atypical cells results in a flat growth pattern.

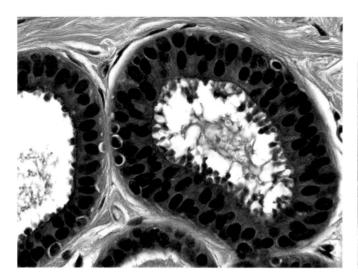

FIGURE 4.21 The atypical cells are of the same height and form a sharply defined luminal border. Apical blebs, or snouts, are common.

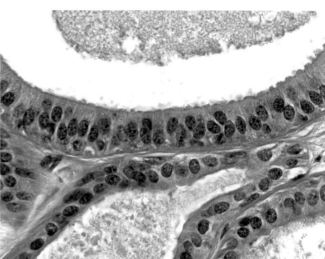

FIGURE 4.22 Atypical cells with variant nuclear morphology have slightly granular chromatin and distinct but small nucleoli.

units; larger ducts sometimes retain a relatively intact myoepithelial cell layer.

Intraluminal secretions are characteristically present, and they may be flocculent and basophilic (Figures 4.2 and 4.26) or more dense and eosinophilic (Figures 4.3–4.4). The secretions have a tendency to calcify (Figures 4.2 and 4.28), resulting in clustered calcifications that raise concern on mammography and lead to biopsy of these lesions.

The earliest recognizable changes of flat epithelial atypia occur in the preterminal ductule adjacent to the lobule (Figure 4.29) (1). The atypical ductal cells first appear here, replacing the normal luminal cells. A transition between normal-appearing and atypical epithelium can sometimes be distinguished (Figure 4.30). As the proliferation progresses, the atypical cells spread into the terminal ductule and then the acini of the lobule (Figures 4.29–4.30). The accumulation of increasing numbers of atypical cells leads to cellular crowding

and pseudostratification and/or compensatory dilatation of the involved glandular spaces. Because the atypical proliferation originates in the preterminal ductule, this structure often shows more well-developed changes than the terminal duct-lobular unit in early examples of flat epithelial atypia (Figures 4.6 and 4.29).

Even in minimally involved lobules, the characteristic features of flat epithelial atypia can still be appreciated, particularly when viewed in comparison with normal lobules from the same patient (Figures 4.8 and 4.31). Slight acinar distension and the presence of mildly enlarged epithelial cells are the first suggestions that an atypical process may be at hand. Closer inspection reveals the presence of monomorphic, hyperchromatic nuclei and increased cytoplasm. These cytologic features contrast with those of normal acinar cells, which are smaller and lack the monomorphism of the atypical cells. Myoepithelial cell layer attenuation is often already present at this stage.

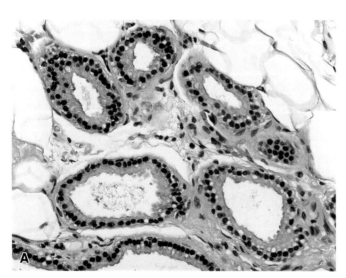

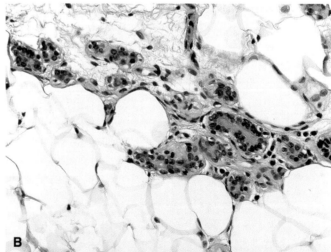

FIGURE 4.23 (A) The cells of flat epithelial atypia are enlarged and have tall apical cytoplasmic compartments. (B) Normal lobule from same patient.

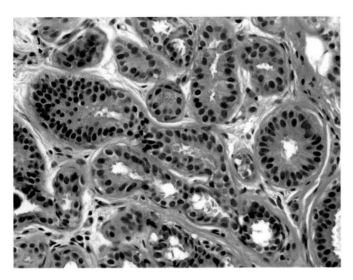

FIGURE 4.24 Atypical ductal cells with uniform, hyperchromatic nuclei and abundant apical cytoplasm have replaced the normal luminal cells of this lobule.

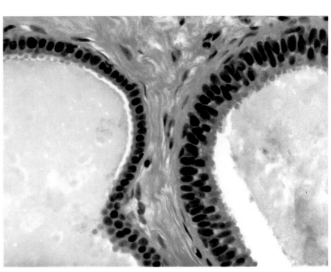

FIGURE 4.25 Atypical ductal cells can be either cuboidal (left) or columnar (right).

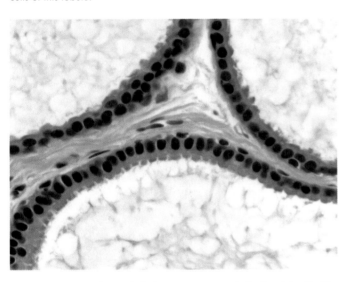

FIGURE 4.26 Flat epithelial atypia composed of cuboidal cells. The presence of low-grade nuclear atypia defines the cells as atypical.

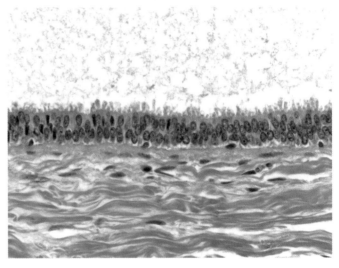

FIGURE 4.27 Myoepithelial cells are widely spaced.

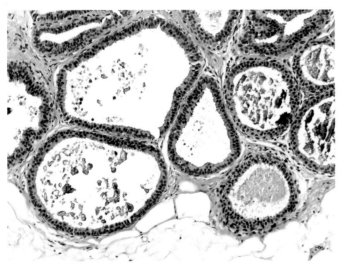

FIGURE 4.28 Clustered intraluminal calcifications are often present in flat epithelial atypia.

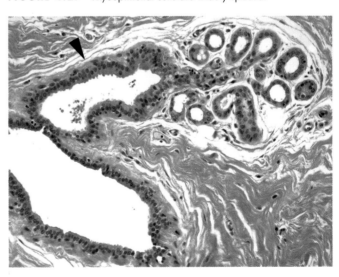

FIGURE 4.29 A single layer of atypical ductal cells lines the preterminal ductule (arrowhead) in this very early example of flat epithelial atypia. Atypical cells have also replaced the luminal cells of the adjacent terminal duct-lobular unit, but the degree of alteration in the lobule is less pronounced than in the extralobular ductule.

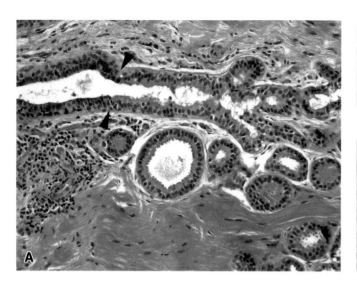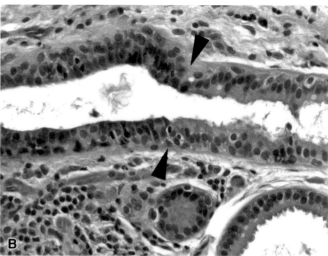

FIGURE 4.30 (A) Early flat epithelial atypia involving the distal preterminal ductule and associated terminal duct-lobular unit. (B) Transition point between normal luminal cells (left of arrowheads) and atypical ductal cells (right of arrowheads).

The study of very early examples of flat epithelial atypia has revealed that it usually develops in otherwise structurally normal ductules and lobules (Figure 4.32) (1). It may occasionally involve lobules previously altered by benign processes, such as sclerosing adenosis. It does not appear to arise, at least in any routine way, as a secondary phenomenon in lobules that are already enlarged and dilated, such as those of blunt duct adenosis. Replacement of the native epithelium by the atypical cells occurs first, with glandular dilatation and lobular expansion representing subsequent alterations.

Flat epithelial atypia encompasses a morphologic spectrum: it can range from small numbers of atypical cells in minimally distorted lobules to thick pseudostratified proliferations in large cystic glands. Histologically, flat epithelial atypia can be simply defined as the presence of low-grade cytologic atypia in the absence of architectural atypia. Although the diagnosis is primarily a cytologic one, alterations to the structure of involved terminal duct-lobular units and accompanying changes in other components, such as the intralobular stroma and the myoepithelial cell layer, can aid in the recognition of this sometimes subtle form of low-grade ductal atypia (Table 4.2).

■ BIOLOGIC SIGNIFICANCE

Flat epithelial atypia represents an early form of low-grade ductal neoplasia. It appears to be a precursor to conventional types of atypical ductal hyperplasia and to certain ductal carcinomas. Early evidence linking flat epithelial atypia to carcinomas of the breast came in the first part of the 20th century, when eminent physicians such as Dr John Collins Warren, Dr Joseph Bloodgood, and

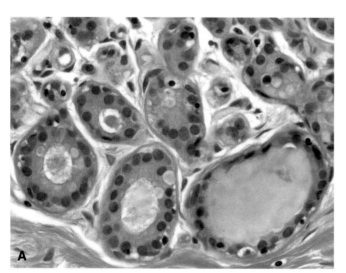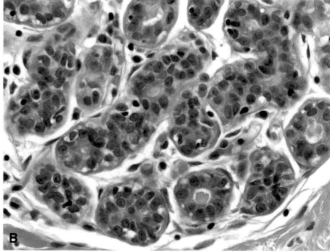

FIGURE 4.31 (A) Early flat epithelial atypia in a lobule. (B) Adjacent normal lobule. Images represent higher power fields from Figure 4.8.

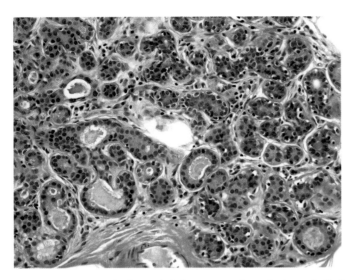

FIGURE 4.32 Early flat epithelial atypia involving the lower half of an otherwise structurally normal lobule. At this magnification, the atypical areas can be identified by the presence of mild acinar dilatation, increased eosinophilic cytoplasm, and basophilic secretions.

■ **Table 4.2** Main histologic features of flat epithelial atypia

1. Terminal duct-lobular units are enlarged and dilated with diminished intralobular stroma

2. Low-grade cytologic atypia of the ductal cells is present

3. The atypical ductal cells grow either as a single or pseudostratified layer; genuine stratification is absent

4. Myoepithelial cells are often diminished in number

Sir G. Lenthal Cheatle described a distinctive columnar cell alteration that was associated with ductal carcinoma in situ (2–4). They considered the changes to be premalignant. A century later, our biologic concept of flat epithelial atypia remains rooted in the fundamental observation that flat epithelial atypia and ductal carcinoma in situ are frequently seen together (Figures 4.33–4.35). Flat epithelial atypia is present in 34% to 36% of cases of low-grade ductal carcinoma in situ and in 23% of cases of intermediate-grade ductal carcinoma in situ (5,6). It is most commonly associated with micropapillary and cribriform patterns of carcinoma (5,6). It is less frequently seen in the background of high-grade ductal carcinoma in situ (<10% of cases) (6), which is not surprising given the dualistic

nature of breast carcinoma development along distinct low- and high-grade pathways (7).

When flat epithelial atypia and low-grade ductal carcinoma in situ coexist in the same specimen, they often directly merge with each other and show identical cytologic characteristics (5,8). The frequent association, intimate spatial relationship, and shared cytologic features of the 2 lesions strongly suggest that they are biologically related. Flat epithelial atypia is favored to be the precursor lesion, with ductal carcinoma in situ arising secondarily through the progressive accumulation of the atypical cells. Alternatively, one might hypothesize that flat epithelial atypia merely represents the leading edge of an established low-grade ductal carcinoma in situ. This view fails, however, to explain the frequent occurrence of flat epithelial atypia in the absence of carcinoma (5,9).

Flat epithelial atypia also often coexists with conventional forms of atypical ductal hyperplasia (Figures 4.36–4.41). The frequency of this association is not well documented but is likely as high as or higher than that seen with low-grade ductal carcinoma in situ. As with low-grade ductal carcinoma in situ, flat epithelial atypia

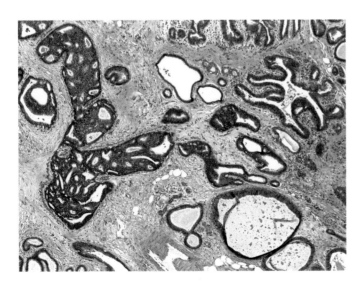

FIGURE 4.33 Flat epithelial atypia merging with low-grade cribriform ductal carcinoma in situ.

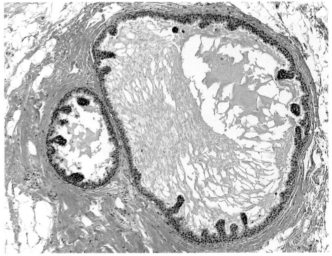

FIGURE 4.34 Low-grade micropapillary ductal carcinoma in situ arising out of a flat, pseudostratified layer of atypical cells.

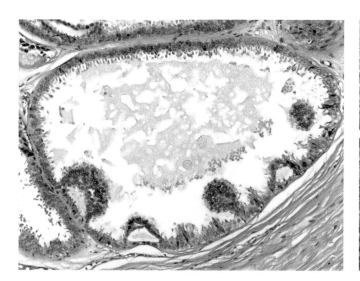

FIGURE 4.35 Micropapillary ductal carcinoma in situ emerging out of a single to minimally pseudostratified layer of atypical cells.

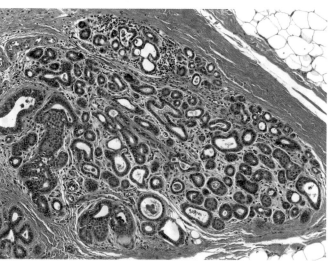

FIGURE 4.36 Lobules involved by flat epithelial atypia merging into atypical ductal hyperplasia (left).

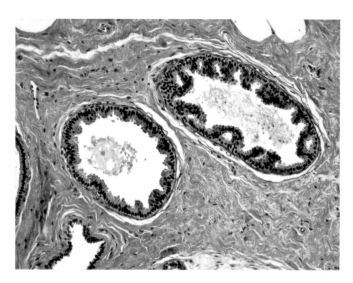

FIGURE 4.37 Atypical ductal hyperplasia (right) and flat epithelial atypia (left) in close proximity.

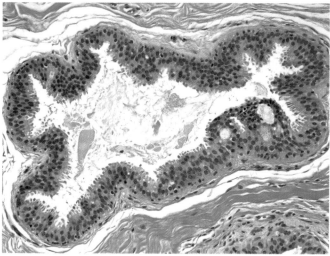

FIGURE 4.38 The presence of even focal areas of genuine stratification warrants a diagnosis of atypical ductal hyperplasia.

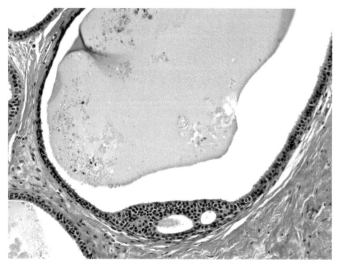

FIGURE 4.39 Focal atypical ductal hyperplasia arising out of a background of flat epithelial atypia.

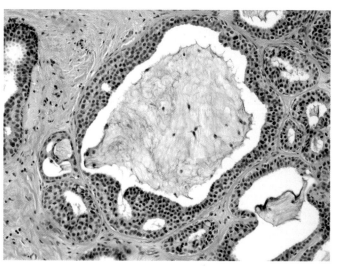

FIGURE 4.40 Flat epithelial atypia seamlessly merging into atypical ductal hyperplasia.

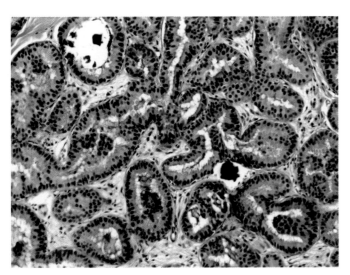

FIGURE 4.41 Although the atypical proliferation is predominately flat, the presence of small micropapillary tufts warrants a diagnosis of atypical ductal hyperplasia.

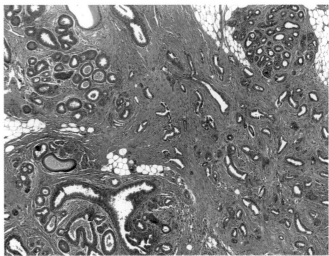

FIGURE 4.42 Invasive tubular carcinoma (right) is frequently associated with flat epithelial atypia (left).

shows a close spatial and cytologic relationship to atypical ductal hyperplasia, indicating a pathogenetic link.

Morphologic observations support that flat epithelial atypia is biologically related to certain invasive carcinomas as well. In particular, there is a strong association with tubular carcinoma: up to 84% of pure tubular carcinomas (composed of at least 90% tubules) are associated with flat epithelial atypia, as are 70% of mixed tubular-invasive ductal carcinomas (composed of 75% to 89% tubules) (10,11). Other studies find slightly lower rates of synchronous flat epithelial atypia and tubular carcinoma (44%–57%) (12–14). Brandt et al (15) document a high prevalence of columnar cell lesions in the setting of pure tubular carcinoma, but their use of an alternate classification system makes it difficult to determine the specific incidence of flat epithelial atypia. The frequent association of flat epithelial atypia with tubular carcinoma does not appear to extend to other forms of low-grade invasive ductal carcinoma: only 4% to 13% of grade 1 invasive ductal carcinomas of no special type contain flat epithelial atypia in the background (12–14).

Invasive tubular carcinoma and flat epithelial atypia generally occur in close proximity when both are present in the same specimen (Figures 4.42–4.43), and the cells of one are morphologically indistinguishable from those of the other. Again, the anatomic and cytologic findings suggest a biologic relationship.

Given the shared cytologic characteristics among flat epithelial atypia and these various forms of low-grade ductal neoplasia, it is not surprising that their immunohistochemical profiles are remarkably similar. Like low-grade ductal carcinoma, flat epithelial atypia is typically strongly positive for estrogen receptor, progesterone receptor, and luminal cytokeratins (cytokeratins 19, 18, and 8) and negative for Her-2/neu and basal-type cytokeratins (cytokeratins

5/6 and 14) (5,8,16–20). The Ki67 proliferative index is characteristically low (0.3%–8%) (8,18,19,21,22). Cyclin D1 and Bcl-2, which are often expressed in breast cancers, are positive in many examples of flat epithelial atypia (5,19,23). Expression patterns of p53 and ataxia telangiectasia mutated have been found to parallel those of associated invasive carcinomas (8,19).

Flat epithelial atypia demonstrates decreased expression of the putative tumor suppressor 14-3-3 sigma, similar to in situ and invasive ductal carcinomas (17). It shows decreased protein expression of the tumor suppressor p16^{INK4a} as a result of increased promoter methylation, akin to what is observed in atypical ductal hyperplasia and low-grade ductal carcinoma in situ (23). microRNA-21, which may play an oncogenic role in mammary neoplasia, is up-regulated in flat epithelial atypia, ductal carcinoma in situ, and invasive ductal carcinoma (24).

Genetic studies further support the theory that flat epithelial atypia is a precursor to low-grade forms of ductal neoplasia. Loss of heterozygosity is frequently seen in flat epithelial atypia and is especially common at loci on the long arm of chromosome 16, a site of recurrent alteration in low-grade ductal carcinomas (11,25,26). Moreover, loss of the same alleles is found in flat epithelial atypia and in synchronous in situ and invasive carcinomas (11,25). Clonality studies of flat epithelial atypia and associated tubular carcinoma reveal a monoclonal pattern in a number of cases and a close genetic relationship in others (11,25). Comparative genomic hybridization analysis demonstrates low numbers of chromosomal alterations and recurrent loss on 16q in flat epithelial atypia, findings that overlap with those observed in atypical ductal hyperplasia and low-grade ductal carcinomas (20,27). In addition, flat epithelial atypia has a gene expression profile that clusters with that seen in low-grade ductal carcinomas, both in situ and invasive (28).

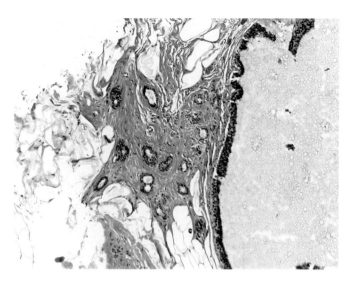

FIGURE 4.43 Minute invasive tubular carcinoma arising in intimate association with flat epithelial atypia. A more advanced intraductal lesion was not identified despite careful sampling. The diagnosis of invasion was confirmed with myoepithelial cell markers.

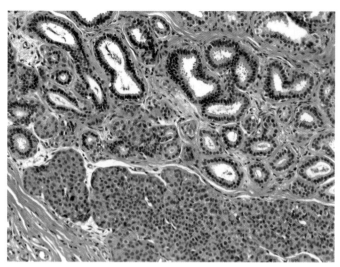

FIGURE 4.44 Flat epithelial atypia and coexistent lobular carcinoma in situ.

These morphologic, immunohistochemical, and molecular observations strongly support that flat epithelial atypia represents one of the earliest recognizable precursors to ductal carcinoma. One model of low-grade ductal neoplasia postulates that flat epithelial atypia evolves into atypical ductal hyperplasia, which then gives rise to ductal carcinoma in situ (29). After the acquisition of additional molecular alterations, ductal carcinoma in situ can progress to invasive carcinoma. Of note, the preinvasive lesions in the pathway are differentiated from each other largely on the basis of quantitative, rather than qualitative, criteria; therefore, they may not represent distinct biologic stages of neoplasia, and progression through a recognized ductal carcinoma in situ phase may not necessarily precede the development of invasion in some cases (Figure 4.43).

Another intriguing association is that of flat epithelial atypia and lobular neoplasia (lobular carcinoma in situ or atypical lobular hyperplasia) (Figures 4.44–4.45). When flat epithelial atypia is the most advanced form of ductal neoplasia in a specimen, coexistent lobular neoplasia is present in 26% of cases (9). More strikingly, when cases of lobular neoplasia (without associated ductal carcinoma in situ or invasive carcinoma) are evaluated, flat epithelial atypia is found in the background in up to 87% (30,31). One can occasionally encounter the 2 lesions in the same lobule or duct (Figure 4.45), but they do not demonstrate any statistically significant anatomic relationship with each other (30–32). Flat epithelial atypia is also found in association with 54% and 86% of invasive lobular and tubulolobular carcinomas, respectively, and the coexistence of lobular neoplasia, columnar cell lesions (including flat epithelial atypia), and invasive tubular carcinoma is a well-recognized phenomenon (10,15,33). The biological

underpinnings of the frequent association of flat epithelial atypia and lobular neoplasia are not clear, but both lesions harbor genetic alterations that indicate a commonality within the low-grade pathway of neoplasia in the breast (7).

■ DIFFERENTIAL DIAGNOSIS

A variety of benign and neoplastic alterations in the breast can superficially mimic flat epithelial atypia (Table 4.3). The benign alterations are distinguished from flat epithelial atypia by their lack of cytologic atypia. The neoplastic considerations in the differential diagnosis, atypical ductal hyperplasia and ductal carcinoma in situ, demonstrate either genuine stratification of atypical cells or higher-

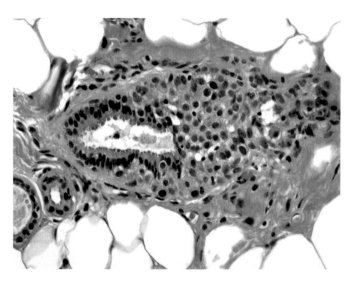

FIGURE 4.45 Flat epithelial atypia and lobular neoplasia involve the same small duct.

■ **Table 4.3** Benign and neoplastic considerations in the differential diagnosis of flat epithelial atypia

Benign entities

- Blunt duct adenosis, proliferative phase
- Blunt duct adenosis, inactive phase
- Early usual ductal hyperplasia
- Activated epithelium in pseudoangiomatous stromal hyperplasia

Neoplastic entities

- Atypical ductal hyperplasia
- Low-grade ductal carcinoma in situ
- High- or intermediate-grade ductal carcinoma in situ with flat growth

grade cytologic atypia than is allowable for flat epithelial atypia.

Benign Entities

Benign alterations that demonstrate cystic change, enlargement of terminal duct-lobular units, or prominent columnar cells may be mistaken for flat epithelial atypia. Fibrocystic changes, blunt duct adenosis, early usual ductal hyperplasia, and certain reactive ductular changes may all exhibit one or more of these features. The absence of cytologic atypia is the key criterion that distinguishes these changes from flat epithelial atypia. Associated architectural, stromal, and myoepithelial findings can provide supportive diagnostic information.

The microcysts of fibrocystic change can mimic the dilated glandular spaces of flat epithelial atypia and vice versa. In microcysts, however, the nuclei are small and slightly variable in their morphologies, and they do not display the mild enlargement, hyperchromasia, and monomorphism

indicative of low-grade ductal atypia. Microcysts are also typically lined by a single layer of flat or low cuboidal cells (Figure 4.46). In contrast, cystic glands in flat epithelial atypia are commonly lined by a pseudostratified layer of tall columnar cells; the epithelium appears thickened rather than flattened, and cellular crowding is evident (Figure 4.47). Occasional cystic glands in flat epithelial atypia may be lined by a single layer of relatively small cuboidal cells. These may be difficult to distinguish from benign microcysts, but more convincing evidence of flat epithelial atypia is usually found in neighboring glands.

Apocrine metaplasia may be a consideration in the differential diagnosis of flat epithelial atypia. Apocrine cells, however, differ from ductal cells with low-grade atypia in several ways. First, apocrine cells have characteristic round nuclei with open chromatin, distinct nuclear membranes, and prominent nucleoli (Figure 4.48A). The nuclei contrast with those of flat epithelial atypia, which are hyperchromatic, contain powdery chromatin, and have inconspicuous nucleoli (Figure 4.48B). Second, the cytoplasm in apocrine cells is notably granular and voluminous, whereas that in ductal cells with low-grade atypia is fine, nongranular, and comparatively lesser in amount. Third, apocrine cells rarely pseudostratify, in contradistinction to the cells of flat epithelial atypia, which characteristically form a pseudostratified layer as they proliferate. Although morphologic features are generally sufficient to distinguish apocrine metaplasia from flat epithelial atypia, it is worth noting that apocrine cells are typically negative for estrogen and progesterone receptors. This is in stark contrast to the strong estrogen and progesterone receptor positivity that is seen in flat epithelial atypia and supports the concept that flat epithelial atypia and apocrine metaplasia are biologically unrelated.

Flat epithelial atypia is more likely to be underdiagnosed as fibrocystic changes than the reverse. Several other

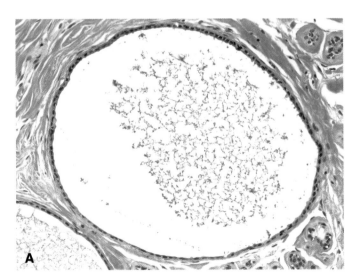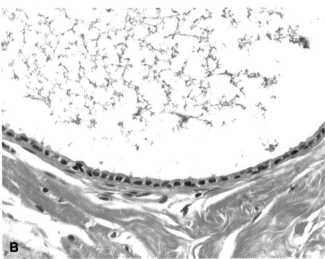

FIGURE 4.46 (A) Simple microcyst of fibrocystic change. (B) The lining is composed of a single layer of flattened to low cuboidal cells without atypia.

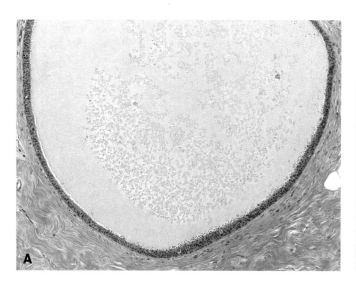
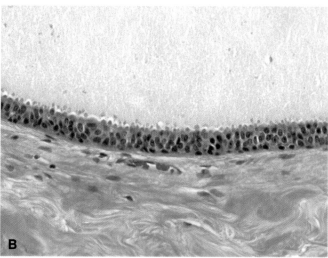

FIGURE 4.47 (A) Cystic flat epithelial atypia with distinctive thickened and cellular epithelium evident even at low power. (B) The lining is composed of a pseudostratified layer of columnar cells with low-grade nuclear atypia.

benign alterations, however, can show a predominance of columnar cells with slightly enlarged nuclei and can easily be misinterpreted as flat epithelial atypia. These include blunt duct adenosis, early benign hyperplastic changes, and activated epithelium in pseudoangiomatous stromal hyperplasia.

Most pathologists use the term *blunt duct adenosis* to refer to a form of benign lobular hypertrophy in which the lobule becomes expanded and the glands become dilated (Figures 4.49–4.50) (34). In the proliferative phase of blunt duct adenosis, the luminal cells are columnar with slightly increased amounts of cytoplasm, and the nuclei are mildly enlarged (Figure 4.51). These findings overlap with those of flat epithelial atypia, but several observations help differentiate the 2 entities (Table 4.4). Although the glands of blunt duct adenosis are dilated, they tend

to have tubular or branching shapes (Figures 4.49–4.50) that contrast with the more globoid, cystically dilated glands seen in flat epithelial atypia (Figures 4.1–4.6). The myoepithelial cells in blunt duct adenosis are especially prominent, often being larger than those in unaltered lobules and forming a continuous ring around the glands (Figures 4.51–4.52). Their prominence markedly differs from the myoepithelial cell layer attenuation that is commonly seen in flat epithelial atypia. The intralobular stroma in blunt duct adenosis is expanded and mildly cellular (Figures 4.49–4.50), contrasting in appearance with the diminished and inconspicuous intralobular stroma in flat epithelial atypia. Blunt duct adenosis shows hypertrophy of all 3 major elements of the terminal duct-lobular unit: luminal epithelium, myoepithelium, and stroma. Flat epithelial atypia, on the other hand, is solely an epithelial

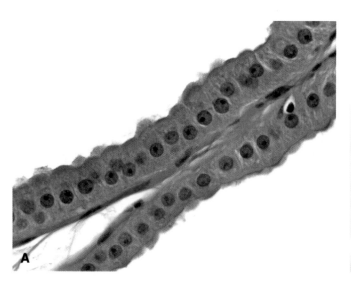
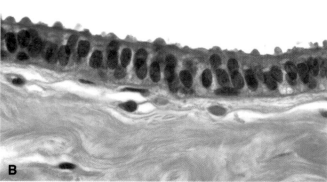

FIGURE 4.48 (A) Apocrine metaplasia. (B) Flat epithelial atypia. Apocrine cells differ in both their nuclear and cytoplasmic characteristics from the cells of flat epithelial atypia.

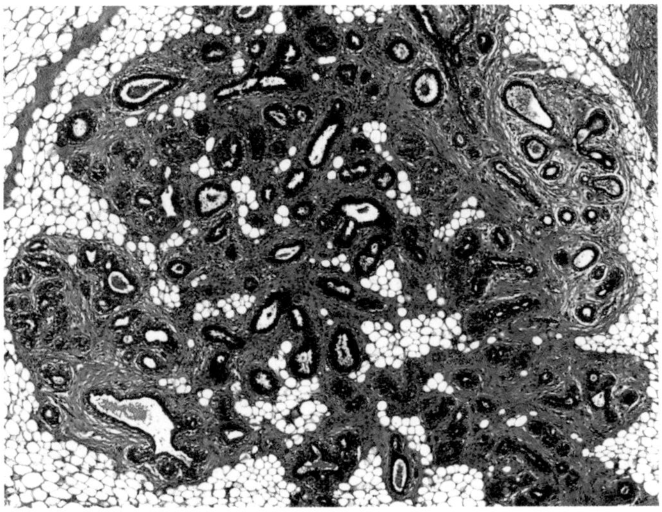

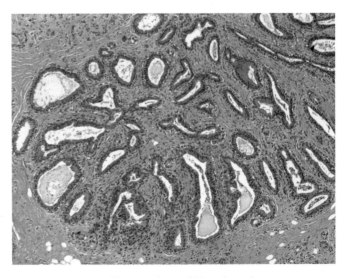

FIGURE 4.49 Proliferative phase of blunt duct adenosis.

proliferation and shows diminution of the other lobular components.

The nuclei in blunt duct adenosis are larger than those in normal luminal cells, and they have slightly granular chromatin and small nucleoli (Figures 4.52–4.54). Their appearance may raise the specter of low-grade atypia, but in actuality, they are morphologically similar to the nuclei in usual ductal hyperplasia. Like the latter, the nuclei in blunt duct adenosis are oval to tapered in shape and have slightly speckled chromatin, small nucleoli, and nuclear grooves; they demonstrate mild morphologic variability from cell to cell. The nuclei also have a tendency to tilt and slightly overlap. Often, the apical borders of the cells are not sharply aligned, creating a somewhat shaggy look to the luminal border. These features differ from those of low-grade ductal atypia, in which the round to oval nuclei have fine powdery chromatin, inconspicuous nucleoli, smooth nuclear contours, consistent radial orientation toward the luminal space, and an overall uniform appearance. The cell apices tend to be evenly aligned, resulting in a sharply defined luminal border.

In the inactive phase of blunt duct adenosis, some glands retain their tubular and branching configurations, but others adopt more rounded profiles (Figures 4.55–4.56). The glands are lined by a simple, single layer of luminal cells; pseudostratification or genuine stratification is not seen. The cells have stubby columnar or cuboidal shapes and minimal cytoplasm, apical or otherwise. The nuclei are hyperchromatic and ovoid with squared-off or tapered ends. The nucleoli are inconspicuous. The myoepithelial cells are numerous and prominent, and they are typically rounded rather than flattened. The cellular intralobular stroma of the proliferative phase is now fibrotic but still expanded. Although the hyperchromatic nuclei may raise concern for atypia, these changes are not observed to merge into atypical proliferations. Taken together, the low-power architecture, stubby cells with

minimal cytoplasm, lack of pseudostratification, increased myoepithelial cell density, and prominent fibrotic stroma allow one to distinguish the inactive phase of blunt duct adenosis from flat epithelial atypia.

Early usual ductal hyperplasia may also superficially resemble flat epithelial atypia. In usual ductal hyperplasia, the cells closest to the basement membrane are columnar and contain nuclei that are larger than those seen centrally. These columnar cells may constitute the sole or dominant cell population in early hyperplasia (Figure 4.57). The enlarged nuclei may at first glance cause concern for atypia, but they do not demonstrate the hyperchromasia or monomorphism that typifies flat epithelial atypia. Instead, the nuclei appear similar to those seen in blunt duct adenosis, both in their cytologic characteristics and their spatial arrangement. A few smaller, more mature hyperplastic cells are often found near the luminal border (Figure 4.58).

Glands within areas of pseudoangiomatous stromal hyperplasia often show reactive proliferative changes. These can range from simple activation and mild enlargement of columnar luminal cells (Figure 4.59) to overt usual ductal hyperplasia. The former changes basically represent early usual ductal hyperplasia and are distinguished from flat epithelial atypia by the histologic features noted above.

If present, areas of early cellular stratification into the lumen can help one differentiate between benign and atypical columnar cell alterations. In blunt duct adenosis and early hyperplasia, the accumulating cells demonstrate the architectural and cytologic characteristics of usual ductal hyperplasia (Figures 4.60–4.61). Conversely, in an atypical process, any cells that amass in the lumen adopt the growth characteristics of atypical ductal hyperplasia or ductal carcinoma in situ: they form architecturally atypical structures such as micropapillae, trabecular bars,

FIGURE 4.50 Proliferative phase of blunt duct adenosis.

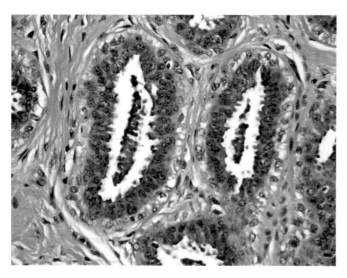

FIGURE 4.51 Active-appearing luminal cells and prominent myoepithelial cells in blunt duct adenosis.

Roman arches, and cribriform spaces (Figures 4.34–4.35 and 4.37–4.41). These polarized structures, in which the cells are radially oriented toward the luminal space, contrast with the randomly distributed cells of usual ductal hyperplasia. The characteristic cytologic features of low-grade atypia are present, and maturation is absent. The combination of bona fide architectural atypia and low-grade cytologic atypia takes the diagnosis into the realm of atypical ductal hyperplasia or ductal carcinoma in situ (discussed in the next section); nevertheless, attention to even small areas where the cells mound up can help clarify the benign or atypical character of the associated columnar cells.

The morphologic differences discussed above generally permit distinction of benign columnar cell alterations from flat epithelial atypia. Occasional cases, however, may still present diagnostic difficulty. Several points are helpful to keep in mind. First, lobules with the classic appearance of blunt duct adenosis—branching and tubular glands, expanded intralobular stroma, and prominent myoepithelial cells—seldom harbor atypical ductal cells. Second, columnar cell lesions associated with proliferative stroma are often benign. Third, oval-shaped nuclei can be seen in both benign changes and low-grade atypia, but smooth round nuclei are usually atypical. Fourth, neighboring epithelial proliferations can aid in the evaluation of ambiguous columnar cell lesions. If straightforward usual ductal hyperplasia or ductal carcinoma in situ is present in adjacent glands and the columnar cells in question have similar cytologic characteristics, then the former is generally a reliable indicator of the benign or atypical nature of the latter.

Immunohistochemistry

Immunohistochemistry plays a negligible role in the distinction of flat epithelial atypia from benign columnar cell

lesions. Although high-molecular-weight cytokeratins, such as 34βE12, 5/6, and 14, can aid in the differentiation of usual ductal hyperplasia from ductal carcinoma in situ (the former shows a mosaic pattern of reactivity, whereas nonbasal examples of the latter are typically negative) (35), they do not reliably distinguish benign from atypical flat proliferations. The cells of flat epithelial atypia, like those of atypical ductal hyperplasia and low-grade ductal carcinoma in situ, are negative for high-molecular-weight cytokeratins (Figure 4.62A) (19,20). The problem lies in the fact that benign columnar cells are also frequently negative (Figure 4.62B). The reactivity that is seen in usual ductal hyperplasia is largely within the intraluminal mass of cells, whereas the peripheral columnar cells tend to be negative. Early usual ductal hyperplasia, which is composed of the peripheral cells, is accordingly often negative

■ **Table 4.4** Comparison of the histologic features of flat epithelial atypia and blunt duct adenosis (proliferative phase)

	Flat Epithelial Atypia	Blunt Duct Adenosis
Terminal duct-lobular unit size	Enlarged	Enlarged
Dilated gland shapes	Round to cystic	Tubular and branching
Cell shape	Columnar or cuboidal	Columnar
Nuclei	Monomorphic low-grade atypia	Polymorphic, similar to benign hyperplastic nuclei
Cytoplasm	Increased, with tall apical cytoplasmic compartments	Modest
Apical snouts	Often present	Often present
Cell borders	Sometimes distinct	Inconspicuous
Luminal borders	Sharp and even	Often shaggy
Myoepithelial cells	Usually diminished	Prominent
Intralobular stroma	Usually diminished	Expanded and often cellular
If cells begin to stratify, the proliferation develops into	Atypical ductal hyperplasia or ductal carcinoma in situ	Usual ductal hyperplasia

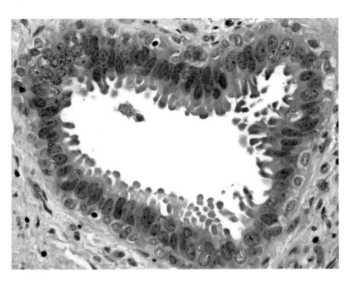

FIGURE 4.52 The nuclei in blunt duct adenosis have slightly granular chromatin, distinct but small nucleoli, and tapering ovoid forms.

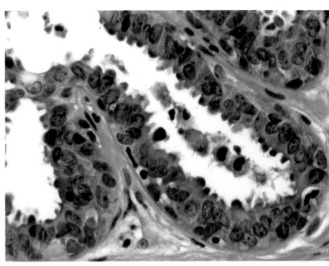

FIGURE 4.53 The nuclei in blunt duct adenosis demonstrate a mild polymorphism and often tilt and overlap.

or only minimally reactive for high-molecular-weight cytokeratins; blunt duct adenosis shows parallel findings. When positivity is seen, it is usually localized to small knots of hyperplastic cells protruding into the lumen. If present in a flat proliferation, reactivity for high-molecular-weight cytokeratins does support a benign diagnosis. Bear in mind, however, that many benign columnar cell lesions are negative for these markers, overlapping with the profile of flat epithelial atypia and effectively limiting the diagnostic utility of these stains. Estrogen receptor also fails to reliably distinguish flat epithelial atypia from benign columnar cell alterations: although flat epithelial atypia shows strong expression of estrogen receptor, blunt duct adenosis and early usual ductal hyperplasia are also often positive. Morphology, in the end, remains the main-

stay for distinguishing flat epithelial atypia from other entities in the differential diagnosis.

Neoplastic Entities

Flat epithelial atypia, atypical ductal hyperplasia, and low-grade ductal carcinoma in situ all share the same low-grade cytologic atypia. The latter 2 entities, however, exhibit architectural atypia in addition to cytologic atypia. If micropapillae, trabecular bars, Roman arches, cribriform spaces, or solid areas are present, the proliferation is no longer flat and a more severe diagnosis is warranted (Table 4.5) (Figures 4.33–4.41). The presence of genuine epithelial stratification therefore distinguishes atypical ductal hyperplasia and low-grade ductal carcinoma in situ from flat epithelial atypia.

Uncommonly, ductal cells with low-grade atypia can be genuinely stratified but still maintain a flat-type

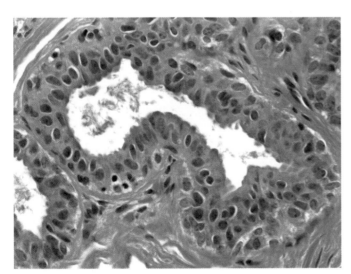

FIGURE 4.54 The epithelial cells in blunt duct adenosis are not as rigidly arrayed as those of flat epithelial atypia (compare with Figures 4.14-4.27).

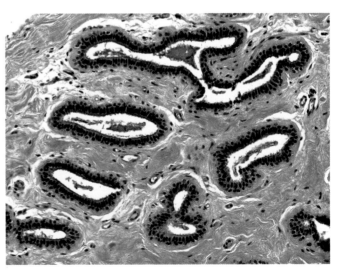

FIGURE 4.55 Inactive phase of blunt duct adenosis.

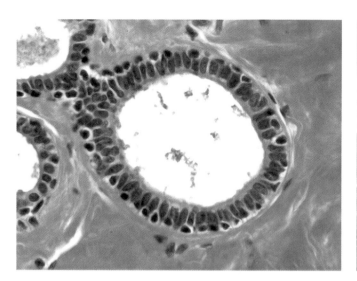

FIGURE 4.56 Short columnar luminal cells and prominent myoepithelial cells in the inactive phase of blunt duct adenosis.

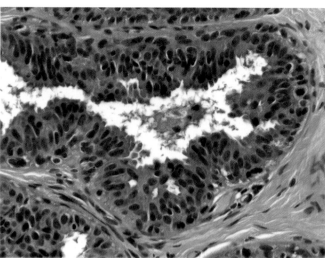

FIGURE 4.57 Early usual ductal hyperplasia with a somewhat disheveled appearance and shaggy luminal border.

growth pattern. In such instances, the epithelium is markedly thickened, and the number of nuclear layers is generally more than 5 (Figure 4.63). These truly stratified but flat atypical proliferations should not be classified as flat epithelial atypia. Flat epithelial atypia consists of a single or pseudostratified layer of cells, whereas these lesions exceed what can reasonably be considered pseudostratified. They are usually found adjacent to more classical patterns of ductal carcinoma in situ, and in such settings, they are best considered part of the ductal carcinoma in situ. When the changes are focal and occur in the absence of more conventional ductal carcinoma in situ, a diagnosis of atypical ductal hyperplasia may be considered.

High-grade ductal carcinoma in situ can also demonstrate a flat pattern of growth. This type of clinging

carcinoma is distinguished from flat epithelial atypia by the presence of high-grade nuclear atypia (Figures 4.64–4.68). The nuclei are notably larger than those of flat epithelial atypia, and they exhibit pleomorphism rather than monomorphism. The chromatin is hyperchromatic and can vary from fine and evenly dispersed to clumped and cleared. Red macronucleoli are typical. The cells are columnar or hobnail in shape and may demonstrate dyshesion. Intraluminal necrotic debris is occasionally seen. Although high-grade clinging carcinomas are descriptively both flat and atypical, they do not fall into the diagnostic category of flat epithelial atypia because the latter is, by definition, exclusively a low-grade lesion. The presence of severe cytologic atypia warrants a diagnosis of high-grade ductal carcinoma in situ regardless of the degree of architectural atypia (Table 4.5).

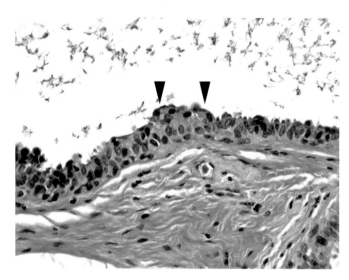

FIGURE 4.58 A few small, mature hyperplastic cells (arrowsheads) lie along the luminal border of this example of early usual ductal hyperplasia.

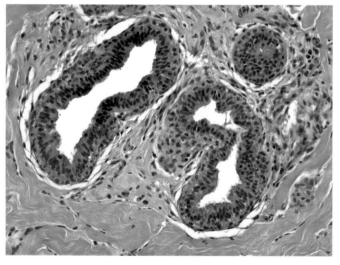

FIGURE 4.59 Benign columnar cells in the setting of pseudoangiomatous stromal hyperplasia. Note the prominent myoepithelial cell layer.

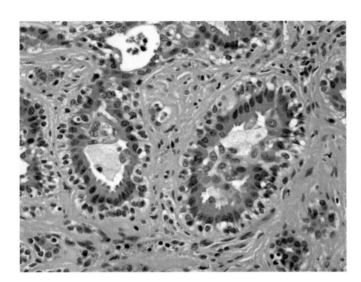

FIGURE 4.60 Conventional usual ductal hyperplasia arising in blunt duct adenosis.

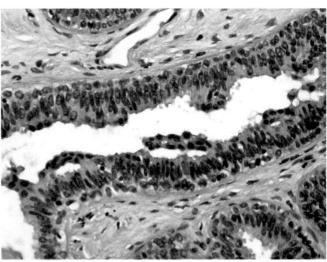

FIGURE 4.61 The presence of small tufts of mature hyperplastic cells is a reassuring sign that the underlying columnar cells are not atypical.

A more difficult challenge lies in flat proliferations that have intermediate-grade nuclei (Figures 4.69–4.70). The nuclei are more atypical than the low-grade nuclei of flat epithelial atypia, yet are not so atypical as to be unequivocally diagnostic of carcinoma on cytologic grounds alone. They do not show the degree of pleomorphism or marked nuclear enlargement seen in overtly high-grade lesions. Nevertheless, the nuclei are quite atypical: they are larger than those of flat epithelial atypia, the chromatin is often coarser and may have areas of clearing, and prominent red nucleoli are common. These intermediate-grade flat proliferations often merge into conventional areas of ductal carcinoma in situ, simplifying the analysis. When they occur in isolation, their classification is more controversial. Some pathologists believe they are best categorized as atypical ductal hyperplasia, whereas others consider them to be intermediate-grade ductal carcinoma in situ.

Regardless, they do not demonstrate the characteristic low-grade cytology of flat epithelial atypia and should not be classified as such.

■ MANAGEMENT

Many important clinical parameters of flat epithelial atypia remain to be elucidated. We do not know the frequency of the lesion in the general population or the demographic characteristics of women with flat epithelial atypia. Even the distribution of flat epithelial atypia in the breasts is not well studied. We do know that flat epithelial atypia frequently coexists with several types of low-grade neoplasia: low-grade ductal carcinoma in situ, atypical ductal hyperplasia, lobular neoplasia, and certain subtypes of invasive carcinoma (Table 4.6). The pathologist must

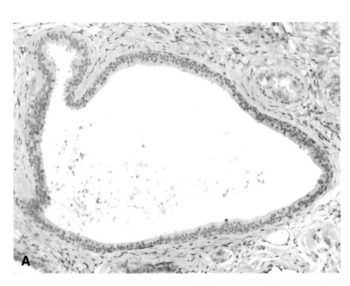

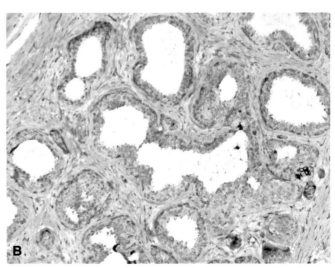

FIGURE 4.62 Negative cytokeratin 5/6 reaction in flat epithelial atypia (A) and blunt duct adenosis (B).

■ Table 4.5 Guide to diagnosis based on degree of cytologic and architectural atypia

Cytologic Atypia	Architectural Atypia	Diagnosis
Low grade	Absent (ie, flat growth)	Flat epithelial atypia
Low grade	Limited	Atypical ductal hyperplasia
Low grade	Well developed	Ductal carcinoma in situ
Intermediate grade	Absent	Atypical ductal hyperplasia vs ductal carcinoma in situ
Intermediate grade	Present	Ductal carcinoma in situ
High grade	Present or absent	Ductal carcinoma in situ

■ Table 4.6 Neoplastic often associated with flat epithelial atypia

- Atypical ductal hyperplasia
- Ductal carcinoma in situ
- Invasive tubular carcinoma
- Lobular neoplasia

well-differentiated clinging carcinoma, a lesion comparable to flat epithelial atypia, remained free of progression or recurrence after a median interval of 5.4 years. Shaaban et al (38) calculated a relative risk for subsequent carcinoma of 2.32 for a group of lesions they termed *blunt duct adenosis with atypical columnar cell metaplasia*; however, the number of cases was small, the confidence interval was broad (0.95–5.62), and the results did not achieve statistical significance. Furthermore, it is not entirely clear which of the 6 morphologic categories of *blunt duct adenosis* in their study corresponds to flat epithelial atypia.

Boulos et al (39) found a mild increase in breast cancer risk associated with columnar cells lesions (relative risk, 1.47); however, no significant difference in risk was observed between columnar cell lesions with atypia (flat epithelial atypia) and those without. One limitation of their study was the small the number of cases containing atypical columnar cell lesions as the most severe abnormality (n = 14). Martel et al (40) found an absolute risk for subsequent invasive carcinoma of 11.1% based on a series of core biopsies in which flat epithelial atypia was retrospectively identified. In their study, 7 of 63 women developed invasive carcinoma in the ipsilateral breast 2 to 9 years (mean, 3.7 years) after the index core biopsy. de Mascarel et al (41) did not identify any subsequent carcinomas in 84 cases of flat epithelial atypia diagnosed on excisional biopsy.

carefully look for these other forms of neoplasia when flat epithelial atypia is discovered.

Little is known about the prognostic significance of flat epithelial atypia. The risk for development of subsequent breast carcinoma and its expected time course have not yet been defined. The literature contains only a small number of studies that address this issue. Eusebi et al (36) evaluated the clinical outcomes for 25 women with lesions equivalent to flat epithelial atypia. None of the women developed invasive breast cancer after an average interval of 19 years, and only 1 (4%) had a recurrence of flat epithelial atypia. Bijker et al (37) found that 59 women with

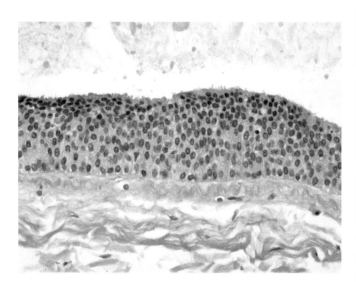

FIGURE 4.63 Flat low-grade ductal carcinoma in situ.

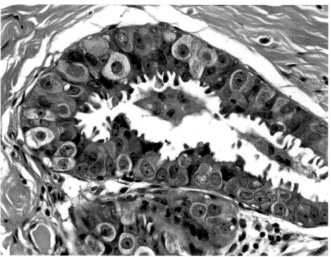

FIGURE 4.64 High-grade ductal carcinoma in situ with flat growth pattern.

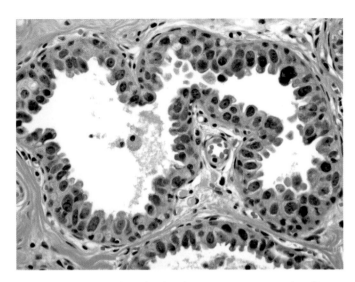

FIGURE 4.65 High-grade ductal carcinoma in situ with a flat, or clinging, growth pattern.

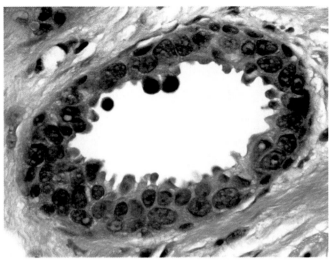

FIGURE 4.66 High-grade ductal carcinoma in situ with a flat growth pattern. Nuclei are too large and too pleomorphic for a diagnosis of flat epithelial atypia.

Although the above data are derived from studies with limited numbers of patients, sometimes short follow-up intervals, and varying methodological designs, they suggest that women with flat epithelial atypia have at most a mildly increased risk for subsequent breast carcinoma. It is likely that flat epithelial atypia represents a relatively indolent, nonobligate precursor to ductal carcinoma. Larger clinical studies with extended follow-up, however, are needed to more fully understand the long-term breast cancer risk in these patients.

A more immediate clinical concern is whether a patient with flat epithelial atypia as the most advanced lesion in a core biopsy needs to have a follow-up excision, akin to the management of atypical ductal hyperplasia diagnosed by core biopsy. Because flat epithelial atypia appears to

have a relatively low risk for progression to carcinoma, the purpose of excision is not to treat the flat epithelial atypia but to detect associated carcinoma that was missed due to sampling error. A number of factors may influence the likelihood of such upgrades to carcinoma and include the radiologist's level of expertise, the nature of the targeted lesion (microcalcifications vs mass), the volume of the tissue removed (dependent on core biopsy gauge and biopsy method), the extent of histologic sampling, the pathologist's level of expertise, and varying pathological thresholds used for diagnosis. Analysis of the literature on this topic is also hampered by the inclusion of apparent atypical ductal hyperplasia in the study cases (42), variant classification schemes (42,43), inconsistent exclusionary

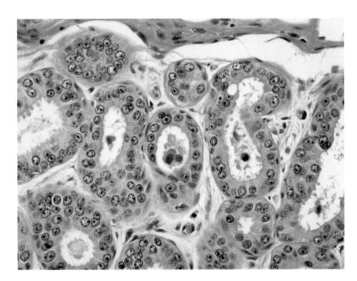

FIGURE 4.67 High-grade ductal carcinoma in situ with a flat growth pattern. The clumped and cleared chromatin, red macronucleoli, and early cellular necrosis are incompatible with a diagnosis of flat epithelial atypia.

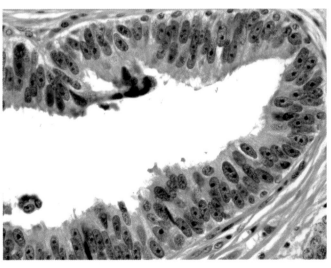

FIGURE 4.68 High-grade ductal carcinoma in situ composed of tall columnar cells. The large size of the nuclei and red macronucleoli are features of high-grade rather than low-grade atypia.

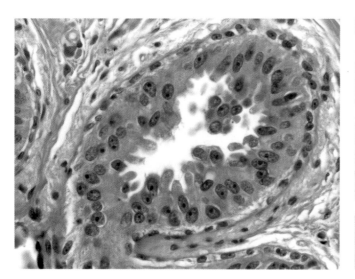

FIGURE 4.69 Columnar cell proliferation with intermediate-grade nuclear atypia.

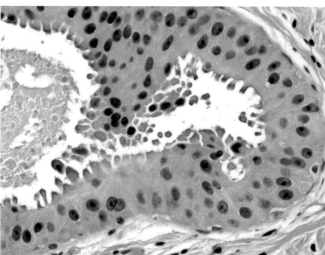

FIGURE 4.70 Columnar cell proliferation with intermediate-grade nuclear atypia.

criteria for lobular neoplasia, limited rates of follow-up excision (44,45), and the relatively small number of core biopsy cases in which flat epithelial atypia is present in the absence of atypical ductal hyperplasia, ductal carcinoma in situ, or invasive carcinoma. Published data indicate that flat epithelial atypia is the most advanced ductal lesion in less than 0.1% to 3.7% of all breast core biopsies (22,40,44–46).

The rate of upgrade to either ductal carcinoma in situ or invasive carcinoma on follow-up excision ranges from 0% to 21% among various studies (Table 4.7) (22,44–49). Although methodological differences exist, summation of the results from these studies indicates an overall 8% upgrade rate. Ductal carcinoma in situ is found as the most significant lesion in 5% of overall excisions and is most often low grade, and invasive carcinoma is found in 3%. Atypical ductal hyperplasia as the most advanced lesion is identified in up to 36% of follow-up excisions (22).

The overall upgrade rates are not strikingly different from those predicted by examining the incidence of associated neoplasia in specimens harboring flat epithelial atypia. Bratthauer and Tavassoli (9) reviewed 1000 cases in which flat epithelial atypia was the most advanced ductal intraepithelial lesion and found that 7% had coexistent invasive carcinoma. de Mascarel et al (41) identified synchronous ductal carcinoma in situ with or without microinvasion in 12% and invasive carcinoma in 5% of surgical excisions containing flat epithelial atypia without atypical ductal hyperplasia (n = 101).

Given the wide range in upgrade rates from individual studies (Table 4.7), it is not surprising that opinions differ as to whether follow-up excision is warranted after a core biopsy diagnosis of flat epithelial atypia. Some investigators find similar upgrade rates for flat epithelial atypia and atypical ductal hyperplasia and therefore recommend excision (22,46). Others find no evidence of malignancy on subsequent excisions and suggest that with careful

clinicopathological correlation, clinical follow-up may be sufficient (40,44,47). Currently, at Massachusetts General Hospital, surgical excision is routinely performed after a core biopsy diagnosis of flat epithelial atypia.

Additional surgery is not considered necessary when flat epithelial atypia is the most significant finding in an excisional biopsy, since the risk for direct progression to carcinoma appears limited. Similarly, the presence of flat epithelial atypia at the surgical margin in cases of carcinoma is not an indication for reexcision. Currently, no data exist regarding the role of tamoxifen for risk reduction in patients with flat epithelial atypia. Some investigators feel that close clinical follow-up after excision may be the most appropriate course of management because the risk for subsequent carcinoma appears low (37). The management of high-risk patients diagnosed with flat epithelial atypia or those with particularly extensive disease remains to be addressed.

■ TERMINOLOGY

The history of flat epithelial atypia is awash in the myriad of terms that have been used to describe it. In the early 20th century, *abnormal involution*, *senile parenchymatous hypertrophy*, and *cystiphorous desquamative epithelial hyperplasia* were all applied to a distinct columnar cell alteration of terminal duct-lobular units that was considered premalignant (2–4). In more recent decades, *clinging carcinoma*, *atypical cystic lobule*, *columnar alteration with prominent apical snouts and secretions with atypia*, *flat ductal intraepithelial neoplasia 1*, *columnar cell change with atypia*, and *columnar cell hyperplasia with atypia*, among others, have been used to refer to the lesion that constitutes flat epithelial atypia (5,34,40,50,51). In 2003, the World Health Organization working group on

■ **Table 4.7** Findings on follow-up excision after diagnosis of flat epithelial atypia as the most advanced lesion in core biopsy

Study	No. of FEA Core Biopsy Cases, n	Core Biopsy Gauge, n	Follow-up Excisions, n (%)	ADH on Excision[a], n (%)	DCIS on Excision[a], n (%)	Invasive Carcinoma on Excision[a], n (%)	Overall Upgrade Rate to Carcinoma (%)
Kunju and Kleer, 2007	14	14	12 (86)	5 (36)	1 (7)	2 (14)	21
Chivukula et al, 2009	39	14, 12	35 (90)	10 (26)[b]	3 (8)	2 (5)	13
Senetta et al, 2009	41	11	36 (88)	(13)[d]	0 (0)	0 (0)	0
Piubello et al, 2009	33	11	20 (61)	1 (3)	0 (0)	0 (0)	0
Ingegnoli et al, 2009	18	11	15 (83)	NA	1 (6)	2 (11)	17
Darvishian et al, 2009	12	NA	12 (100)[c]	NA	2 (17)	0 (0)	17
Noske et al, 2010	43	14, 11	30 (70)	1 (2)	2 (5)	0 (0)	5
Total	200		160 (80)		9 (5)	6 (3)	8

ADH, atypical ductal hyperplasia; DCIS, ductal carcinoma in situ; FEA, flat epithelial atypia; NA, not available.
[a]Categorized by the most advanced lesion in the excision specimen; for example, a specimen demonstrating both ADH and DCIS would be categorized as DCIS.
[b]Flat epithelial atypia and ADH were grouped together into 1 category in the excision results.
[c]Only cases with follow-up excisions were selected for analysis.
[d]Only the % is given in the reference.

breast tumors proposed the term *flat epithelial atypia* (52), which has since become increasingly used in clinical practice. Nevertheless, the columnar cell change/hyperplasia classification system remains popular and widely used, leading to inevitable questions about which columnar cell categories are equivalent to flat epithelial atypia.

Rosen (53) first categorized columnar cell lesions into 2 general groups: columnar cell change and columnar cell hyperplasia. Columnar cell change has only 1 or 2 layers of cells, whereas hyperplasia has more than 2 layers. Schnitt and Vincent-Salomon (51) further subdivided the 2 groups into those without and with cytologic atypia, thereby creating 4 categories: columnar cell change, columnar cell hyperplasia, columnar cell change with atypia, and columnar cell hyperplasia with atypia. The 2 categories of columnar cell change with atypia and columnar cell hyperplasia with atypia are equivalent to flat epithelial atypia. Those lesions without atypia constitute a relatively diverse group of benign alterations and include blunt duct adenosis, early usual ductal hyperplasia, and activated luminal cells in the setting of stromal hyperplasia. *Columnar cell*

change and *columnar cell hyperplasia* without atypia are therefore descriptive umbrella terms and are not indicative of specific entities.

■ CONCLUSION

As Azzopardi (34) noted in his comprehensive description of this "orderly form of clinging carcinoma," flat epithelial atypia may be difficult to recognize, but "careful study of the cytology of the breast lesions in question, and comparison with known cases of adenosis and other benign lesions, will reveal distinct though frequently subtle differences." The monomorphism, hyperchromasia, fine chromatin, smooth nuclear contours, and inconspicuous nucleoli of flat epithelial atypia distinguish it from reactive epithelial cells in various benign columnar cell alterations, as well as from higher-grade neoplastic entities with flat growth. Although cytologic features remain the key to diagnosis, attention to the architecture of involved lobules, the prominence of the myoepithelial cell layer, and the character of the surrounding stroma can provide helpful diagnostic information in difficult cases.

Morphologic and molecular evidence support that flat epithelial atypia is part of the low-grade pathway of neoplasia in the breast. Its presence should prompt one to look for associated invasive carcinoma, ductal carcinoma in situ, atypical ductal hyperplasia, and lobular neoplasia. Additional levels and, if applicable, submission of additional sections can be helpful for identifying these associated forms of neoplasia. Our understanding of its biologic behavior remains incomplete, but flat epithelial atypia does not appear to be a particularly aggressive lesion. It is likely that many examples of flat epithelial atypia do not progress to carcinoma or do so only very slowly. The optimal clinical management of patients with flat epithelial atypia as the most severe pathologic finding remains to be defined.

■ KEY POINTS

- Flat epithelial atypia is morphologically defined by the presence of low-grade cytologic atypia in the absence of architectural atypia.
- Benign lesions in the differential diagnosis are distinguished by their lack of distinctive low-grade cytologic atypia.
- Low-grade ductal carcinoma in situ and atypical ductal hyperplasia are differentiated from flat epithelial atypia by the presence of both cytologic and architectural atypia.
- High-grade cytologic atypia is not part of the spectrum of flat epithelial atypia.
- Flat epithelial atypia is part of the low-grade pathway of neoplasia in the breast, and it is frequently associated with low-grade ductal carcinoma, atypical ductal hyperplasia, and lobular neoplasia.
- When flat epithelial atypia is the most severe finding, the risk for the development of carcinoma appears to be relatively low.

■ REFERENCES

1. Koerner FC, Oyama T, Maluf H. Morphological observations regarding the origins of atypical cystic lobules (low-grade clinging carcinoma of flat type). *Virchows Arch.* 2001;439:523–530.
2. Warren JC. The surgeon and the pathologist. A plea for reciprocity as illustrated by the consideration of the classification and treatment of benign tumors of the breast. JAMA. 1905;45:149–165.
3. Bloodgood JC. Senile parenchymatous hypertrophy of female breast. Its relation to cyst formation and carcinoma. Surg Gynecol Obstet. 1906;3:721–730.
4. Cheatle SGL, Cutler M. Tumours of the Breast: Their Pathology, Symptoms, Diagnosis and Treatment. Philadelphia, PA: J. B. Lippincott Company; 1931.
5. Oyama T, Maluf H, Koerner F. Atypical cystic lobules: an early stage in the formation of low-grade ductal carcinoma in situ. Virchows Arch. 1999;435:413–421.
6. Collins LC, Achacoso NA, Nekhlyudov L, et al. Clinical and pathologic features of ductal carcinoma in situ associated with the presence of flat epithelial atypia: an analysis of 543 patients. Mod Pathol. 2007;20:1149–1155.
7. Simpson PT, Reis-Filho JS, Gale T, Lakhani SR. Molecular evolution of breast cancer. J Pathol. 2005;205:248–254.
8. Kusama R, Fujimori M, Matsuyama I, et al. Clinicopathological characteristics of atypical cystic duct (ACD) of the breast: assessment of ACD as a precancerous lesion. Pathol Int. 2000;50:793–800.
9. Bratthauer GL, Tavassoli FA. Assessment of lesions coexisting with various grades of ductal intraepithelial neoplasia of the breast. Virchows Arch. 2004;444:340–344.
10. Abdel-Fatah TM, Powe DG, Hodi Z, Lee AH, Reis-Filho JS, Ellis IO. High frequency of coexistence of columnar cell lesions, lobular neoplasia, and low grade ductal carcinoma in situ with invasive tubular carcinoma and invasive lobular carcinoma. Am J Surg Pathol. 2007;31:417–426.
11. Aulmann S, Elsawaf Z, Penzel R, Schirmacher P, Sinn HP. Invasive tubular carcinoma of the breast frequently is clonally related to flat epithelial atypia and low-grade ductal carcinoma in situ. Am J Surg Pathol. 2009;33:1646–1653.
12. Goldstein NS, O'Malley BA. Cancerization of small ectatic ducts of the breast by ductal carcinoma in situ cells with apocrine snouts: a lesion associated with tubular carcinoma. Am J Clin Pathol. 1997;107:561–566.
13. Fernandez-Aguilar S, Simon P, Buxant F, Simonart T, Noel JC. Tubular carcinoma of the breast and associated intra-epithelial lesions: a comparative study with invasive low-grade ductal carcinomas. Virchows Arch. 2005;447:683–687.
14. Kunju LP, Ding Y, Kleer CG. Tubular carcinoma and grade 1 (well-differentiated) invasive ductal carcinoma: comparison of flat epithelial atypia and other intra-epithelial lesions. Pathol Int. 2008;58:620–625.
15. Brandt SM, Young GQ, Hoda SA. The "Rosen triad": tubular carcinoma, lobular carcinoma in situ, and columnar cell lesions. Adv Anat Pathol. 2008;15:140–146.
16. De Potter CR, Foschini MP, Schelfhout AM, Schroeter CA, Eusebi V. Immunohistochemical study of neu protein overexpression in clinging in situ duct carcinoma of the breast. Virchows Arch A Pathol Anat Histopathol. 1993;422:375–380.
17. Simooka H, Oyama T, Sano T, Horiguchi J, Nakajima T. Immunohistochemical analysis of 14-3-3 sigma and related proteins in hyperplastic and neoplastic breast lesions, with particular reference to early carcinogenesis. Pathol Int. 2004; 54:595–602.
18. Dessauvagie BF, Zhao W, Heel-Miller KA, Harvey J, Bentel JM. Characterization of columnar cell lesions of the breast: immunophenotypic analysis of columnar alteration of lobules with prominent apical snouts and secretions. Hum Pathol. 2007;38:284–292.
19. Abdel-Fatah TM, Powe DG, Hodi Z, Reis-Filho JS, Lee AH, Ellis IO. Morphologic and molecular evolutionary pathways of low nuclear grade invasive breast cancers and their putative precursor lesions: further evidence to support

the concept of low nuclear grade breast neoplasia family. Am J Surg Pathol. 2008;32:513–523.

20. Simpson PT, Gale T, Reis-Filho JS, et al. Columnar cell lesions of the breast: the missing link in breast cancer progression? A morphological and molecular analysis. Am J Surg Pathol. 2005;29:734–746.

21. Noel JC, Fayt I, Fernandez-Aguilar S, Buxant F, Boutemy R. Proliferating activity in columnar cell lesions of the breast. Virchows Arch. 2006;449:617–621.

22. Kunju LP, Kleer CG. Significance of flat epithelial atypia on mammotome core needle biopsy: should it be excised? Hum Pathol. 2007;38:35–41.

23. Liu T, Niu Y, Feng Y, et al. Methylation of CpG islands of p16INK4a and cyclinD1 overexpression associated with progression of intraductal proliferative lesions of the breast. Hum Pathol. 2008;39:1637–1646.

24. Qi L, Bart J, Tan LP, et al. Expression of miR-21 and its targets (PTEN, PDCD4, TM1) in flat epithelial atypia of the breast in relation to ductal carcinoma in situ and invasive carcinoma. BMC Cancer. 2009;9:163.

25. Moinfar F, Man YG, Bratthauer GL, Ratschek M, Tavassoli FA. Genetic abnormalities in mammary ductal intraepithelial neoplasia-flat type ("clinging ductal carcinoma in situ"): a simulator of normal mammary epithelium. Cancer. 2000;88:2072–2081.

26. Dabbs DJ, Carter G, Fudge M, Peng Y, Swalsky P, Finkelstein S. Molecular alterations in columnar cell lesions of the breast. Mod Pathol. 2006;19:344–349.

27. Reis-Filho JS, Lakhani SR. The diagnosis and management of pre-invasive breast disease: genetic alterations in pre-invasive lesions. Breast Cancer Res. 2003;5:313–319.

28. Ma XJ, Salunga R, Tuggle JT, et al. Gene expression profiles of human breast cancer progression. Proc Natl Acad Sci USA. 2003;100:5974–5979.

29. Sgroi DC. Preinvasive breast cancer. Annu Rev Pathol. 2010;5: 193–221.

30. Brogi E, Oyama T, Koerner FC. Atypical cystic lobules in patients with lobular neoplasia. Int J Surg Pathol. 2001;9:201–206.

31. Leibl S, Regitnig P, Moinfar F. Flat epithelial atypia (DIN 1a, atypical columnar change): an underdiagnosed entity very frequently coexisting with lobular neoplasia. Histopathology. 2007;50:859–865.

32. Gopalan A, Hoda SA. Columnar cell hyperplasia and lobular carcinoma in situ coexisting in the same duct. Breast J. 2005;11:210.

33. Rosen PP. Columnar cell hyperplasia is associated with lobular carcinoma in situ and tubular carcinoma. Am J Surg Pathol. 1999;23:1561.

34. Azzopardi JG. Problems in Breast Pathology. London: W.B. Saunders; 1979.

35. Lerwill MF. Current practical applications of diagnostic immunohistochemistry in breast pathology. Am J Surg Pathol. 2004;28:1076–1091.

36. Eusebi V, Feudale E, Foschini MP, et al. Long-term follow-up of in situ carcinoma of the breast. Semin Diagn Pathol. 1994;11:223–235.

37. Bijker N, Peterse JL, Duchateau L, et al. Risk factors for recurrence and metastasis after breast-conserving therapy for ductal carcinoma-in-situ: analysis of European organization for research and treatment of cancer trial 10853. J Clin Oncol. 2001;19:2263–2271.

38. Shaaban AM, Sloane JP, West CR, et al. Histopathologic types of benign breast lesions and the risk of breast cancer: case-control study. Am J Surg Pathol. 2002;26:421–430.

39. Boulos FI, Dupont WD, Simpson JF, et al. Histologic associations and long-term cancer risk in columnar cell lesions of the breast: a retrospective cohort and a nested case-control study. Cancer. 2008;113:2415–2421.

40. Martel M, Barron-Rodriguez P, Tolgay Ocal I, Dotto J, Tavassoli FA. Flat DIN 1 (flat epithelial atypia) on core needle biopsy: 63 cases identified retrospectively among 1,751 core biopsies performed over an 8-year period (1992-1999). Virchows Arch. 2007;451:883–891.

41. de Mascarel I, MacGrogan G, Mathoulin-Pelissier S, et al. Epithelial atypia in biopsies performed for microcalcifications. Practical considerations about 2,833 serially sectioned surgical biopsies with a long follow-up. Virchows Arch. 2007;451:1–10.

42. Guerra-Wallace MM, Christensen WN, White RL. A retrospective study of columnar alteration with prominent apical snouts and secretions and the association with cancer. Am J Surg. 2004;188:395–398.

43. Tomasino RM, Morello V, Gullo A, et al. Assessment of "grading" with ki-67 and c-kit immunohistochemical expressions may be a helpful tool in management of patients with flat epithelial atypia (FEA) and columnar cell lesions (CCLs) on core breast biopsy. J Cell Physiol. 2009;221: 343–349.

44. Piubello Q, Parisi A, Eccher A, Barbazeni G, Franchini Z, Iannucci A. Flat epithelial atypia on core needle biopsy: which is the right management? Am J Surg Pathol. 2009;33:1078–1084.

45. Noske A, Pahl S, Fallenberg E, et al. Flat epithelial atypia is a common subtype of B3 breast lesions and is associated with noninvasive cancer but not with invasive cancer in final excision histology. Hum Pathol. 2010;41:522–527.

46. Chivukula M, Bhargava R, Tseng G, Dabbs DJ. Clinicopathologic implications of "flat epithelial atypia" in core needle biopsy specimens of the breast. Am J Clin Pathol. 2009; 131:802–808.

47. Senetta R, Campanino PP, Mariscotti G, et al. Columnar cell lesions associated with breast calcifications on vacuum-assisted core biopsies: clinical, radiographic, and histological correlations. Mod Pathol. 2009;22:762–769.

48. Ingegnoli A, d'Aloia C, Frattaruolo A, et al. Flat epithelial atypia and atypical ductal hyperplasia: carcinoma underestimation rate. Breast J. 2010;16:55–59.

49. Darvishian F, Singh B, Simsir A, Ye W, Cangiarella JF. Atypia on breast core needle biopsies: Reproducibility and significance. Ann Clin Lab Sci. 2009;39:270–276.

50. Fraser JL, Raza S, Chorny K, Connolly JL, Schnitt SJ. Columnar alteration with prominent apical snouts and secretions: a spectrum of changes frequently present in breast biopsies performed for microcalcifications. Am J Surg Pathol. 1998;22:1521–1527.

51. Schnitt SJ, Vincent-Salomon A. Columnar cell lesions of the breast. Adv Anat Pathol. 2003;10:113–124.

52. Tavassoli, FA, Hoefler H, Rosai J, et al. Intraductal proliferative lesions. In: Tavassoli FA, Devilee P, eds. Pathology and Genetics of Tumours of the Breast and Female Genital Organs. Lyon: IARC Press; 2003.

53. Rosen PP. Rosen's Breast Pathology. 2nd ed. Philadelphia, PA: Lippincott Williams & Wilkins; 2001.

5

Adenosis: Mimickers of Carcinoma

JUAN P. PALAZZO

JOSE PALACIOS CALVO

In all breast biopsies, it is very important to correlate the biopsy findings with the clinical and imaging features. There should always be concordance between the microscopic and the imaging findings. This correlation is crucial when dealing with adenosis of the breast. In many biopsies, adenosis may represent the main lesion or may be a component of other lesions such as fibrocystic changes or cancer.

The diagnosis of adenosis of the breast has become particularly important because the initial evaluation of breast lesions is frequently done with the use of core biopsies. The amount of representative tissue is limited and the diagnosis becomes more challenging for the pathologist.

The two steps to follow when examining breast biopsies are to identify the proliferation as adenosis and to differentiate it from invasive well-differentiated carcinoma. The low-magnification appearance of the proliferation is very important to evaluate the pattern of growth and the relationship between the proliferating acini and the surrounding breast. A proliferation that is well circumscribed and lacks an infiltrative pattern is always suggestive of adenosis rather than carcinoma. There are, however, exceptions with cases of adenosis characterized by the lack of circumscription.

In addition to the morphologic findings, immunohistochemical markers to identify myoepithelial cells can help in the differential diagnosis between adenosis and carcinoma. These markers can be very useful to make this distinction, but they need to be interpreted in conjunction with the morphologic findings. Several markers are currently available and can be used as single markers or as a panel. Among the most useful and reliable markers to identify myoepithelial cells, CD10, p63, calponin, and alpha smooth muscle actin can be used as single antibodies or as a panel. Some of these markers, such as alpha smooth muscle actin, can also stain myofibroblasts; therefore, they have to be interpreted with caution.

The literature that includes studies with follow-up information supports the specific diagnosis of certain subtypes of breast adenosis given their premalignant potential and association with carcinoma. Adenosis of the breast may represent a spectrum of lesions rather than a specific entity, and as such, it is not uncommon to find morphologic diversity present in a single breast biopsy. Therefore, overlapping features of the different types of adenosis can be present in a single breast biopsy.

Table 5.1 summarizes the main pathologic and immunohistochemical features that are useful to differentiate adenosis from carcinoma.

■ SCLEROSING ADENOSIS

Pathologic Features

Sclerosing adenosis (SA) can be the predominant component of a biopsy or be associated with other benign or malignant lesions.

At low magnification, SA has a lobulocentric growth pattern. The proliferating acini show both open and close ("slit-like") spaces. Although in SA both epithelial and myoepithelial cells are seen, the epithelial cells are atrophic, whereas the myoepithelial cells frequently become more abundant and prominent with spindle cell morphology and they may acquire a myoid phenotype. The proliferating acini of SA show a well-demarcated pushing margin and single glands that usually do not infiltrate between the normal breast (Figures 5.1 and 5.2). However, in some lesions, the proliferating acini have

■ **Table 5.1** Comparative pathologic features between adenosis and tubular carcinoma

	Shape of Acini	Acinic/Stromal Interface	Intraluminal Material	Epithelial Lining	Stroma	Myoepithelial Cells	Risk of Cancer
Sclerosing Adenosis	Round and slit like	Well demarcated lobulocentric	No	Flat and cuboidal Myoepithelial cells	Hypocellular Hyalinized	Present	Very low
Microglandular Adenosis	Round	Infiltrating	Yes	Flat and cuboidal lack of myoepithelial cells	Hypocellular	Absent	Low
Cancerization of Adenosis	Round and slit like	Well demarcated infiltrating	No	Atypical:ductal, lobular, apocrine	Hypocellular Hyalinized	Present; Decreased	High
Tubular Carcinoma	Round; tear drop shaped	Infiltrating	No	Cuboidal, apocrine snouts, lack of myoepithelial cells	Desmoplastic	Absent	N/A

an infiltrative pattern into the surrounding stroma and adipose tissue that can closely resemble a well-differentiated invasive ductal carcinoma (Figures 5.3–5.5). The lobular stroma in SA is frequently fibrotic, similar to the surrounding breast stroma, and lacks the desmoplasia seen in most invasive carcinomas (Figures 5.6). Sclerosing adenosis frequently contains microcalcifications. When SA is well circumscribed with a nodular shape and

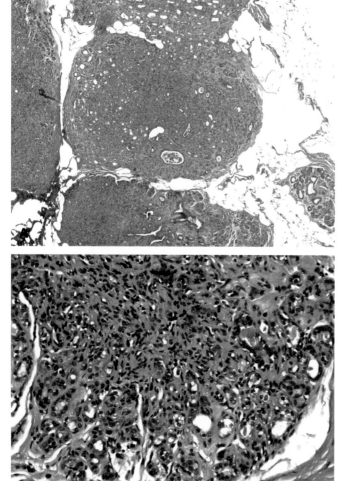

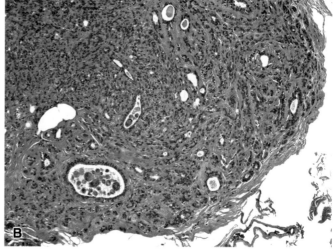

FIGURE 5.1 (A–C) Sclerosing adenosis showing a well-demarcated proliferation of open and slit-like glandular spaces.

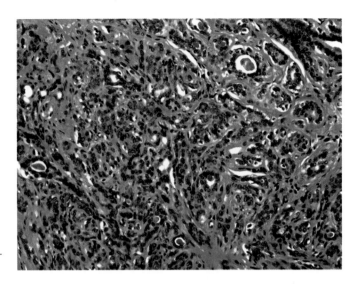

FIGURE 5.2 Sclerosing adenosis with a predominance of close glandular spaces and streaming of the cell proliferation.

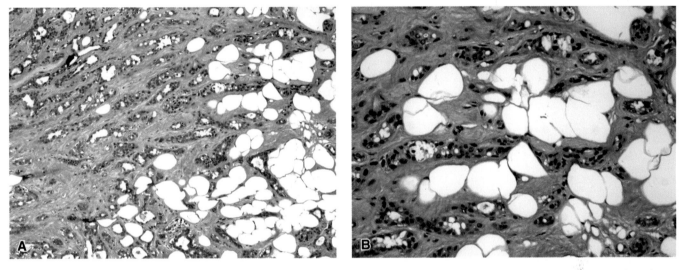

FIGURE 5.3 (A and B) Sclerosing adenosis with open acini that simulate invasive carcinoma. (B) Whereas some acini have a teardrop shape, others form slit-like spaces.

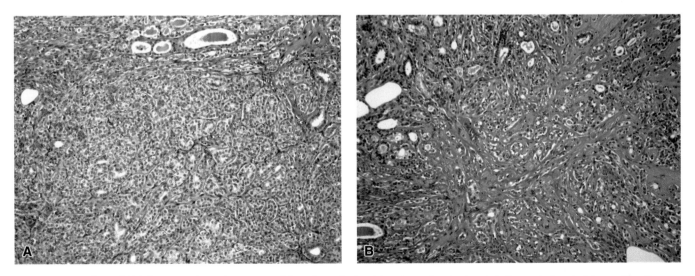

FIGURE 5.4 (A and B) Adenosis with predominance of densely packed acini and prominent sclerosis in the central part of the proliferation.

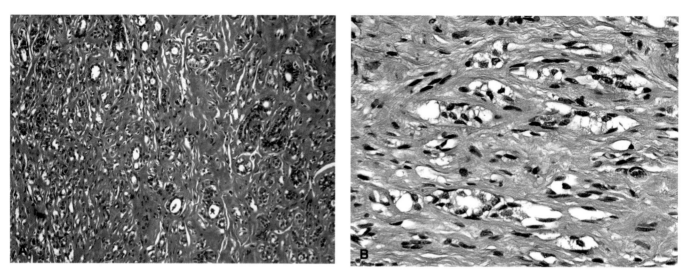

FIGURE 5.5   (A and B) Sclerosing adenosis that shows a less circumscribed growth pattern with acini that infiltrate into the surrounding tissue. Note the lack of desmoplasia. (B) Some of the cells lining the acini have clear cytoplasms.

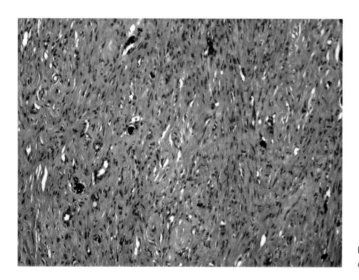

FIGURE 5.6   Sclerosing adenosis with slit-like acini with microcalcifications and lacking desmoplasia.

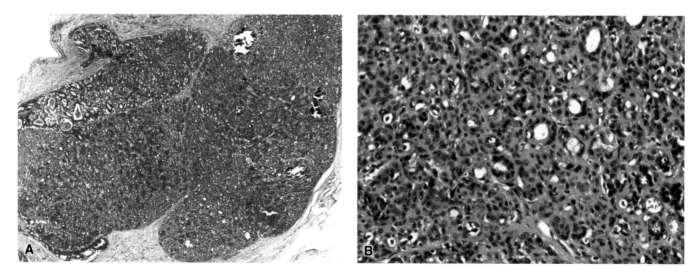

FIGURE 5.7   (A and B) Adenosis with a proliferation of acini with almost no intervening stroma and well-circumscribed sharp margins. (B) Some open, round acini are admixed with more cellular acini with no clearly discernible lumens.

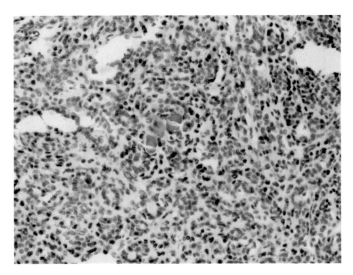

FIGURE 5.8 Immunohistochemistry for p63 demonstrates multiple myoepithelial cells surrounding the acini.

FIGURE 5.10 Sclerosing adenosis with acini surrounding intrammammary nerves.

swirling of the proliferating acini, the term *nodular SA* can be used (Figures 5.7 and 5.8). Sclerosing adenosis can involve fibroadenomas, and the pattern of involvement can closely simulate invasive carcinoma (Figure 5.9). The presence of more typical areas of SA or carcinoma outside the fibroadenoma should help make this distinction.

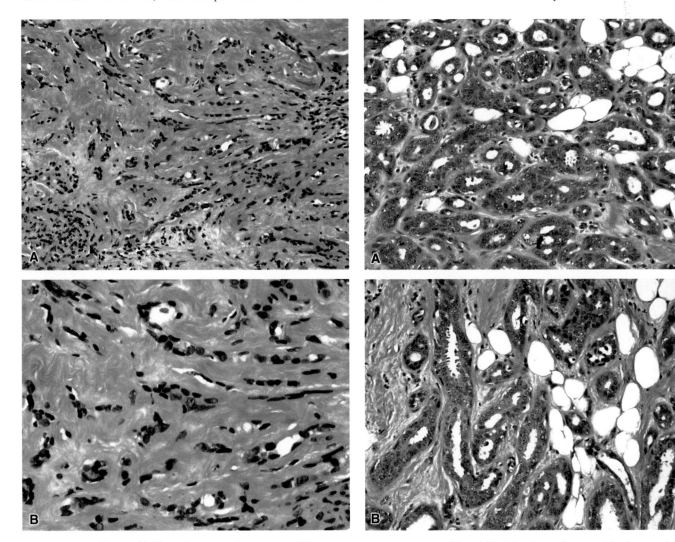

FIGURE 5.9 (A and B) Fibroadenoma with prominent SA is composed of slit-like acini and single cells simulating lobular carcinoma.

FIGURE 5.11 (A and B) Sclerosing adenosis with elongated and tubular acini infiltrating the adipose tissue.

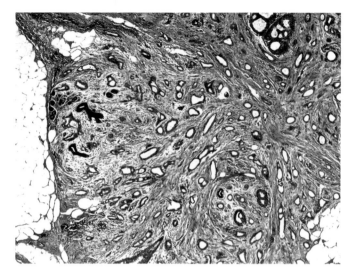

FIGURE 5.12 Tubular carcinoma with a haphazard proliferation of acini with round and teardrop shapes. The malignant acini infiltrate between the breast parenchyma. There is minimal stromal desmoplasia.

In addition, some SA can show perineural infiltration (Figure 5.10).

Within the morphologic spectrum of breast adenosis, some cases can show tubular structures, most often as a component of more classic SA. At low magnification, the proliferating acini form elongated branching tubular structures that infiltrate between the normal breast and the adipose tissue (1) (Figure 5.11).

Sclerosing adenosis should be differentiated from invasive carcinoma. Microscopically, tubular carcinoma, which can closely resemble SA, is characterized by open acini with a "teardrop" appearance and a haphazard growth pattern infiltrating normal breast and adipose tissue. The cells lining the neoplastic acini in tubular carcinoma may contain apocrine snouts, and the stroma surrounding the acini is usually but not always desmoplastic. In some cases, the stroma can show more of a keloid-like appearance, making the diagnosis of carcinoma more difficult (Figures 5.12–5.15).

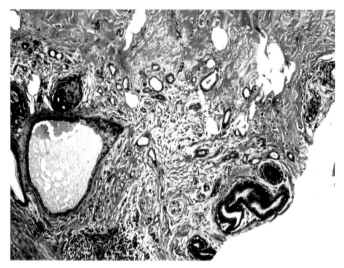

FIGURE 5.13 A small focus of tubular carcinoma in a core biopsy characterized by round acini and desmoplastic stroma.

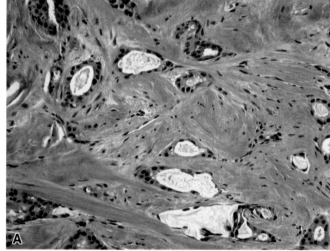

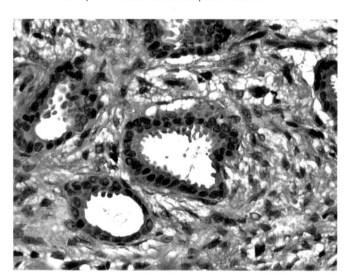

FIGURE 5.14 Tubular carcinoma with desmoplastic stroma and glands showing prominent cytoplasmic snouts.

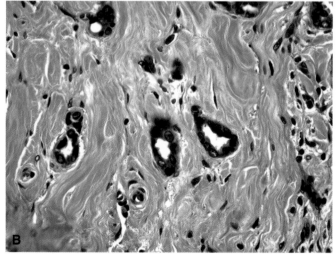

FIGURE 5.15 (A and B) Tubular carcinoma with a hyalinized/keloid-like stroma.

Immunohistochemistry

In most cases of SA, there is no need to use immunohistochemical stains, and the diagnosis can be rendered based on the classical morphologic features. By immunohistochemistry, some of the cells within the proliferating acini express myoepithelial markers. The most common myoepithelial markers available for the identification of myoepithelial cells are alpha smooth muscle actin, p63, calponin, and CD10. These markers will highlight the presence of myoepithelial cells in SA and the lack of them in invasive carcinoma.

Management

If SA represents the main lesion and there is good correlation with the imaging findings, there is no need to recommend reexcision (2). The decision to reexcise a biopsy showing SA should be based on the presence of a different lesion such as atypical hyperplasia and carcinoma in situ or a lack of correlation between imaging findings and pathology.

There is a reported mild increased risk of developing cancer in patients diagnosed with SA (3). However, SA per se is not an indication for reexcision unless there is no correlation between the imaging findings and the pathology.

■ MICROGLANDULAR ADENOSIS

Pathologic Features

This is an uncommon variant of adenosis but very important to identify because it can closely mimic grossly and microscopically invasive ductal carcinomas. By imaging, microglandular adenosis (MA) can also simulate invasive carcinoma. Moreover, MA can pose additional diagnostic difficulties due to its morphologic and immunohistochemical profiles resembling well-differentiated invasive ductal carcinoma.

Microscopically, MA is composed of open, round acini that infiltrate haphazardly the breast and adipose tissue. The acini typically contain intraluminal eosinophilic secretions and are lined by vacuolated clear cells. There is no desmoplastic stroma surrounding the acini as typically seen in tubular carcinoma (4). The acini of MA are more round, less irregular, and elongated compared with those seen in tubular carcinoma (5) (Figure 5.16).

An unusual variant of MA is atypical MA, which is characterized by more irregular glands, back-to-back growth, and cells lining the acini, sometimes filling the

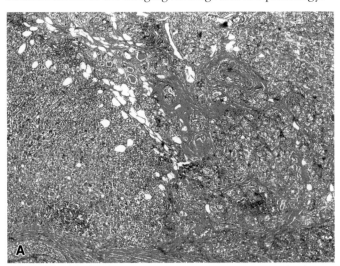

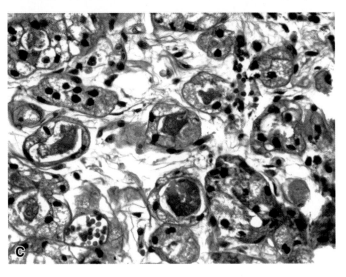

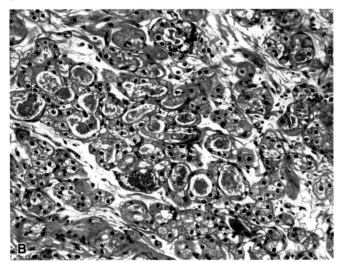

FIGURE 5.16 (A–C) Microglandular adenosis showing a proliferation of round acini infiltrating haphazardly the adipose tissue. (B) The acini are lined by cells with clear cytoplasms and contain eosinophilic secretions. Note the lack of desmoplastic stroma. (C) The acini are lined by single cuboidal cells with hyperchomatic nuclei without nucleoli.

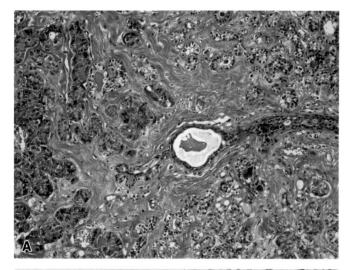

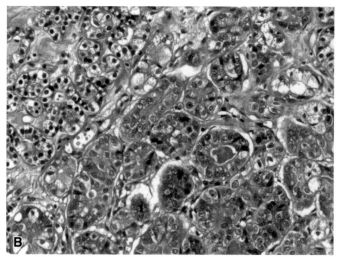

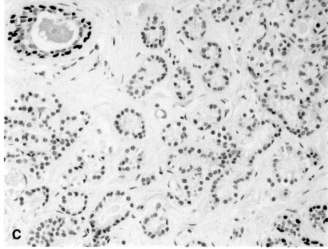

FIGURE 5.17 (A–C) Atypical microglandular adenosis with a component of acini with larger nuclei lining round glands with intraluminal secretions. (B) The atypical acini are lined by cells with larger vesicular nuclei. Some of the cells lining the atypical acini show single prominent nucleoli. (C) There is no p63 staining in the proliferating acini.

acini and showing enlarged nuclei, pleomorphism, and prominent nucleoli with occasional mitotic figures. Transition from MA, atypical MA and in situ and invasive carcinomas can be seen in a single biopsy. There is morphologic and molecular evidence of MA evolving into invasive carcinoma (6–9) (Figures 5.17).

Immunohistochemistry

By immunohistochemistry, myoepithelial cell markers are absent in MA, and the cells lining the acini express S-100 protein. These cells are negative for ER, PR, and HER2, and interestingly, the carcinomas arising in association with MA maintain this immunohistochemical profile (10).

Management

All cases of MA diagnosed in core biopsies should be reexcised to obtain clear margins and to exclude the possibility of an associated invasive carcinoma. Atypical MA also needs to be completely excised to obtain negative margins.

■ ATYPICAL ADENOSIS AND CANCERIZATION OF ADENOSIS

Pathologic Features

All the subtypes of adenosis can be involved by atypical hyperplasias and carcinoma cells of ductal and lobular origin (11,12). When the atypical cells involve the adenosis, excluding invasive carcinoma becomes very difficult. If no obvious areas of carcinoma are present in the biopsy, an effort should be made to identify the presence of a reference lesion that may coexist with the atypical adenosis. However, atypical adenosis may represent the only lesion in the biopsy. Ductal, lobular, and apocrine atypical lesions can involve adenosis.

The low-magnification appearance shows the preserved lobulocentric growth of the proliferating acini as seen in typical SA. The acini are expanded and replaced by a proliferation of small round cells in cases of cancerization by lobular carcinoma or by larger atypical cells when involved by ductal carcinoma cells. The stroma surrounding the adenosis lacks the desmoplastic features seen in most invasive carcinomas. In between and adjacent to the

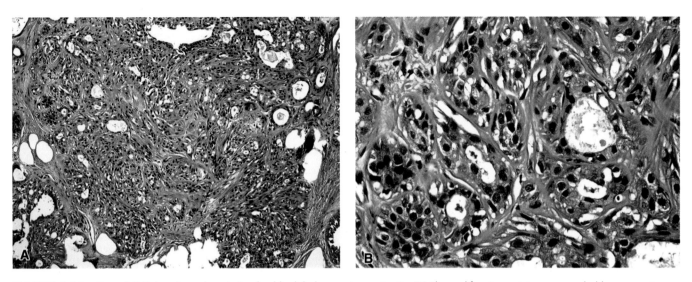

FIGURE 5.18 (A and B) Sclerosing adenosis involved by lobular carcinoma in situ. (B) The proliferating acini are expanded by a monotonous population of cells with hyperchromatic round nuclei.

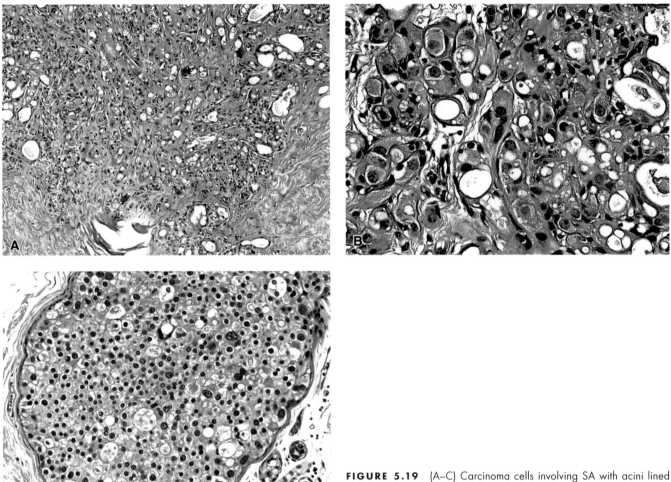

FIGURE 5.19 (A–C) Carcinoma cells involving SA with acini lined by cells with large nuclei, abundant cytoplasm, and prominent nucleoli. (B) The acini are lined by both atypical and nonatypical cells. (C) Ductal carcinoma in situ present within the same lesion.

acini with the atypical cells, there are areas of more classical adenosis. In addition, the single file of tumor cells as seen in classic lobular carcinoma is not seen (Figures 5.18–5.21).

All apocrine lesions ranging from metaplasia to carcinoma can involve adenosis (13,14). The distension of the proliferating acini by apocrine cells can be confused with invasive carcinoma. It has been proposed that the

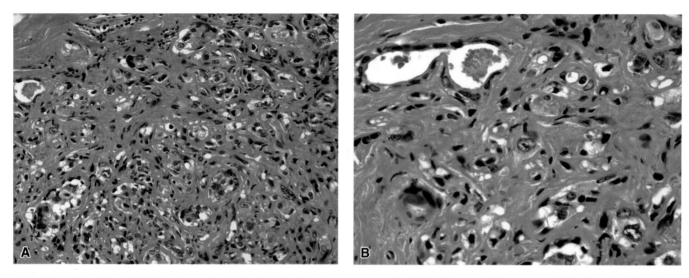

FIGURE 5.20 (A and B) Sclerosing adenosis involved by ductal carcinoma cells. (B) The lumens of the acini are difficult to identify and are involved by atypical cells.

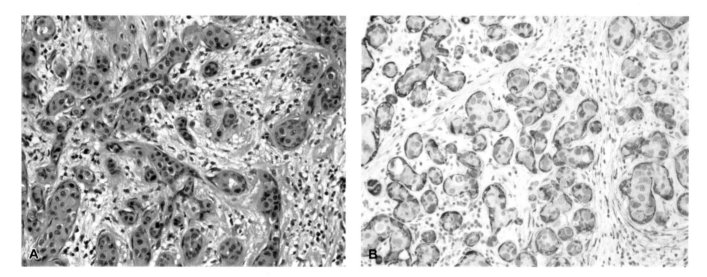

FIGURE 5.21 (A and B) Sclerosing adenosis involved by atypical cells. Invasive carcinoma was present next to this area. (B) Calponin stain is positive for myoepithelial cells in all the acini.

term should be used for adenosis, especially SA, in which more than 50% of the lesion shows apocrine metaplasia of the epithelial cells. Atypical adenosis shows apocrine cells lining the acini. These cells have large nuclei, prominent nucleoli, and abundant eosinophilic cytoplasm and can show marked nuclear pleomorphism and mitotic figures. Apocrine lesions including atypical apocrine lesions can involve also papillomas and sclerosing lesions.

When nuclear pleomorphism amounts to a 3-fold variation in nuclear size, the diagnosis of "atypical apocrine adenosis" is recommended. These lesions can be extremely difficult to distinguish from cancerization by apocrine carcinoma in situ, and there is an overlap between atypical apocrine proliferations and apocrine carcinoma. Indeed, some cases of atypical apocrine adenosis may represent apocrine carcinomas in situ. Apocrine carcinoma cells show irregular nuclear membranes, enlarged nuclei, and coarse chromatin. In the absence of apocrine carcinoma outside the area of adenosis, the distinction between atypical apocrine adenosis and carcinoma involving adenosis may not be possible (Figures 5.22–5.24).

Immunohistochemistry

Immunohistochemical stains can help identify myoepithelial cells to confirm the diagnosis of adenosis, but they may be markedly decreased or replaced by the atypical cells present in the distorted and expanded acini. The decreased

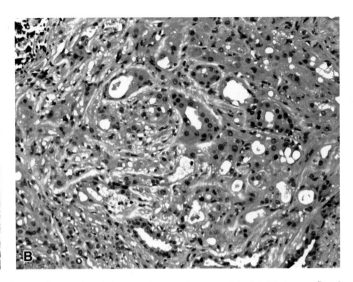

FIGURE 5.22 (A and B) Apocrine adenosis with acini lined by cells with abundant eosinophilic cytoplasm and enlarged nuclei. (B) A more florid example of apocrine adenosis; notice the variability in the size of the nuclei.

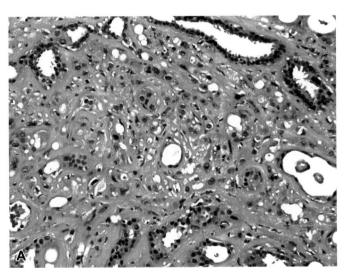
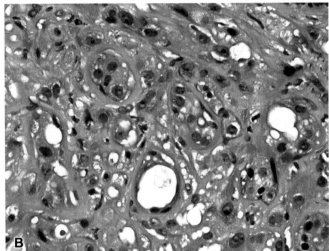

FIGURE 5.23 (A and B) Atypical apocrine adenosis with cells lining the proliferating acini with abundant eosinophilic cytoplasms and large vesicular nuclei. (B) The cells have large nuclei, and some of them show a prominent nucleoli.

number of myoepithelial cells can make the distinction with invasive carcinoma even more difficult. An E-cadherin stain is useful to distinguish involvement by lobular or ductal cells. In ductal lesions, E-cadherin shows membranous staining and is negative in lobular cells. One has to be aware that frequently residual ductal cells can be present, and therefore, the E-cadherin stain can show a mixed population of cells as detected by immunohistochemistry.

Immunohistochemical stains are valuable to identify apocrine differentiation. Apocrine cells are usually ER- and PR-negative and positive for androgen receptor and GCDFP-15 (Gross Cystic Disease Fluid Protein-15). Myoepithelial cells are identified in adenosis involved by atypical and nonatypical apocrine cells, but they may be decreased in number and difficult to identify even with the use of immunohistochemical markers.

Management

Reexcision is recommended in all cases of atypical adenosis and carcinomas involving adenosis. For some authors, apocrine adenosis is a risk factor for the development of carcinoma, and it should also be reexcised when diagnosed in core biopsies to exclude associated apocrine carcinoma in situ or invasive carcinoma.

■ KEY POINTS

1. Adenosis of the breast and invasive carcinomas can show overlapping features that are most difficult to distinguish in core biopsies.

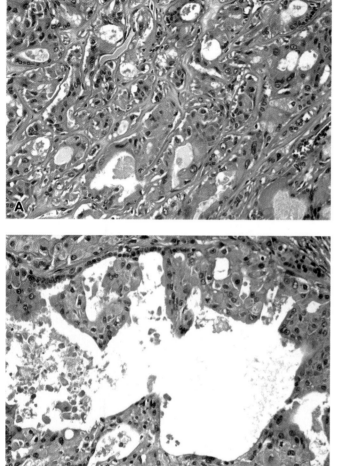

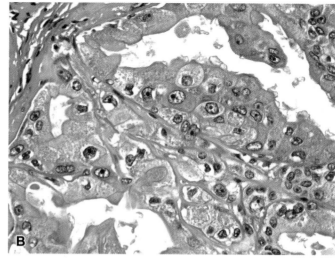

FIGURE 5.24 (A–C) Adenosis involved by apocrine carcinoma cells showing abundant eosinophilic cytoplasm. (B) There is variation in the size of the vesicular nuclei, most of which have prominent nucleoli. (C) Apocrine carcinoma in situ next to the adenosis involved by the carcinoma cells.

2. Attention should be directed to the proliferating acini, their growth pattern, and the characteristics of the surrounding stroma.

3. The use of immunohistochemistry can help in the differential diagnosis; however, stains should always be interpreted in conjunction with the morphologic features of the lesion.

■ REFERENCES

1. Lee KC, Chan JK, Gwi E. Tubular adenosis of the breast. A distinctive benign lesion mimicking invasive carcinoma. *Am J Surg Pathol.* 1996;20:46–54.
2. Gill HK, Ioffe OB, Berg WA. When is a diagnosis of sclerosing adenosis acceptable at core biopsy? *Radiology.* 2003;228:50–57.
3. Jensen RA, Page DL, Dupont WD, Rogers LW. Invasive breast cancer risk in women with sclerosing adenosis. *Cancer.* 1989;64:1977–1983.
4. Rosen PP. Microglandular adenosis: a benign lesion simulating invasive mammary carcinoma. *Am J Surg Pathol.* 1983;7:137–144.
5. Clement PB, Azzopardi JG. Microglandular adenosis of the breast—a lesion simulating tubular carcinoma. *Histopathology.* 1983;7:169–180.
6. Salarieh A, Sneige N. Breast carcinoma arising in microglandular adenosis. A review of the literature. *Arch Pathol Lab Med.* 2007;131:1397–1399.
7. Shin SJ, Simpson PT, Da Silva L, et al. Molecular evidence for progression of microglandular adenosis (MGA) to invasive carcinoma. *Am J Surg Pathol.* 2009;33:496–504.
8. Khalifeh IM, Albarracin C, Diaz LK, et al. Clinical, histopathologic, and immunohistochemical features of microglandular adenosis and transition into in situ and invasive carcinoma. *Am J Surg Pathol.* 2008;2:544–552.
9. Resetkova E, Flanders DJ, Rosen PP. Ten year follow-up of mammary carcinoma arising in microglandular adenosis treated with breast conservation. *Arch Pathol Lab Med.* 2003;127:77–80.
10. Koenig C, Dadmanesh F, Bratthauer GL, Tavassoli FA. Carcinoma arising in microglandular adenosis: an immunohistochemical analysis of 20 intraepithelial and invasive neoplasms. *Int J Surg Pathol.* 2000;8:303–315.

11. Oberman HA, Markey BA. Noninvasive carcinoma of the breast presenting in adenosis. *Mod Pathol*. 1991;4: 31–35.

12. Rasbridge SA, Millis RR. Carcinoma in-situ involving sclerosing adenosis: a mimic of invasive breast carcinoma. *Histopathology*. 1995;27:269–273.

13. Seidman JD, Ashton M, Lefkowitz M. Atypical apocrine adenosis of the breast. A clinicopathologic study of 37 patients with 8.7 year follow-up. *Cancer*. 1996;77:2529–2537.

14. Carter DJ, Rosen PP. Atypical apocrine metaplasia in sclerosing lesions of the breast: a study of 51 patients. *Mod Pathol*. 1991;4:1–5.

6

Microinvasive Carcinoma: Diagnosis and Pitfalls

DILIP GIRI

Microinvasive carcinoma (MIC) is defined per the current Union for International Cancer Control (UICC) classification (pTNM staging, 1997) as any invasive focus no greater than 1 mm (1). If there are multiple invasive foci, the lesion may still qualify as MIC by this definition, provided that none of the individual foci exceed 1 mm. Adding the individual foci is not accepted in this classification scheme. Before making the diagnosis of MIC, adequate and thorough sampling of the tumor is required. Since the diagnosis of MIC has therapeutic implications, it is inappropriate to classify a tumor seen in a core biopsy specimen as MIC. The core biopsy specimen may not always represent the true dimension of the invasive component of a tumor, and although the dimension in such specimens may be less than 1 mm, in excisions, the carcinoma may be larger (2). Thus, it would be erroneous and misleading to classify a tumor as an MIC based on the size obtained in such a specimen. A more appropriate term would be *microinvasion* or *focus of microinvasion* or *microscopic focus of invasion* followed by documentation of the size estimate if possible.

There is some confusion in the published literature on the subject of MIC. In some reports, the term *MIC* is used to designate tumors in which the invasive carcinoma comprises less than 10% of the tumor volume (3). In others, the entity is defined as carcinoma in situ with any stromal invasion (4). Some authors have included in this category tumors that are less than 0.5 cm (5). Although several studies have shed light on various aspects of this entity (6–10), due to lack of universally acceptable definition, the early literature on this subject is difficult to evaluate.

Microinvasive carcinoma is now diagnosed with increasing frequency, probably as a result of extensive screening of the population and the early detection of breast cancer. Microinvasive foci may not only be detected in the main excision specimens or mastectomy specimen but also in specimens submitted as excised margins after lumpectomy. Clearly, in surgical pathology, knowing the definition alone of MIC is not enough. Rather, it is critically important not to miss these foci in the course of histologic examination of a specimen. Indeed, in some occasions, invasion may be present in the form of a few isolated tumor cells in the stroma. Therefore, it helps if there is awareness of the circumstances in which there is an increased likelihood of encountering MIC. Recognizing this fact will minimize errors in the diagnosis of MIC. This chapter attempts to address these and some other practical issues as they relate to MIC.

■ PATHOLOGIC FEATURES

The recognition of microinvasion can be challenging at times. On the other hand, architectural distortion can be misleading and may easily lead to erroneous diagnosis of MIC. A useful strategy is to be aware of the situations where microinvasion or invasion is likely to be present. Similarly, it is important to be aware of the typical lesional settings that may lead to a false diagnosis of invasion or microinvasion. The following list is not meant to be all inclusive; however, it illustrates examples of some situations when microinvasion is likely to occur and could be missed if not sought and situations that represent common pitfalls leading to misdiagnosis of microinvasion.

1. Extensive ductal carcinoma in situ (DCIS) with lymphocytic infiltrates and typically forming a mass-like lesion: This is one of the most common presentations of microinvasion in association with DCIS. Typically, the DCIS is high grade, although on some occasions, this pattern may be seen with lower-grade DCIS. The invasion classically occurs in the form of either single cells or small clusters of cells in the stroma adjacent to the ducts involved by DCIS. The infiltrating cells are present in the midst of lymphoid cells, and there may or may not be a fibrous stromal reaction. Invasion may be present at multiple foci, and careful screening of the slides is essential to detect it especially because the dense lymphoid infiltrates

may obscure the invasive cells. Keratin immunohistochemistry is very useful in this situation because it lights up the infiltrating tumor cells. However, the keratin stain should be interpreted in the context of the assessment made by morphology. Myoepithelial markers that are helpful to delineate the DCIS will not help identify single cells or minute tumor clusters in the stroma. These antibodies help resolve the dilemma posed by cell processes emerging from the duct wall of DCIS units in a "sprouting" fashion. It is also important to remember that sometimes tumor cells may be positive for myoepithelial markers such as 4A4/p63; thus, one needs to be sure that the cells that are positive are not tumor cells before considering them to be myoepithelial cells. The most important element in the assessment of these lesions is the careful screening of the hematoxylin and eosin (H&E)–stained slides and being aware

that microinvasion may be present in this situation. Figures 6.1 to 6.7 illustrate the various patterns of microinvasion associated with DCIS and also show the application of immunohistochemical markers in the elucidation of microinvasion.

2. Invasive carcinoma associated with lobular carcinoma in situ (LCIS): Invasion seen in this setting is easy to miss especially in core biopsy specimens. The small infiltrating cells with low-grade nuclei may be present as minute microscopic foci. Careful scrutiny of the sections is the key. Cytokeratin stain, preferably a cocktail (such as AE1:AE3), is often very helpful to detect the presence of single cells. However, routine use of keratin stains in all cases that show LCIS will have low yield of positivity. In addition, myoepithelial markers are of little use in such a situation because the issue is not the distortion of architecture but rather the recognition of the few infiltrative

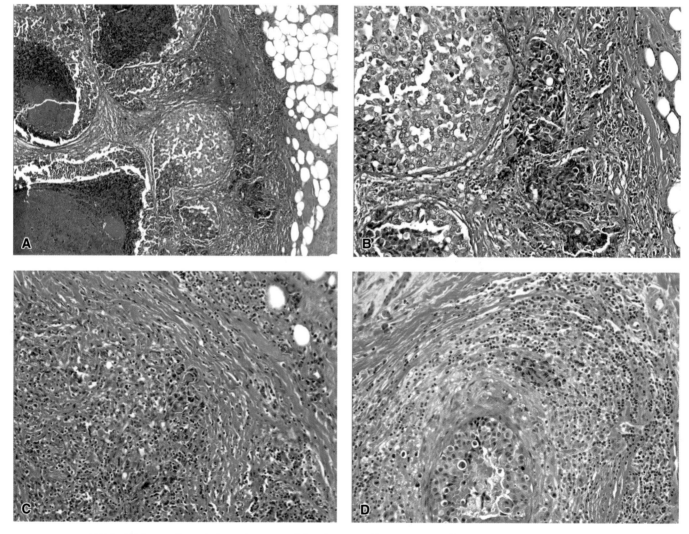

FIGURE 6.1   (A) The H&E stain shows high-grade DCIS with lymphocytic infiltrates and a confluent cluster of tumor cells in the adjacent stroma representing microinvasion. (B) Higher-power view demonstrates the invasive cluster. Note the lymphocytic infiltrates in the stroma.

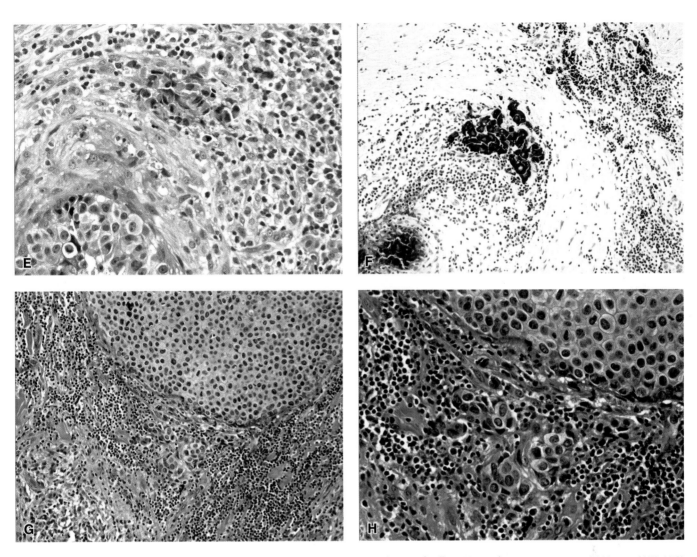

FIGURE 6.1 (*Continued*) (C–E) The H&E stain shows single cells and minute clusters of cells in MIC within reactive stroma. (F) Keratin (AE1:AE3) immunostain shows the MIC cell clusters brightly lit up and easy to recognize. (G) The H&E stain shows lower-grade DCIS with MIC. (H) A higher magnification view of the tumor cells.

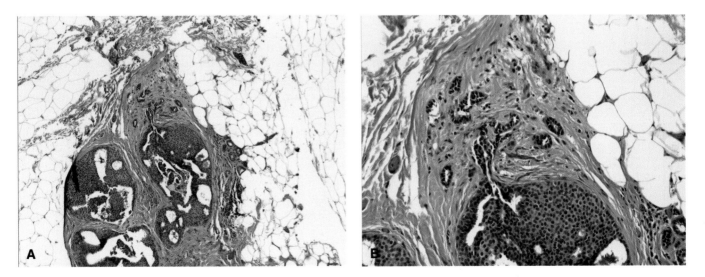

FIGURE 6.2 (A) The H&E stain scanning view of low-grade DCIS with MIC. There is a breach in the basement membrane of the duct wall with sprouting of the invasive focus. (B) Higher magnification view.

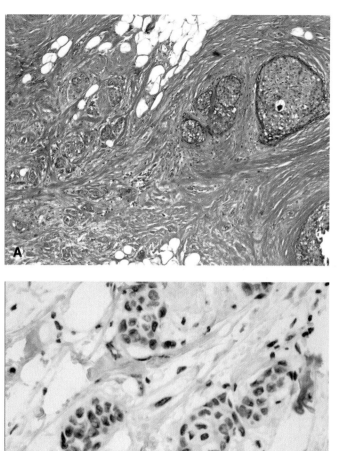

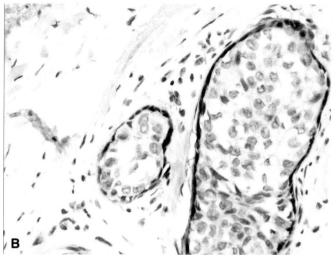

FIGURE 6.3 (A) The H&E stain shows low-grade DCIS with nests of infiltrating tumor cells. The growth pattern resembles sclerosing adenosis–like growth pattern. (B) Calponin immunostain shows peripheral positive stain. (C) The nests of tumor cells are negative, supporting the diagnosis of microinvasion.

tumor cells. In my experience, the likelihood of invasion is greater in cases with unusual variants of LCIS (such as large cell LCIS with necrosis or pleomorphic LCIS); thus, a heightened alertness is indicated in core biopsy specimens that show those variants of LCIS. Invasive carcinoma may also be missed in excision specimens for similar reasons (low nuclear grade and low cellularity). Postbiopsy changes with exuberant stromal reactive changes may on occasion obscure the presence of invasive cells. If it is known that the core biopsy had invasive lobular carcinoma and no obvious invasion is noted in the excised specimen, then the use of keratin stains facilitates the detection of residual invasive carcinoma. Images illustrating the various issues described above are shown in Figures 6.8 to 6.13. As shown in Figure 6.13, it is important to be aware of unusual growth patterns of invasive lobular carcinoma, especially when they present as minute lesions. Such awareness will usually prompt further investigation with immunostains and lead to the correct diagnosis. Figures 6.8 to 6.13

illustrate various examples of lobular lesions with microinvasion.

3. In situ carcinoma involving sclerosing adenosis/radial scar lesion: This is another instance where invasion may be missed. Ductal carcinoma in situ or LCIS can sometimes involve sclerosing adenosis or radial scar lesions. The difficulty arises when the neoplastic cells involve the small tubules that are native to these proliferative lesions. This pattern of neoplastic involvement of an existing lesion that has a "pseudoinfiltrative" pattern now becomes apparently invasive. Myoepithelial markers such as calponin and 4A4 (p63) will confirm the noninvasive nature of these glands.

Sometimes, extensive involvement of such lesions by LCIS with reactive stromal changes will create cords of neoplastic cells, which can easily be misinterpreted as invasive carcinoma cells. However, myoepithelial markers will show a myoepithelial layer confirming the absence of invasion. Figures 6.14 and 6.15 show 2 such examples where the involvement of adenosis can simulate invasive carcinoma.

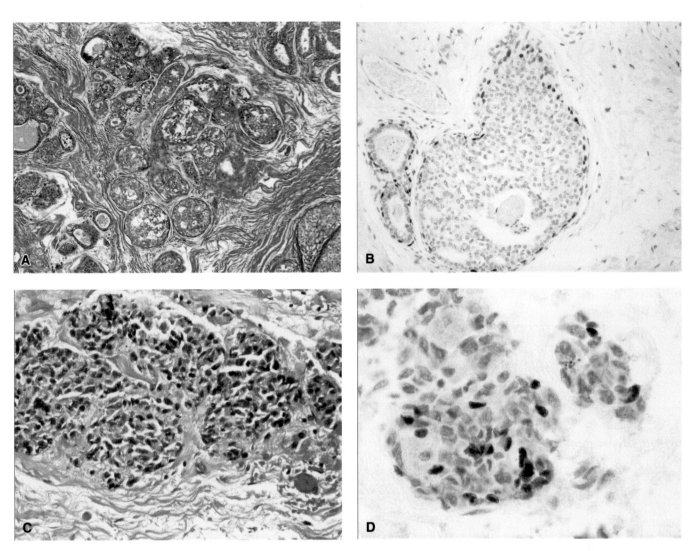

FIGURE 6.4 (A) The H&E stain shows DCIS with lobular extension. Note the smooth contours of the lobular units involved by DCIS. (B) Nuclear staining of myoepithelial cells stained with 4A4/P63. (C) The H&E stain shows a suspicious invasive area composed of somewhat crushed and distorted focus. (D) Staining with 4A4/P63 of this focus. The positive myoepithelial cells are peripherally oriented and are distorted mechanically due to crushing. This should not be interpreted as invasion.

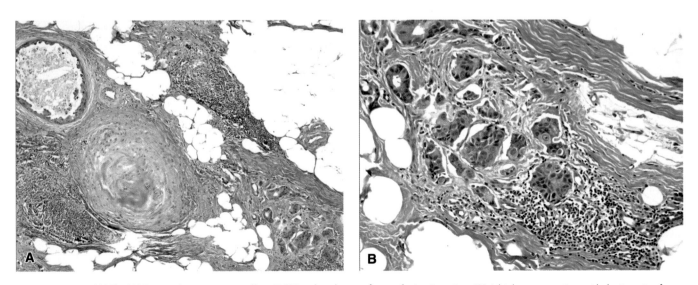

FIGURE 6.5 (A) The H&E stain shows micropapillary DCIS with a discrete focus of microinvasion. (B) A higher-power view with the invasive focus with micropapillary features.

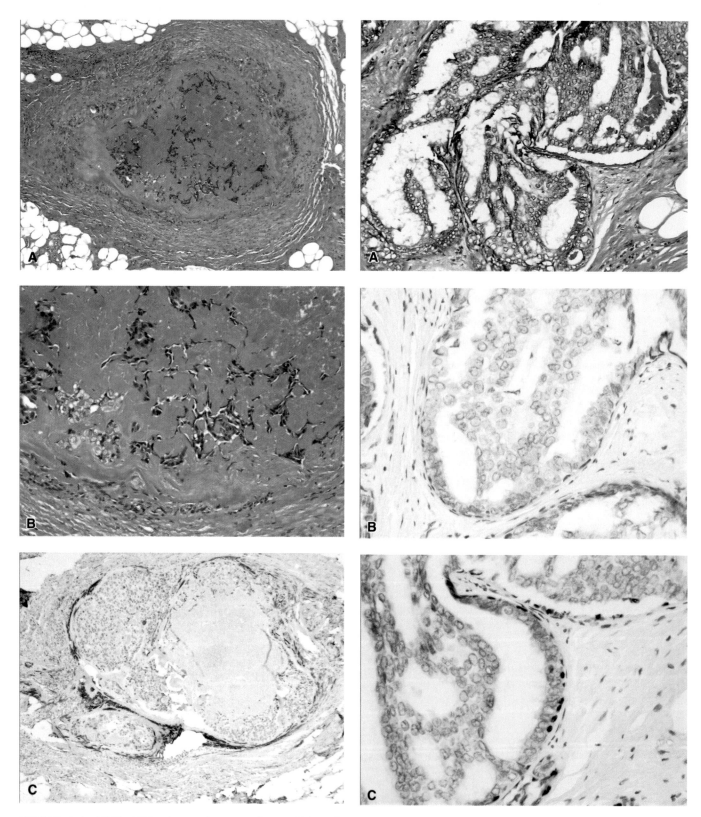

FIGURE 6.6 (A) The H&E stain scanning power shows a high-grade DCIS-like lesion with marked necrosis and architectural distortion. (B) The lesion at higher-power view suspicious for invasion. (C) Calponin stain showing peripheral band staining. Although no obvious myoepithelial cell layer is seen, the pattern suggests a duct wall with marked hyalinization and is best regarded as in situ carcinoma.

FIGURE 6.7 (A) The H&E stain shows an intermediate-grade DCIS with cribriform and micropapillary features and focal necrosis. (B) Negative calponin stain. (C) The same focus stained with 4A4/P63. There is crisp peripheral nuclear staining confirming that this is DCIS.

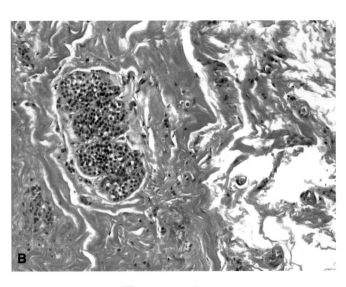

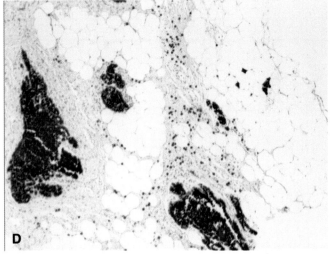

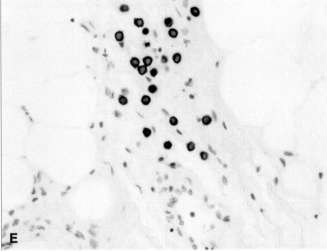

FIGURE 6.8 (A) The H&E stain scanning view shows LCIS. (B) A higher-power view that shows a few isolated atypical cells in the stroma, which on higher power, as seen in panel (C) have vacuolated cytoplasm and round nuclei representing invasive lobular carcinoma. (D) A scanning view of a keratin (AE1:AE3) stain showing numerous positive cells. (E) A high-power view of the tumor cells.

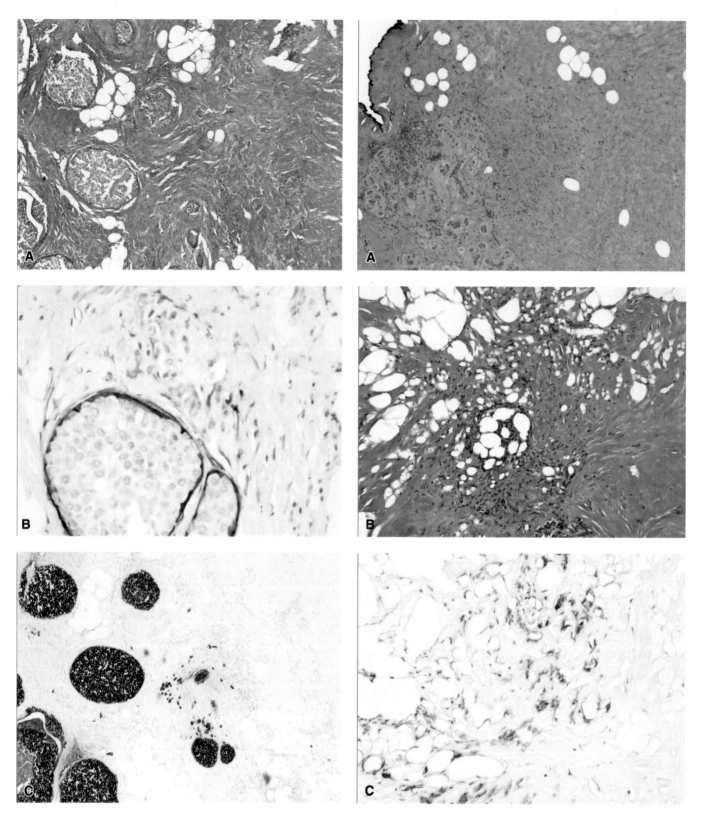

FIGURE 6.9 (A) The H&E stain shows LCIS in an excision specimen in a case that in core biopsy had invasive lobular carcinoma. No obvious invasion is seen. (B) A negative E-cadherin stain confirming the lobular phenotype. (C) A keratin (AE1:AE3) stain showing isolated keratin-positive infiltrating tumor cells.

FIGURE 6.10 (A) The H&E stain shows a microscopic focus of invasive lobular carcinoma. (B) A focus of crushed cells with a suspicious growth pattern for invasive carcinoma. (C) The cells are positive for keratin (AE1:AE3) confirming the presence of invasive carcinoma.

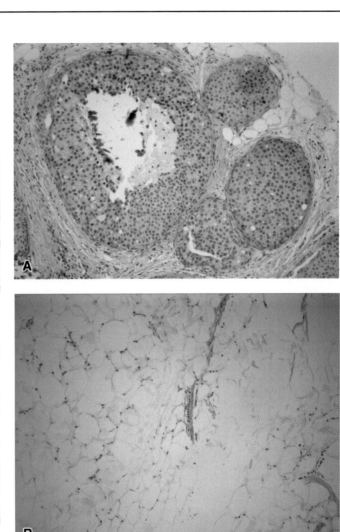

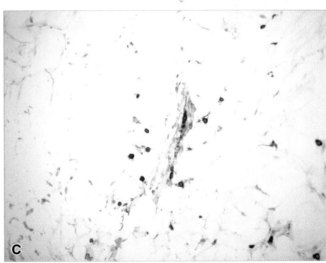

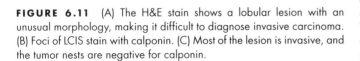

FIGURE 6.11   (A) The H&E stain shows a lobular lesion with an unusual morphology, making it difficult to diagnose invasive carcinoma. (B) Foci of LCIS stain with calponin. (C) Most of the lesion is invasive, and the tumor nests are negative for calponin.

FIGURE 6.12   (A) The H&E stain shows an unusual form of LCIS with acini that are large and expanded with necrosis and calcifications. (B) Very few atypical single cells scattered in the adipose tissue. (C) The cells are keratin (AE1:AE3)-positive, confirming the presence of invasive carcinoma.

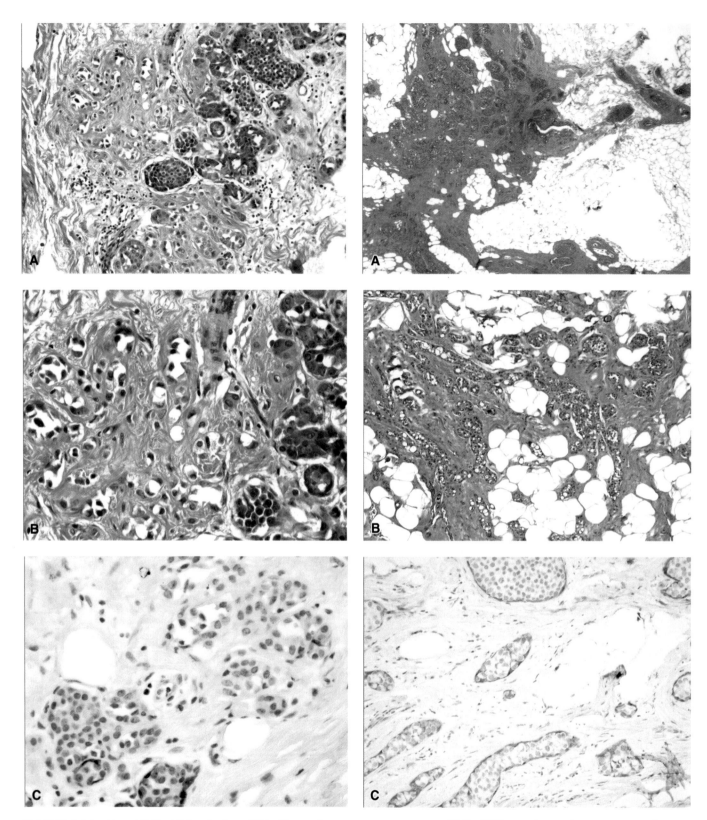

FIGURE 6.13   (A and B) The H&E stain shows LCIS with an adjacent proliferation of neoplastic cells. These cells are suspicious but do not have the usual diagnostic features of invasive lobular carcinoma. (C) Staining of the myoepithelial layer in LCIS, whereas the rest of the lesion is negative, confirming the presence of invasive carcinoma.

FIGURE 6.14   (A) The H&E stain shows a low-power view of a complex LCIS lesion involving sclerosing adenosis. (B) An area with LCIS involvement of adenosis simulating invasive carcinoma. (C) Calponin stain positivity, confirming the noninvasive nature of the lesion.

4. Microinvasion in association with precancerous lesion atypical ductal hyperplasia (ADH) and flat epithelial atypia (FEA): Similar to its association with DCIS and LCIS as illustrated above, microinvasion may be present in sections that primarily show ADH or FEA. Oftentimes, the invasive foci are of low grade (tubular carcinoma or classical invasive lobular carcinoma) and may be missed in the absence of meticulous examination of the sections. Immunostains may not be necessary to diagnose these lesions, as once recognized on the slide, the interpretation of invasion is usually obvious. It is important to note that on some occasions, the foci of invasion may be extremely small and easy to miss by oversight, and thus, awareness of the possibility of associated invasion should always be considered. Figure 6.16 shows one such example.

5. Mucinous carcinoma: Mucinous carcinoma is characterized by nests of infiltrating tumor cells with low-grade nuclei floating in pools of mucin. The

difficulty arises when there is DCIS in association with extravasated stromal mucin. The mere presence of mucin in the stroma should not lead to the diagnosis of invasive carcinoma or microinvasion. For invasion to be diagnosed, nests of tumor cells should be present within the mucin pools. In an otherwise benign mucocele-like lesion, there may be mucin extravasation due to rupture of the ducts and subsequent spillage of mucin into the stroma. In addition, nests of ductal cells may be mechanically transported within the mucin, and the presence of myoepithelial cells will confirm their benign nature. Similarly, it is possible that DCIS elements may be mechanically displaced into the mucin, and such a question would be resolved by the use of myoepithelial stains. Figure 6.17 illustrates one such example.

6. Invasion in solid/cystic papillary lesions: Assessment of invasion in papillary lesions, particularly the solid/cystic papillary carcinomas, can be particularly difficult. When unequivocal stromal invasion

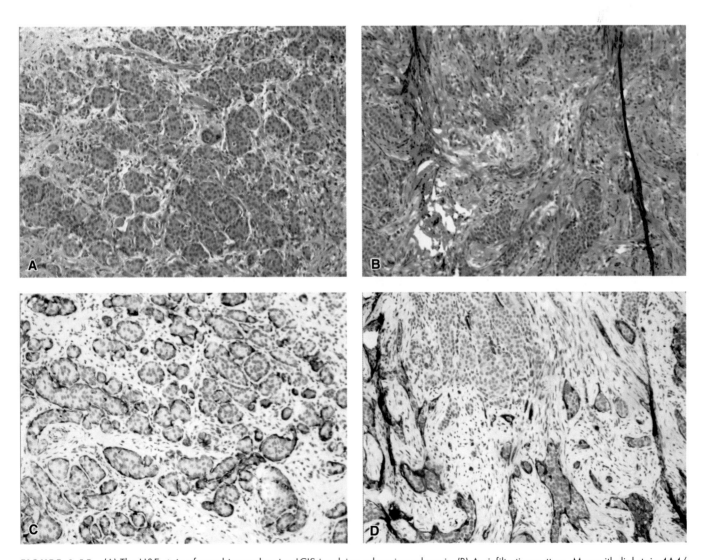

FIGURE 6.15 (A) The H&E stain of core biopsy showing LCIS involving sclerosing adenosis. (B) An infiltrative pattern. Myoepithelial stain 4A4/P63 reveals the noninvasive nature of this lesion as shown in panels (C) and (D).

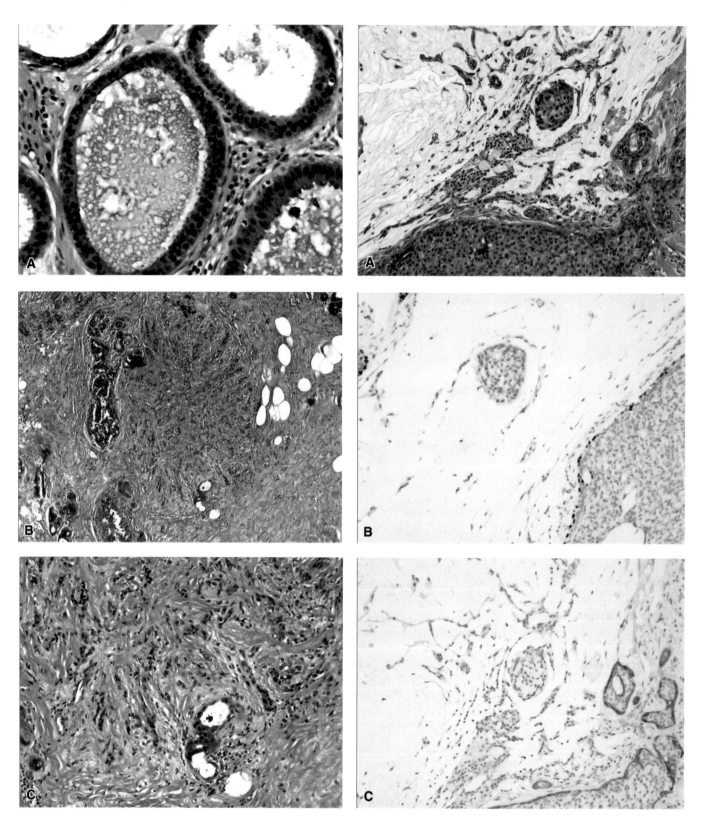

FIGURE 6.16 (A) The H&E stain shows a focus of FEA. (B and C) A focus of invasion in the same section.

FIGURE 6.17 (A) The H&E stain shows a mucin-producing lesion with a component of DCIS. A minute cluster of cells in the mucin pool are suspicious for invasion. (B) A 4A4/P63 stain that demonstrates that the cells are negative, supporting the diagnosis of invasion while the DCIS has a layer of myoepithelial cells. (C) Another area where the contour of the DCIS is irregular and would lead to suspect invasion with conventional stain; however, the 4A4 stain shows a layer of myoepithelial cells confirming absence of invasion in this area.

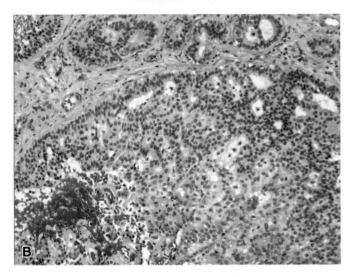

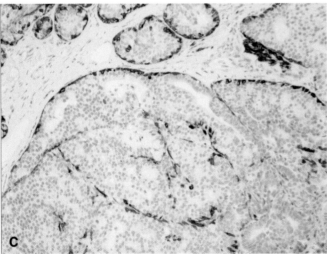

FIGURE 6.18 (A and B) The H&E stain shows a papillary lesion with a complex architecture and cytologic atypia consistent with a papillary carcinoma. (C) Calponin stain positivity in the peripheral layer of myoepithelial cells confirming the lack of invasion.

is present, the diagnosis is usually straightforward. Myoepithelial cell markers may be used to confirm invasion. Absence of staining with these markers around nests or cords of tumor cells within the reactive stroma at the periphery of the papillary lesion will support the diagnosis of invasion.

The difficulty arises when there is no obvious stromal invasion in the vicinity of the lesion that essentially has a circumscribed, solid, or cystic architecture. With myoepithelial stains, if a peripheral layer of myoepithelial cells can be demonstrated, then it is easy to confirm absence of invasion. Oftentimes however, lesions that appear to be noninvasive by conventional stains may not show a peripheral myoepithelial layer. On closer examination, such lesions may show irregular or "pushing" borders. Some regard these lesions as invasive and reserve the diagnosis of noninvasive papillary carcinoma for those lesions in which a peripheral layer of myoepithelial cells is present. Figures 6.18 to 6.20 illustrate examples of papillary lesions.

7. Nipple adenoma/florid adenomatosis of nipple: This is a benign proliferative lesion, and yet due to considerable architectural distortion, it may be misdiagnosed as invasive ductal carcinoma. Myoepithelial stains are of great value in these cases because they will reveal the presence of a peripheral myoepithelial layer and help confirm the diagnosis. In addition, the cells in these lesions lack atypical features. Figure 6.21 illustrates an example of nipple adenoma.

8. Sclerosing adenosis/radial scar lesion: These lesions may be misdiagnosed as invasive lesions, especially in core biopsies. Familiarity with the architectural features of these lesions is important to avoid this pitfall. Myoepithelial stains typically resolve the diagnostic dilemma. Figure 6.22 shows an example of sclerosing adenosis.

9. Tubular carcinoma versus adenosis: The individual glands in tubular carcinoma have sharp angulated edges in contrast to the somewhat blunted edges seen in the glands that compose adenosis. Myoepithelial stains will almost always make the distinction clear so their use is recommended to confirm the diagnosis. However, the use of such stains may not always be necessary because the morphologic features are usually sufficiently typical. Figure 6.23 shows an example of tubular carcinoma.

10. Tubular carcinoma versus microglandular adenosis: As discussed above, the morphologic features of tubular carcinoma are fairly distinct. In contrast, individual acini in microglandular adenosis are rounded and usually contain intraluminal eosinophilic secretions at least in some acini. Myoepithelial markers are of little use in the distinction because

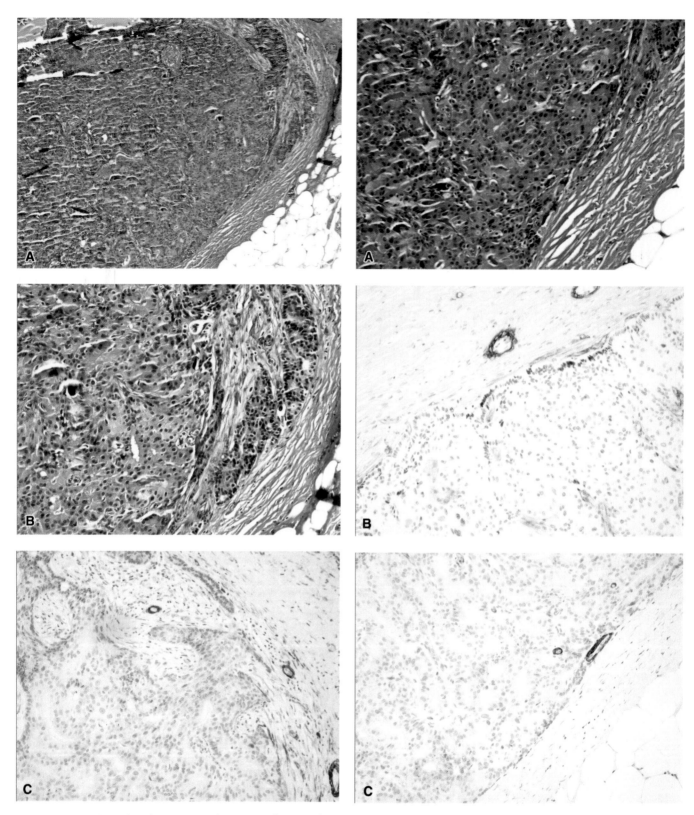

FIGURE 6.19 (A and B) The H&E stain shows a papillary neoplasm with an area suggestive of stromal microinvasion. (C) A calponin stain that is negative for a peripheral myoepithelial layer supporting the presence of unequivocal stromal invasion.

FIGURE 6.20 (A) The H&E stain shows a papillary neoplasm with a rather smooth contour at its interface with the stroma. However, panels (B) (calponin) and (C) (collagen IV) show no evidence of myoepithelial layer or basement membrane at the periphery of this lesion supporting the presence of invasive carcinoma.

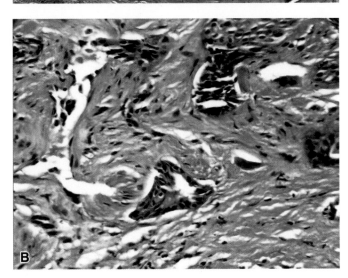

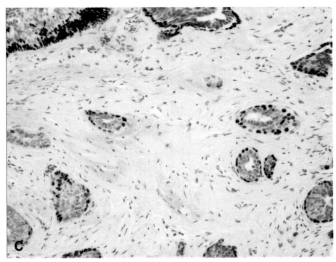

FIGURE 6.21 (A) The H&E stain of a nipple adenoma. Note the infiltrative growth pattern simulating invasive carcinoma. (B) A higher-power view of glandular structures with angulated edges reminiscent of tubular carcinoma. The glandular structures are benign and show a peripheral myoepithelial layer as seen in panel (C) (4A4/P63 stain).

the myoepithelial layer is absent in the acini of microglandular adenosis. Instead, the cells lining the microglandular adenosis are S-100–positive and have a collagen layer surrounding the acini.

11. Mechanical displacement of ductal epithelium in biopsy tract: This is an important pitfall to remember. Significantly, the use of myoepithelial markers may not help, as even benign clusters of ductal cells trapped within the scarred stroma of the biopsy tract may be devoid of a myoepithelial layer. It is therefore important to recognize the biopsy tract and avoid the diagnosis of microinvasion/microscopic invasion. On some occasions, the malignant epithelium may also be mechanically transported into the tract, and the presence of such clusters does not equate to invasion.

■ IMMUNOHISTOCHEMISTRY

Immunohistochemistry using myoepithelial markers is a standard practice in the evaluation of lesions where there is a suspicion of microinvasion.

Rather than using only one marker, it is important to use a panel of such markers or at least 2 markers. This will help minimize the possibility of false-negative results. Various myoepithelial markers have been described, such as S-100 protein, glial fibrillary acidic protein (GFAP), smooth muscle actin, smooth muscle myosin, CD10, calponin, and 4A4 (p63). S-100 protein, GFAP, and smooth muscle actin are not used as frequently as the others due to either lack of sensitivity or specificity. It is best to test these antibodies in the laboratory and to include them in the panel that gives the best results. The use of myoepithelial markers is particularly helpful in the evaluation of lesions such as sclerosing adenosis, radial scar, and papillary lesion to exclude invasion.

In some situations, keratin antibodies such as AE1:AE3 can help in highlighting scattered single cells. These antibodies are particularly useful in the evaluation of lobular lesion or in cases where there is extensive DCIS with dense lymphocytic infiltrates.

■ MANAGEMENT

The prognosis of MIC is excellent. Currently, MIC is treated by surgery (usually lumpectomy or in some occasions with mastectomy), followed by radiation in cases treated with lumpectomy. Generally, patients with MIC are not treated with chemotherapy, except for Tamoxifen in cases where the tumor is ER-positive. Patients with a diagnosis of MIC will get a sentinel node biopsy as part of their management.

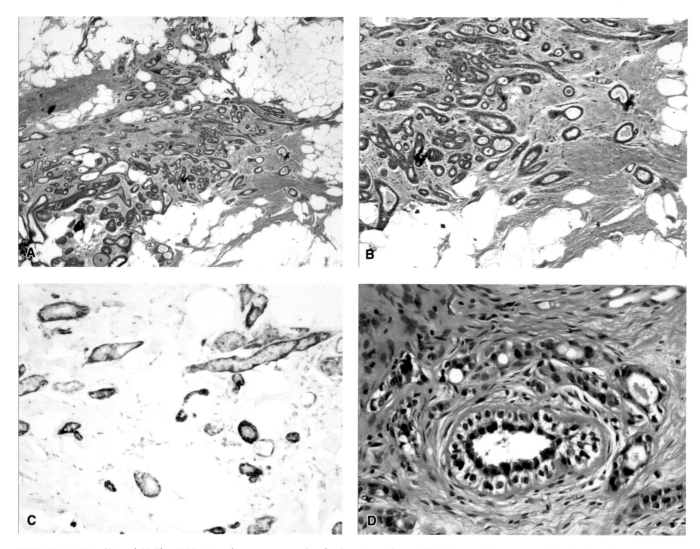

FIGURE 6.22 (A and B) The H&E stain shows an example of sclerosing adenosis that in core biopsy may simulate invasive carcinomas. (C) Calponin stain with complete peripheral layer of myoepithelial cells. (D) A rather prominent myoepithelial cell layer lining a duct, however, in the acini arranged circumferentially around the duct in a "targetoid" fashion; the bilayering, a hallmark of benignancy, is not obvious.

■ KEY POINTS

1. Microinvasive carcinoma is defined as an invasive carcinoma that measures 1 mm or less. When multiple foci are noted, they should not be greater than 1 mm, and the measurements of individual foci may not be added.

2. A lesion may be classified as MIC on excision or mastectomy specimens. The diagnosis should be avoided in core biopsy specimens. Other terms such as *microscopic foci of invasion*, *microscopic invasion*, or *microinvasion* may be used to describe the minimal invasion seen in such specimens.

3. Careful and meticulous examination of the sections is the most important prerequisite in the diagnosis of MIC.

4. Extensive high-grade DCIS with dense lymphocytic infiltrates: microinvasion typically occurs in the form of single cells or minute tumor clusters in the inflamed stroma. The use of keratin stains enhances the detection of microinvasion unless there is distortion of the duct architecture in which case myoepithelial cell markers should be used.

5. Microinvasion in lobular carcinoma may be difficult to detect, and the pathologist should be alert when examining foci of LCIS.

6. Remain alert to the possibility of microinvasion when precancerous changes such as ADH or FEA appear to be the dominant lesional change.

7. Mechanically displaced benign epithelial elements may mimic microinvasion.

8. Lesions such as sclerosing adenosis, radial scar lesions, and nipple adenoma may cause diagnostic difficulties leading to misdiagnosis of invasion especially in core biopsies.

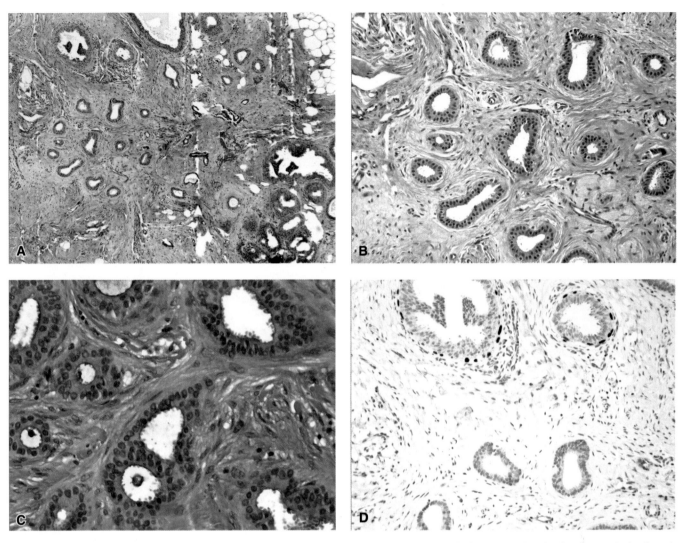

FIGURE 6.23 (A) The H&E stain illustrates an atypical tubular proliferation in the background of ADH. (B) The glands composed of cells with atypical low-grade nuclei. The differential diagnosis is between a small tubular carcinoma and adenosis. (C) An example of a typical tubular carcinoma with the classical glandular configuration. (D) A 4Aa/P63 stain, whereas the atypical hyperplasia shows a myoepithelial layer and the atypical glands are negative confirming the diagnosis of carcinoma.

9. When required, more than one myoepithelial marker should be routinely used. Keratin immunostains are in some instances very useful; however, these stains should be interpreted in the context of changes seen in sections stained with H&E.

■ REFERENCES

1. Bianchi S, Vezzosi V. Microinvasive carcinoma of the breast. *Pathol Oncol Res.* 2008;14:105–111.
2. Renshaw AA. Minimal (< or =0.1 cm) invasive carcinoma in breast core needle biopsies. Incidence, sampling, associated findings and follow-up. *Arch Pathol Lab Med.* 2004;128:996–999.
3. Solin LJ, Fowble BL, Yeh IT, et al. Microinvasive ductal carcinoma of the breast treated with breast conserving surgery and definitive irradiation. *Int J Radiat Oncol Biol Phys.* 1992;23:961–968.
4. Schuh ME, Nemoto T, Penetrante RB, et al. Intraductal carcinoma. Analysis of presentation, pathologic findings, and outcome of disease. *Arch Surg.* 1986;121:1303–1307.
5. Nevin JE, Pinz AG, Moran TJ, Baggerly JT. Minimal breast carcinoma. *Am J Surg.* 1980;139:357–359.
6. Yang M, Moriya T, Oguma M, et al. Microinvasive ductal carcinoma (T1mic) of the breast. The clinicopathological profile and immunohistochemical features of 28 cases. *Pathol Int.* 2003;53:422–428.
7. Prasad ML, Osborne MP, GiriDD, Hoda SA. Microinvasive carcinoma (T1mic) of the breast: clinicopathologic profile of 21 cases. *Am J Surg Pathol.* 2000;24:422–428.
8. Ellis IO, Lee AH, Elstom CW, Pinder SE. Microinvasive carcinoma of the breast: diagnostic criteria and clinical relevance. *Histopathology.* 1999;35:470–472.
9. Prasad ML, Osborne MP, Hoda SA. Observations on the histopathologic diagnosis of microinvasive carcinoma of the breast. *Anat Pathol.* 1998;3:209–212.
10. Schnitt SJ. Microinvasive carcinoma of the breast: a diagnosis in search of a definition. *Adv Anat Pathol.* 1998;5:367–372.

7

Carcinomas With Good Prognosis

MELINDA E. SANDERS

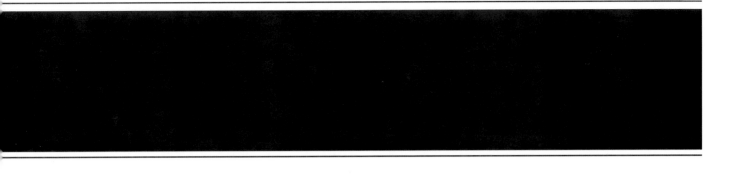

Recognition of specific constellations of histologic features defining "special types" of invasive breast carcinoma allows for the identification of women with good to excellent prognoses, often approaching or equaling that of women in the general population, from among those with "no special type" aka infiltrating ductal carcinomas. Most special-type carcinomas have indolent behavior warranting less-aggressive treatment (with special problems for medullary), compared with no special type carcinomas of similar grade and stage. The distinguishing features of special-type breast cancers are present in "classic" form in the "pure" examples of these cases. It is equally important to recognize that these features may be present in lesser degrees in many carcinomas of no special type, where they do not portend the same excellent prognosis but still have important clinical correlates.

■ PURE TUBULAR CARCINOMA

Pathologic Features

The morphologic features of tubular carcinoma were first described over a century ago by Cornil and Ranvier but received little attention until the last 20 years because they are rarely symptomatic. Only recently, with the advent of mammographic screening programs, have these usually small, indolent, nonpalpable tumors regularly reached clinical attention (1). Tubular carcinomas are usually detected by their spiculated appearance and occasionally by the presence of microcalcifications but may have subtle mammographic findings (2,3). They are usually incidental findings on screening mammography and not associated with a palpable mass on physical examination. Pure tubular carcinoma accounts for 1% to 2% of invasive cancers in the premammographic era series (4,5). The frequency of cases now reported by mammographic screening is 9% to 19% (1,6–11). Grossly, no specific features, except small size, distinguish tubular cancer from other tumor types. Tubular carcinomas usually measure between 2.0 mm and 2.0 cm, with most measuring less than 1.0 cm (5,12,13). Occasional cases can reach 3.0 cm.

Because tubular areas are found focally in many breast cancers, specific criteria for the diagnosis of tubular carcinoma must be used so that the excellent prognosis applies. Pure tubular carcinoma should be diagnosed when greater than 90% of the lesion demonstrates a haphazard infiltration of distinctly tubular structures lined by a single layer of epithelial cells with the remainder of the tumor showing the same well-differentiated morphology (14) (Figure 7.1). The tubules may be round, oval, or "bent teardrop" shaped (Figure 7.2). The epithelial cells lining the tubules are small and round with minimal pleomorphism. Mitotic figures are essentially absent. Apical snouts are seen in at least one third of cases (15) but are not specific (Figure 7.3).

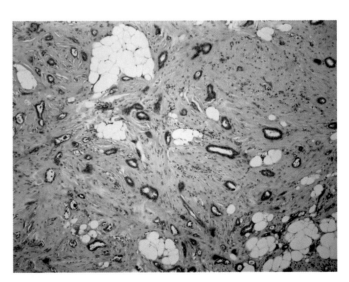

FIGURE 7.1 Pure tubular carcinoma showing a haphazard arrangement of very low grade tubules lined by a single layer of myoepithelial cells.

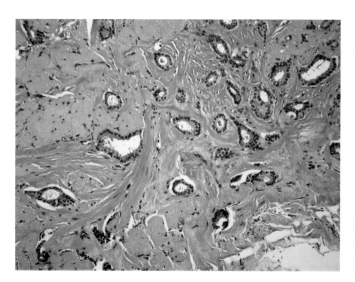

FIGURE 7.2 Pure tubular carcinoma with bent teardrop and ovoid glands admixed with elastosis and densely collagenized stroma.

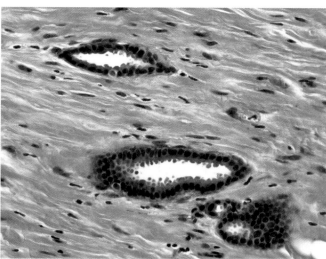

FIGURE 7.3 High-power view of the typical angulated tubules present in tubular carcinomas characterized by a single-cell layer and apical snouts.

Fine calcifications may be present in the lumina in occasional cases (12,16). This is in agreement with the current World Health Organization classification (17). We regard tumors containing between 70% and 89% tubules as tubular variant carcinomas, and we designate tumors containing less than 70% of the classic tubules as "no special type tumors" with tubular features. Multiple studies indicating that tubular histology is of prognostic value and that the greater the purity of the pattern, the more favorable the prognosis justifies these divisions (4,18–20). Several studies have now demonstrated that when greater than 90% purity of pattern is observed, an excellent prognosis can be expected, even in the presence of a positive lymph node (18–20). Patients with pure tubular carcinoma can expect survival rates similar to the general population (20).

An additional diagnostic consideration is the coexistence of mixed tubular and invasive cribriform carcinomas (ICCs) (14,21). Essentially, any combination of these 2 elements conveys the same excellent prognosis as a pure tubular carcinoma (Figure 7.4). This is an important consideration, as many such cases may be assigned to the no special type group by an inexperienced pathologist or clinician and this potentially useful prognostic information may be lost.

Low-grade cribriform or micropapillary ductal carcinoma in situ and atypical ductal hyperplasia are usually found in association with tubular carcinoma and are usually centrally located within the lesion (Figure 7.5). Occasionally, tubular carcinoma is associated with atypical lobular hyperplasia or lobular carcinoma in situ (13).

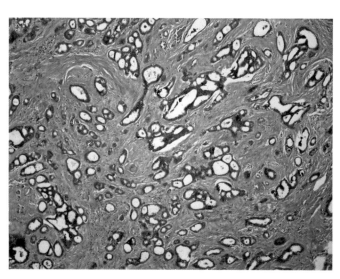

FIGURE 7.4 Invasive carcinoma showing a mixture of invasive tubular and ICC. These 2 patterns in any proportion portend the same excellent prognosis as pure tubular carcinoma.

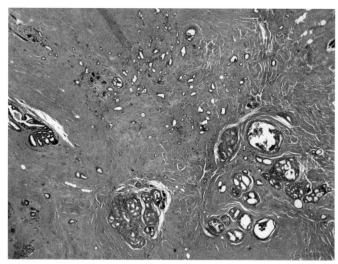

FIGURE 7.5 Low-grade cribriform ductal carcinoma in situ is commonly associated with pure tubular carcinoma.

In some cases, the tumor may be seen in association with a radial scar or complex sclerosing lesion. In such cases, tumor involvement is usually focal, with neoplastic tubules surrounding normal structures associated with the radial scar/complex sclerosing lesion and infiltration of the neoplastic tubules into the adjacent adipose tissue.

Immunohistochemistry

Tubular carcinoma is essentially always estrogen receptor– (Figure 7.6) and progesterone receptor–positive, has a low growth fraction as demonstrated by Ki-67 staining, rare, if any, mitoses, and is HER2/neu- and epidermal growth factor receptor (EGFR)-negative (20,22). Distinction of tubular carcinoma from adenosis or entrapped benign tubules in a radial scar may be facilitated by immunohistochemical staining for myoepithelial cells. In our practice, we use p63 (Figure 7.7) and smooth muscle actin. These stains are negative in tubular carcinomas but should be interpreted with caution because they may occasionally be negative in benign glands entrapped in sclerosis.

Management

For pure tubular carcinomas, the excellent prognosis indicates that conservative but complete surgical excision is adequate therapy for the overwhelming majority of cases (16). Since the addition of radiation or chemotherapy does not improve disease-free survival or overall survival, they should not be advocated (18,23,24). Similarly, involvement of axillary lymph nodes is an uncommon finding and does not adversely affect outcome (25). We would advocate performance of a sentinel node biopsy at the time of definitive surgery only for large tumors, which may not have been adequately sampled at the time of core biopsy (22). Because pure tubular carcinomas are estrogen receptor–positive, endocrine therapy with tamoxifen or aromatase

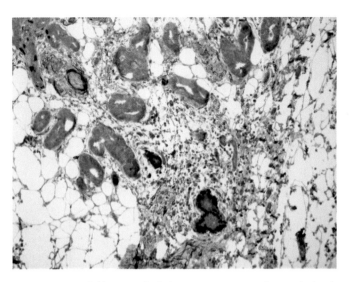

FIGURE 7.7 Infiltration of tubular carcinoma around normal glands is common and can be distinguished by the use of immunohistochemical stains for myoepithelial cells. Note in this case the absence of p63 staining in the invasive tubules.

inhibitors (for postmenopausal women) is usually considered, although it should be recognized that such therapy likely benefits most women by reducing the incidence of subsequent contralateral tumors rather impacting their survival. Based on limited series and long-term follow-up data, there seems to be no role for adjuvant chemotherapy in the treatment of pure tubular carcinomas, regardless of tumor size or lymph node involvement (20).

Key Points

- The frequency of tubular carcinoma now reported by mammographic screening series is between 9% and 19%.
- A diagnosis of pure tubular carcinoma should be reserved for cases where greater than 90% of the lesion demonstrates a haphazard infiltration of distinctly tubular structures lined by a single layer of epithelial cells with the remainder of the tumor showing the same well-differentiated morphology.
- Using this definition, an excellent prognosis can be expected, even in the presence of a positive lymph node.
- Tumors showing a mixture of pure tubular and pure ICC in any ratio convey the same excellent prognosis as pure tubular carcinoma.
- Tubular carcinoma is essentially always estrogen receptor– and progesterone receptor–positive and negative for HER2/neu overexpression.
- Distinction of tubular carcinoma from adenosis or entrapped benign tubules in a radial scar may be facilitated by immunohistochemical staining for myoepithelial cells.
- Conservative but complete surgical excision without a sentinel node biopsy is adequate therapy for the overwhelming majority of cases.

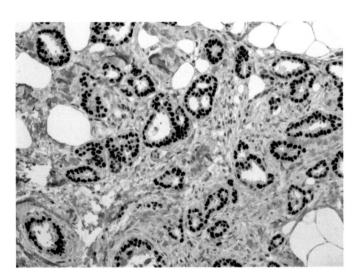

FIGURE 7.6 Tubular carcinomas are essentially 100% estrogen receptor–positive as seen in this case.

■ INVASIVE CRIBRIFORM CARCINOMA

Pathologic Features

Invasive cribriform carcinoma is uncommon, representing approximately 0.08% to 3.5% of invasive breast carcinomas (26–28), and is closely related to tubular carcinoma. Most women presenting with ICC are in their sixth decade (26–27). Radiologically, these tumors have a spiculated appearance and are associated with microcalcifications. The average size at presentation ranges from 2.5 to 3.0 cm, and there are no distinctive gross findings.

Histologically, pure ICC is composed of infiltrating islands of tumor cells with a cribriform architecture (Figure 7.8), which may on some occasions be difficult to distinguish from cribriform ductal carcinoma in situ (Figure 7.9). By definition, these tumors are of low combined Nottingham grade. The tumor cells have low- to intermediate-grade nuclei and scant to moderate pale cytoplasm. Individual tumor islands contain bars and arches of cells creating well-defined spaces (Figure 7.10). To make a diagnosis of pure ICC, more than 90% of the tumor must have a cribriform architecture, unless the noncribriform areas represent less than 50% of the tumor and have a tubular morphology (17,27). Mixed tubular and cribriform carcinomas in any proportion have the same excellent prognosis as pure tubular carcinomas (14,21). There is usually a desmoplastic stromal response that is occasionally associated with a giant cell reaction accompanied by hemosiderin (Figure 7.11), which is of no known clinical significance (14). Associated cribriform ductal carcinoma in situ is present in 50% to 80% of cases.

Similar to tubular carcinoma, the prognosis is excellent despite the presence of lymph node metastases in approximately 14% of patients (27). Similar to pure tubular

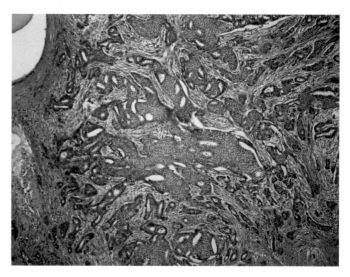

FIGURE 7.9 Pure ICC with a large branching island of tumor. It cannot be determined with certainty whether this island represents in situ or invasive carcinoma. Fortunately, in this case, this distinction is unimportant.

carcinoma, metastases tend to involve a single node and rarely up to 3 nodes. In Page's original series, none of the patients died from ICC of the breast during an average of 14.5 years of follow-up (27). A 100% 5-year survival rate was also confirmed in a subsequent study (26).

The differential diagnosis for ICC includes adenoid cystic carcinoma (ACC), cribriform ductal carcinoma in situ, and no special type carcinoma with cribriform features. Adenoid cystic carcinoma can be excluded by demonstrating lack of a dual-cell population utilizing immunohistochemical stains for myoepithelial markers throughout the tumor, whereas the presence of a surrounding myoepithelial layer

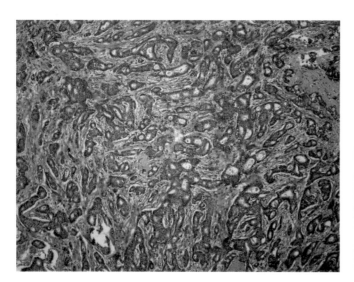

FIGURE 7.8 Pure ICC showing infiltrating islands of tumor cells with a cribriform architecture.

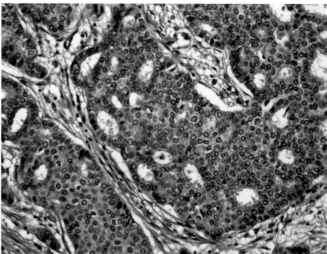

FIGURE 7.10 High-power view of ICC showing well-differentiated cribriform spaces with tumor cells polarized around the intercellular lumina. Note the intermediate-grade nuclei in this case.

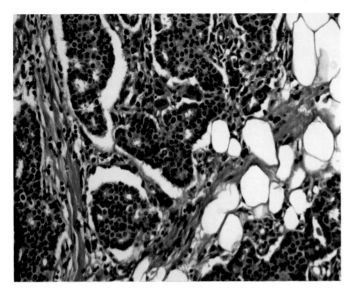

FIGURE 7.11 Occasionally, pure ICC will be associated with hemosiderin and osteoclast-like giant cells. This phenomenon is of no known significance.

and maintenance of a normal ductal and lobular architectural arrangement can be useful in distinguishing cribriform ductal carcinoma in situ from ICC. No special type invasive carcinomas show greater than 50% noncribriform/nontubular areas.

Immunohistochemistry

Virtually 100% of cases are estrogen receptor–positive, and 70% are progesterone receptor–positive. HER-2/neu is negative.

Management

Complete surgical excision accompanied by sentinel node biopsy is the usual surgical approach. Subsequent treatment with adjuvant hormone therapy is standard.

Key Points

- Invasive cribriform carcinoma is uncommon, representing approximately 0.08% to 3.5% of invasive breast carcinomas.
- Histologically, pure ICC is of low combined Nottingham grade and composed of infiltrating islands of tumor cells with a cribriform architecture.
- A diagnosis of pure ICC should be reserved for low combined histologic grade tumors where greater than 90% of the tumor has a cribriform architecture, unless the noncribriform areas represent less than 50% of the tumor and have a tubular morphology.
- Mixed tubular and cribriform carcinomas in any proportion have the same excellent prognosis as pure tubular carcinomas.

- Virtually 100% of ICC are estrogen receptor–positive, and 70% are progesterone receptor–positive; there is no overexpression of HER-2/neu.
- Similar to tubular carcinoma, the prognosis is excellent despite the presence of lymph node metastases in approximately 14% of patients.

■ PURE INVASIVE LOBULAR CARCINOMA

Pathologic Features

Pure invasive lobular carcinoma accounts for 4% of all invasive breast carcinomas (29), and its variants account for another 5% to 10% (26) depending on the stringency of the criteria. This problem of definition has lead to significant confusion regarding the prognostic implication for invasive lobular carcinoma, which varies in the literature from better (29–35), no different (36-38), to worse than no special type (ductal) carcinomas. Very stringent criteria should be used for the diagnosis of pure or classic invasive lobular carcinoma, which must be by definition of low Nottingham combined histologic grade and show a greater than 90% single-file cellular infiltration pattern by bland-appearing tumor cells with exclusively low-grade nuclei (14,26,29) (Figures 7.12 and 7.13). These features identify an excellent prognosis (39) as carefully reported by Wheeler et al (29) and repeated by several other investigators utilizing well-characterized cohorts (29–35), especially when the tumor is less than 1.0 cm. This prognosis lies somewhere between the prognosis of pure tubular carcinoma and no special type tumors in general (39). Variant patterns were carefully defined in the 1970s, 1980s, and early 1990s, which include

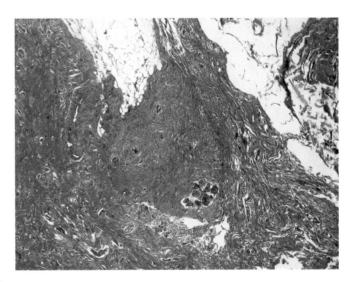

FIGURE 7.12 Low-power view of a small pure invasive lobular carcinoma is identified in the center of the photomicrograph as a subtle increase in cellularity in a background of dense fibrosis.

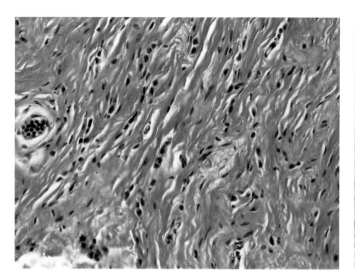

FIGURE 7.13 High-power view of pure invasive lobular carcinoma characterized by small, bland, regular nuclei infiltrating in a subtle single-file fashion with essentially no cellular nesting or desmoplastic response.

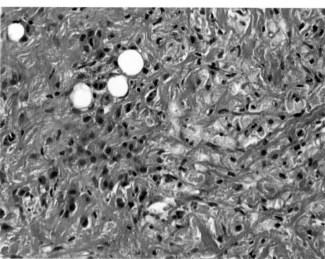

FIGURE 7.14 The cytoplasm of pure invasive lobular carcinoma is usually scant and basophilic (left), but occasionally, it may have a foamy to granular appearance, which could be mistaken for a granular cell tumor (right).

solid, alveolar, mixed, and pleomorphic types (40–45). Recognition that these variants identify intermediate and even high combined histologic grade tumors is critical because they imply a prognosis generally similar to no special type carcinomas of similar grade and stage (40,46,47), contrasting them with the excellent prognosis of pure invasive lobular carcinoma (29–35). Thus, grading of invasive lobular carcinoma and recognition that one is dealing with a lobular variant carcinoma are paramount, whereas diagnosis of specific variants is of historic rather than practical importance.

The average age of women presenting with invasive lobular carcinoma is 63 years (range, 54–67 years). Some reported series implicate postmenopausal hormone therapy as increasing risk for these tumors (48,49). Invasive lobular carcinoma may present mammographically as an assymetric density or as a discrete mass. The only abnormality, if any, detectable on physical examination may be a poorly defined, often subtle, thickening without discrete margins. Invasive lobular carcinoma is often multicentric in the ipsilateral breast and more commonly bilateral than other breast cancer types (46,50,51).

Grossly invasive lobular carcinoma varies from a poorly defined fibrous area to a firm, gritty tumor indistinguishable from no special type carcinomas. Histologically, lobular carcinomas show considerable variabilty, with the pure or classic invasive lobular carcinoma characterized by small, regular nuclei and a diffuse single-cell infiltration pattern as discused above (Figures 7.12 and 7.13). These must be low combined histologic grade, with a score of 3 for tubules, 1 for nuclear pleomorphism, and 1 for rare if any detectable mitoses. The cells may contain intracytoplasmic lumina, which may become large enough to have a signet ring cell appearance in the tubular variant

carcinomas. Pure lobular carcinoma usually has scant basophilic cytoplasm; however, occasionally, it may have a foamy to granular appearance (Figure 7.14), which may be mistaken for a granular cell tumor. Tumor cells frequently create a targetoid pattern around mammary ducts (Figure 7.15). Atypical lobular hyperplasia and lobular carcinoma in situ coexist in 70% to 80% of cases (29,46,52) (Figure 7.16). Especially in the case of pure lobular carcinoma, the tumor cells frequently do not incite a desmoplastic stromal response, invading the mammary parenchyma in an insidious manner (Figure 7.13). Occasionally, pure invasive lobular carcinoma is associated with a myxoid stroma (Figure 7.17). Among the approximately 10% of invasive carcinomas, which we call lobular variant carcinomas, most are

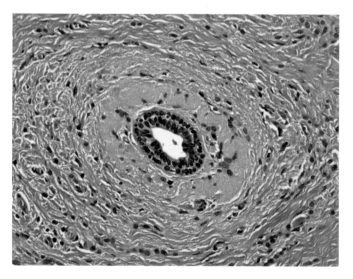

FIGURE 7.15 Pure invasive lobular carcinoma often creates a targetoid pattern as it encircles benign mammary ducts.

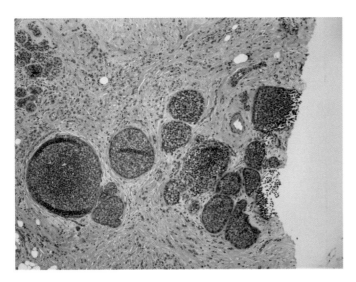

FIGURE 7.16 Invasive lobular carcinoma associated with lobular carcinoma in situ (center) and atypical lobular hyperplasia (upper left).

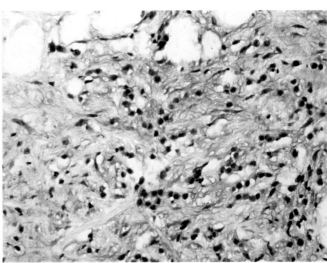

FIGURE 7.17 Pure invasive lobular carcinoma with associated myxoid stroma.

grade 2 using the Nottinghan combined histologic grade, with a score of 2 or 3 for nuclear pleomorphism (Figure 7.18). Although still discohesive, the cells of lobular variant carcinomas demonstrate prominent nesting (Figure 7.19) and occasionally solid (Figure 7.20A–B), trabecular, and alveolar growth patterns.

Tubulolobular carcinoma, first recognized by Fisher et al (53), is best considered a rare variant of invasive lobular carcinoma consisting of a mixture of pure tubular and pure lobular carcinoma (Figure 7.21). Histologically, single-file and often nested lobular carcinoma cells are admixed or separated regionally within the same tumor mass. All the nuclei must be low grade (14). The prognosis is intermediate between a pure tubular carcinoma and a low-grade, no special type carcinoma.

The designation pleomorphic invasive lobular carcinoma (44,45) has been used for bizarre, high-grade neoplasms with large nuclei and high mitotic rates (Figure 7.22). These tumors have been shown to have a poor prognosis (44,45,54,55) and share molecular features with atypical lobular hyperplasia and pure invasive lobular carcinoma, as well as with high-grade ductal carcinoma in situ and high-grade, no special type invasive carcinomas (56–57). These findings further highlight the wide spectrum of the disease, which may be grouped by inexperienced pathologists under the diagnosis

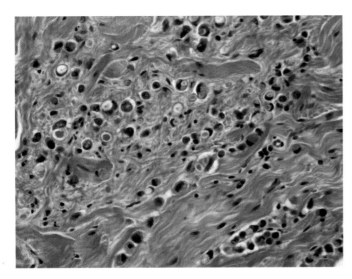

FIGURE 7.18 Invasive lobular variant carcinoma with grade 2 and a few grade 3 nuclei.

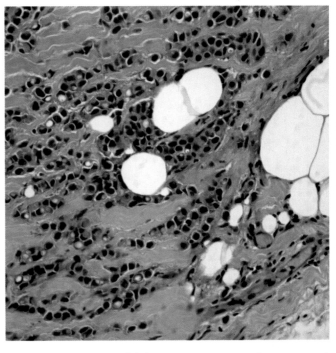

FIGURE 7.19 Invasive lobular variant carcinoma with prominent cellular nesting, grade 2 nuclei, and scattered signet ring cells.

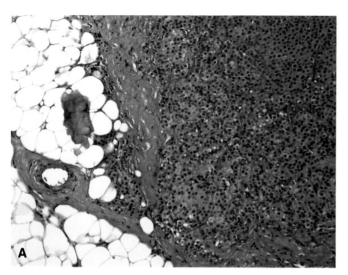
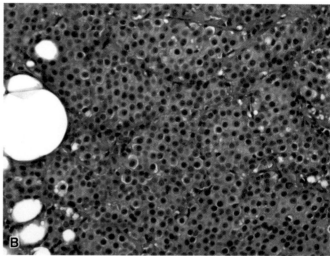

FIGURE 7.20 (A) Solid variant of invasive lobular carcinoma at low power shows a solid, circumscribed mass of invasive lobular carcinoma cells. (B) The discohesive lobular carcinoma cells and occasional intracytoplasmic vacuoles can be seen at higher power.

of invasive lobular carcinoma, obscuring the excellent prognosis of pure invasive lobular carcinoma.

A final special feature of invasive lobular carcinoma worth mentioning is its association with particular patterns of distant metastases. Extensive involvement of bone, peritoneal surfaces, and the gastrointestinal tract is most often seen with invasive lobular carcinomas, pure and variant (26,51).

Immunohistochemistry

Pure invasive lobular carcinomas are strongly estrogen receptor– and progesterone receptor–positive and are

negative for HER2 overexpression. The loosely cohesive phenotype of invasive lobular carcinoma (as well as atypical lobular hyperplasia and lobular carcinoma in situ) is attributed to the loss of expression of E-cadherin as a result of mutation, loss of heterozygosity at 16q22.1, or silencing of expression by promotor methylation (58–62). Approximately 95% of invasive lobular carcinomas show loss of E-cadherin expression (63); however, expression of E-cadherin does not exclude a diagnosis of lobular carcinoma in the presence of the typical diagnostic features. The pleomorphic variant usually shows a less intense expression of estrogen and progesterone receptors and may demonstrate HER2/neu overexpression (64).

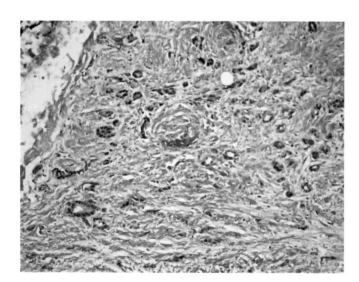
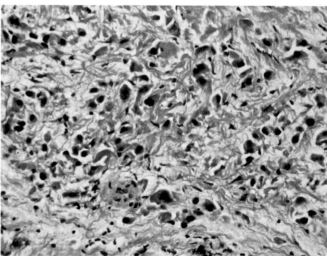

FIGURE 7.21 Tubulolobular carcinoma shows the classic angulated tubules of tubular carcinoma admixed with single-file invasive lobular carcinoma cells.

FIGURE 7.22 Pleomorphic lobular carcinoma shows the typical discohesive histology of lobular carcinoma but by definition has grade 3 nuclei and an intermediate to high proliferative rate.

Management

Breast conservation with sentinel node biopsy may be an adequate treatment for smaller lobular carcinomas, whereas women with multifocal disease and or large tumors may require mastectomy to ensure complete excision. Approximately 40% of patients develop axillary node metastases, and 8% have distant metastases (51). Contralateral mastectomy should be considered prophylactic in the absence of biopsy-proven in situ or invasive carcinoma.

Key Points

- Pure invasive lobular carcinoma accounts for 4% of all invasive breast carcinomas, and its variants account for another 5% to 10% depending on the stringency of the criteria.
- Very stringent criteria should be used for the diagnosis of pure or classic invasive lobular carcinoma, which must be by definition of low Nottingham combined histologic grade and show a greater than 90% single-file cellular infiltration pattern by bland-appearing tumor cells with exclusively low-grade nuclei.
- Accurate reporting of the Nottingham combined histologic grade for all lobular variant carcinomas is critical to ensure proper treatment and assignment of prognosis.
- Pure invasive lobular carcinomas are strongly estrogen receptor– and progesterone receptor–positive and are negative for HER2 overexpression.
- Breast conservation with sentinel node biopsy may be an adequate treatment for smaller lobular carcinomas, whereas women with multifocal disease and or large tumors may require mastectomy to ensure complete excision.

■ PURE MEDULLARY CARCINOMA

Pathologic Features

Pure medullary carcinoma is rare, representing approximately 1% of all invasive breast carcinomas, when strict diagnostic criteria are applied (65). Node-negative pure medullary carcinoma predicts a good prognosis; otherwise, the predictive utility is unclear (14).

Most women with medullary carcinoma present at a younger age than those with no special type carcinomas. The average age at presentation is 52 years; however, 50% of patients are younger than 50 years old, and these women are more commonly BRCA1 mutation carriers (66–71). In such women, a diagnosis of medullary carcinoma should prompt investigation for a family history and genetic counseling/testing.

The average size of a medullary carcinoma in a non-screening population is 2.7 cm. Radiologically, medullary carcinomas are circumscribed masses. Grossly, they are well circumscribed with a tan-brown to gray cut surface. Foci of hemorrhage, necrosis, or cystic degeneration may be seen. Microscopically, the diagnosis of pure medullary carcinoma requires grade 3 nuclei, microscopic circumscription, greater than 90% syncytial growth pattern, absence of glandular differentiation, and moderate to marked lymphoplasmacytic infiltrate that surrounds but is not admixed with the tumor islands (Figures 7.23A–B and 7.24A–B). This is in agreement with recent World Health Organization classification, with the exception of requiring a larger percentage of syncytial growth (17). The syncytial growth pattern consists of sheets or serpentine cords of epithelioid tumor cells with prominent nuclei and indistinct cell borders rimmed by a dense lymphoplasmacytic infiltrate. Focal squamous metaplasia, necrosis, and

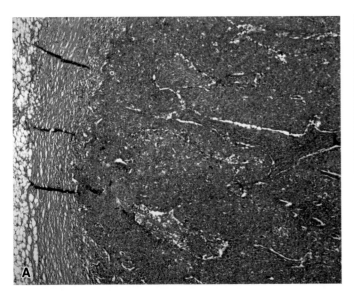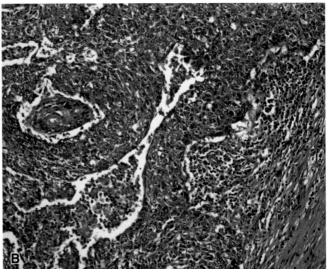

FIGURE 7.23 (A) This medullary carcinoma is well circumscribed with a pushing border and large syncytial islands. (B) On higher power, the highly pleomorphic nuclei and associated lymphocytic infiltrate are appreciated.

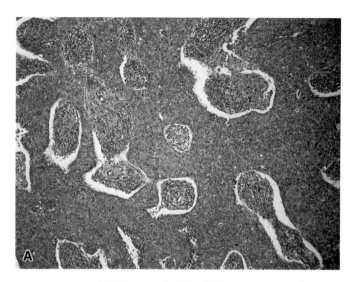 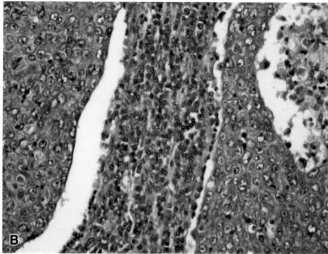

FIGURE 7.24 (A) This example of medullary carcinoma is characterized by broad anastomosing syncytial cords of tumor and a prominent peritumoral lymphocytic infiltrate. (B) The borders distinguishing individual tumor cells forming the syncytial islands cannot be identified. Also note that the lymphocytes are characteristically peritumoral and not admixed with tumor cells.

a giant cell reaction are all compatible with a diagnosis of medullary carcinoma. Rarely, the presence of an intraductal component is seen. Axillary lymph adenopathy is often noted clinically but is usually found to be reactive histologically, although in the study of Ridolfi et al (65), 23% of patients with typical medullary carcinoma developed regional lymph node metastases.

The differential diagnosis includes intermediate- to high-grade invasive carcinomas of no special type arranged largely in solid nests but with a nonsyncytial growth pattern, which is associated with varying degrees of lymphocytic response. Features incompatible with a diagnosis of medullary carcinoma include foci of invasive tumor without associated lymphocytic response and foci with an infiltrative pattern of growth. Some authors recognize an

atypical medullary carcinoma as defined by greater than 75% syncytial growth pattern with either focal or prominent margin infiltration, mild to minimal inflammatory infiltrate, low nuclear grade, or glandular differentiation; however, in our practice, we designate such tumors as no special type tumors with medullary features (Figures 7.25A–B and 7.26A–B). This ensures that these tumors are treated as no special type tumors appropriate to grade and stage and maintains the prognostic significance of pure medullary carcinoma.

Immunohistochemistry

Medullary carcinomas are estrogen receptor– and progesterone receptor–negative and do not overexpress HER2/

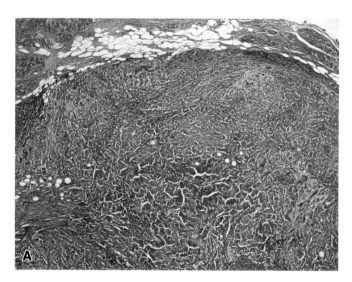 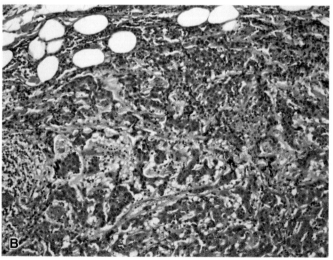

FIGURE 7.25 (A) On low power, this high-grade, well-circumscribed no special type carcinoma has medullary features with its pushing border. (B) Higher-power examination shows small infiltrative tumor nests and a mild lymphocytic response, which is admixed with the tumor cells, both inconsistent with a diagnosis of pure medullary carcinoma.

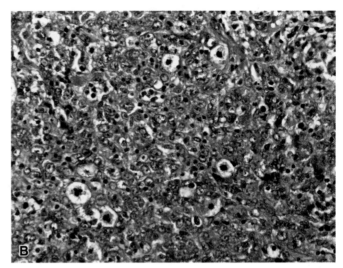

FIGURE 7.26 (A) This high-grade no special type carcinoma has medullary features given the syncytial appearance of the high-grade tumor nests; however, the border is infiltrative and the lymphocytic infiltrate is mild and not intimately associated with the invasive tumor. (B) High-power examination shows admixture of the inflammatory cells with tumor.

neu. p53 overexpression occurs at an increased level in medullary carcinoma.

Management

Excision to negative margins and sentinel node biopsy are adequate therapies for node-negative pure medullary carcinomas meeting the above criteria. This recommendation is based on the fact that node-negative patients with medullary carcinoma have a 10-year survival rate of 84% (92% 5-year survival) (26,65). Most deaths occur within the first 5 years after diagnosis, as might be expected for grade 3 carcinomas. A more recent study with long-term follow-up found that the prognosis of medullary carcinomas is similar to all no special type tumors collectively and better than the high-grade tumors (72).

Key Points

- Pure medullary carcinoma is rare, representing approximately 1% of all invasive breast carcinomas.
- Fifty percent of patients are younger than 50 years, and these women are more commonly BRCA1 mutation carriers.
- Histologically, the diagnosis of pure medullary carcinoma requires grade 3 nuclei, microscopic circumscription, greater than 90% syncytial growth pattern, absence of glandular differentiation, and moderate to marked lymphoplasmacytic infiltrate that surrounds but is not admixed with the tumor islands.
- Medullary carcinomas are estrogen receptor– and progesterone receptor–negative and do not overexpress HER-2/neu.
- Node-negative pure medullary carcinoma predicts a good prognosis; otherwise, the predictive utility is unclear.

- Excision to negative margins and sentinel node biopsy are adequate therapies for node-negative pure medullary carcinomas meeting the above criteria.

■ PURE MUCINOUS CARCINOMA

Pathologic Features

Using strict criteria, pure mucinous carcinomas represent about 2% if invasive mammary carcinomas. Most patients are postmenopausal women with a mean age of 65 years. Although some women present with a palpable mass, most are well-circumscribed, mammographically detected lesions that are associated with microcalcifications in 18% of cases. The median size of mucinous carcinoma is 2.0 cm (range, 0.3–12 cm). Grossly mucinous carcinoma is well circumscribed and has a gelatinous appearance on cross section.

The hallmark histologic appearance of mucinous carcinoma is small nests, trabeculae, or sheets of epithelial cells, with smooth borders and usually with some glandular lumen formation, entirely surrounded by pools of extracellular mucin (14) (Figures 7.27 and 7.28). Sometimes, the tumor nests may be extensively interconnected (73). The nuclei are low to intermediate grade, and the cytoplasm is pale to eosinophilic. The amount of mucin varies among tumors, as does the cellularity, which ranges from paucicellular to highly cellular (14) (Figure 7.29).

The designation of pure mucinous carcinoma should be used only when mucinous morphology is present in greater than 90% of the tumor, which is of low Nottingham grade (14,17,26). Tumors with 50% to 90% mucinous morphology and/or intermediate to high Nottingham grade should be designated as invasive mammary carcinoma of

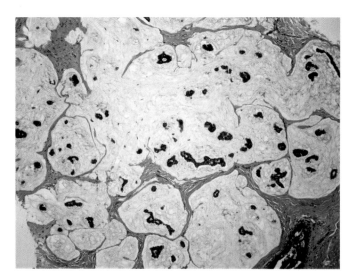

FIGURE 7.27 The tumor islands in this example of mucinous carcinoma show free-floating tumor cell aggregates with low-grade nuclei.

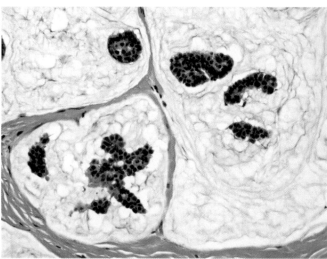

FIGURE 7.28 In pure mucinous carcinoma, the free-floating tumor cell clusters show round to ovoid hyperchromatic nuclei, which are low to intermediate grade and eosinophilic cytoplasm.

no special type with mucinous features (Figure 7.30) to maintain the excellent prognosis of the pure mucinous category.

Patients with pure mucinous carcinomas have 10-year survival rates of 80% to 100%, with the best rates associated with small and node-negative tumors (20,74). This survival rate is intermediate between that of tubular carcinomas and no special type carcinomas (75). Approximately 15% of patients have metastases to axillary lymph nodes at the time of diagnosis, with the frequency correlating with tumor size. Nodal involvement is very rare if the tumor size is less than 1.0 cm (26). The 5-year disease-free survival rate for pure mucinous carcinoma ranges from

81% to 90% (94% for node-negative patients), with the corresponding disease-specific survival rate of 95.3% and an overall 5-year survival of 80% (86% for node-negative patients) (20). The later corresponds favorably with age-matched patients from the general population.

The differential diagnosis for pure mucinous carcinoma is a mucocele-like lesion (MLL) or no special type carcinoma. An MLL may be associated with both benign and atypical epithelial lesions (Figure 7.31). A biopsy procedure or varying degrees of trauma to the breast causes extrusion of mucin from ductal or lobular structures into the surrounding parenchyma. Displaced epithelium may also accompany the mucin simulating a mucinous carcinoma (76–78).

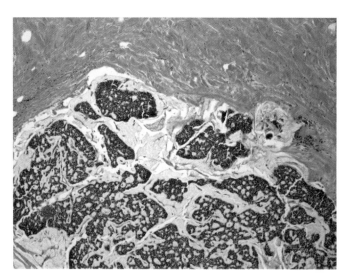

FIGURE 7.29 Occasionally, mucinous carcinoma demonstrates a proportionally larger epithelial component but is still entirely surrounded by mucin and contains low- to intermediate-grade nuclei.

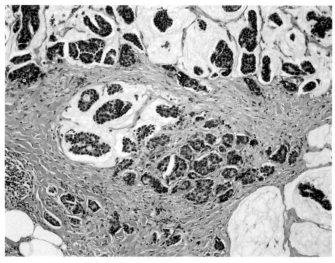

FIGURE 7.30 In addition to areas with mucinous differentiation, this no special type carcinoma with mucinous features shows foci of invasive tumor without accompanying mucin.

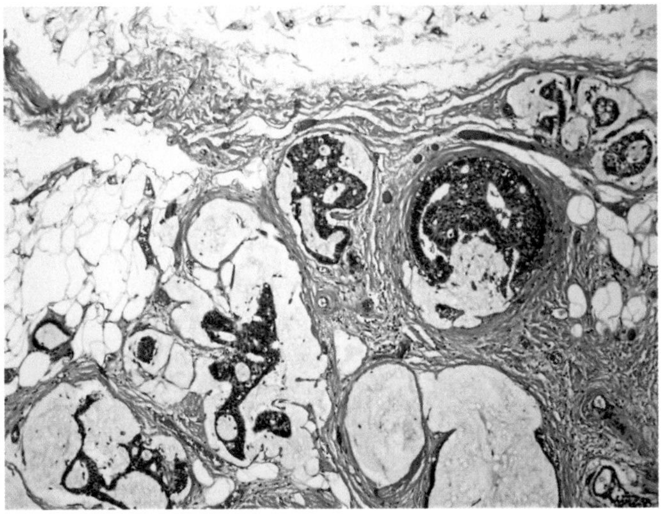

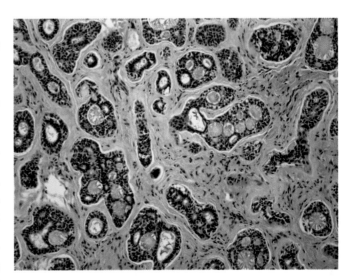

FIGURE 7.31 Disruption of a low-grade, mucin-producing, cribriform ductal carcinoma at the time of core biopsy created a MLL characterized by extrusion of mucin and cribriform islands of atypical epithelium into the adjacent parenchyma simulating invasive mucinous carcinoma.

Immunohistochemistry

Estrogen receptor positivity is seen in approximately 95% of pure mucinous carcinoma, and progesterone receptor positivity is seen in about 80% of cases. Pure mucinous carcinomas are negative for HER2.

Management

Breast conservation without sentinel node biopsy is adequate treatment for pure mucinous carcinomas, especially if less than 1.0 cm. Women with larger tumors whose core biopsy may not be entirely representative of the tumor or with clinically suspicious lymph nodes should undergo a sentinel node biopsy. Subsequent treatment with adjuvant hormone therapy is standard.

Key Points

- Pure mucinous carcinomas represent about 2% if invasive mammary carcinomas.
- Histologically, a diagnosis of pure mucinous carcinoma requires a tumor of low combined Nottingham histologic grade in which greater than 90% of the tumor is composed of small nests or sheets of epithelial cells with glandular lumina entirely surrounded by pools of extracellular mucin.
- Pure mucinous carcinoma is estrogen receptor–positive in approximately 95% of cases and positive for progesterone receptor in about 80% of cases, but all are negative for HER2/neu overexpression.
- Patients with pure mucinous carcinomas have 10-year survival rates of 80% to 100%, with the best rates associated with small and node-negative tumors. This survival rate is intermediate between that of tubular carcinomas and no special type carcinomas.

- Breast conservation without sentinel node biopsy is adequate treatment for pure mucinous carcinomas, especially if smaller than 1.0 cm.

■ ADENOID CYSTIC CARCINOMA

Pathologic Features

Adenoid cystic carcinoma of the breast, when properly and rigidly defined, accounts for about 0.1% of all invasive breast malignancies. Strict criteria were identified in the 1970s, aided by the use of electron microscopic features and histochemistry (52). Adenoid cystic carcinoma of the breast is so named because of its microscopic similarity to tumors of the major and minor salivary glands. Among the several carefully defined special types of breast cancer, ACC is a prime example of the importance of recognizing a cluster of unique pathologic features that guarantee a usually excellent prognosis (79–82). This is exemplified by the greatly increased representation of women with ACC among 20-year survivors of invasive breast cancer (39).

Reported age at diagnosis for ACC varies from 31 to 90 years. These women typically present with a mobile, slowly growing (81,83,84) breast mass, which may be present for years before diagnosis (85,86) and is usually in the region of the nipple or areola (87–89). However, unlike typical mammary carcinoma, the breast mass may be painful or tender (85,86,90–91). The size of these tumors at diagnosis may be large but is with in the range typical of invasive breast cancers in general. Current cases are usually diagnosed by mammography and average approximately 2 cm. However, in circumstances where the breast

FIGURE 7.32 Adenoid cystic carcinoma showing circumscribed tumor islands with rigid cribriform spaces filled with blue-tinged, basement membrane–like material interspersed with occasional true lumina.

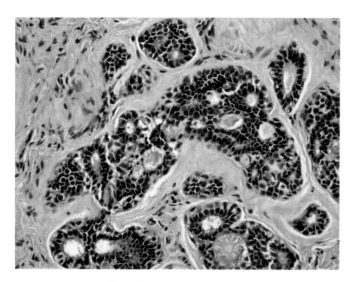

FIGURE 7.33 Adenoid cystic carcinoma at high power shows evidence of a dual-cell population with myoepithelial cells surrounding pseudolumens filled with basement membrane–like material and luminal epithelial cells surrounding true lumina.

mass was neglected, tumors as large as 10 cm have been documented (87,92). Bilaterality has not been reported.

The histologic hallmark of ACC is the presence of a dual-cell population consisting of islands of admixed epithelial and myoepithelial cells forming small, sharply defined glandular and pseudoglandular structures (Figures 7.32 and 7.33), with true glands filled with brightly eosinophilic mucin and pseudolumens filled with more basophilic basement membrane–like material (14,21). Another common pattern is the formation of interanastomosing serpentine cords of tumor; however, the dual-cell population and presence of basement membrane–like material usually remain obvious (Figure 7.34A–B). In some cases, the basement membrane–like material may predominate forming

irregular islands (Figure 7.35). Nodular and diffusely infiltrating smaller, usually rounded collections of infiltrating tumors may coexist, but maintenance of the same cytology and intercellular arrangements is the defining feature. Although not often mentioned in the literature, in situ patterns may be occasionally present in conjunction with areas of invasive tumor (93). Rarely, ACC may be intermixed with or appear to arise from a benign but infiltrative and equally rare condition, microglandular adenosis (94).

Shin and Rosen (93) have recently described a solid variant of ACC that exhibits a greater than 90% solid growth pattern composed of basaloid cells with moderate to occasionally marked nuclear atypia and rare to brisk mitotic activity (Figure 7.36). These tumors show the same immunohistochemical profile as a typical ACC and an excellent prognosis (93,95). Despite the presence of a single lymph node metastasis in 2 of the 9 described patients, no patient developed recurrent or distant disease after initial treatment (93). Kleer additionally found that nuclear grade and proliferative activity did not predict capacity for local recurrence or distant metastasis (93,95).

The differential diagnosis for ACC includes collagenous spherulosis, pure ICC, low-grade cribriform ductal carcinoma in situ, and invasive mammary carcinoma of no special type. Collagenous spherulosis is an important mimicker of mammary ACC, usually easily recognized as bounded by the basement membrane of lobular units and consisting of aggregates of well-circumscribed eosinophilic spherules composed of basement membrane–related collagen (96). Superficially, ACC is similar to ICC (27,28,97), as both of these special types of breast carcinoma are characterized by small sharply defined, rounded spaces within islands of epithelial cells; however, pure ICC does not include a dual-cell population. In addition to lacking a dual-cell population, cribriform ductal carcinoma in situ shows an intact myoepithelial cell layer,

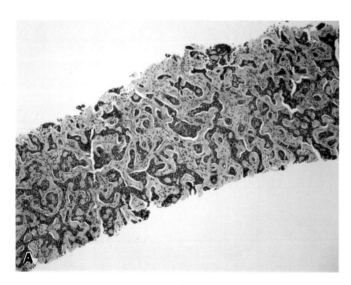
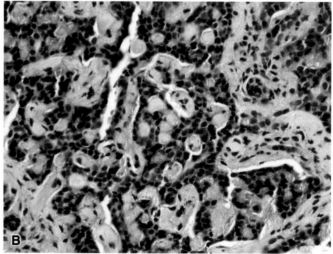

FIGURE 7.34 (A) An example of ACC in core biopsy shows a complex network of interanastomosing cords of tumor within a sclerotic stroma. (B) This higher-power view shows numerous small true lumens and pseudolumens within an irregular island of predominantly myoepithelial cells.

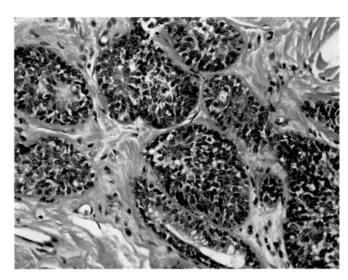

FIGURE 7.35 Adenoid cystic carcinoma forming solid islands of basement membrane–like material bordered by myoepithelial cells.

FIGURE 7.36 Solid variant of ACC shows a solid growth pattern with moderate to occasionally marked nuclear atypia and mitotic activity.

and no special type invasive carcinomas show greater than 50% noncribriform and nontubular areas.

Histochemistry and Immunohistochemistry

Periodic acid–Schiff stains the contents of the "true" lumens pink as is typical of epithelial mucins, which are of near neutral pH, whereas the basement membrane material or "stromal mucin" of the "pseudolumens" is more acidic and stains pale pink or blue (Figure 7.37) (52,98). The main proliferating element in ACC is a population of modified myoepithelial cells as demonstrated by positive staining for smooth muscle actins, vimentin (99), and p63

(100) (Figure 7.38). These cells are grouped in nests outlining the pseudolumens or more irregular islands of basement membrane–like material. The true epithelial lumens, also referred to as the glandular or adenoid component, are lined by cytokeratin and epithelial membrane antigen–positive cells that demonstrate conserved basolateral markers of normal epithelial polarity as exemplified by positivity for fodrin, E-cadherin, and β-catenin (99) expression. Strictly defined ACC are estrogen receptor– and progesterone receptor–negative (101–105). However, this finding should not be used as an indicator of poor outcome. In fact, the detailed study of markers of epithelial polarity in ACC by Kasami et al (99) demonstrating near-normal

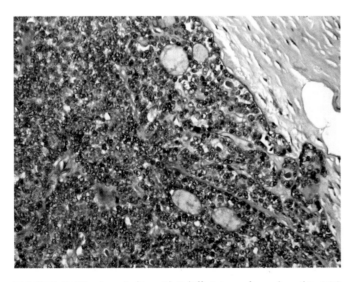

FIGURE 7.37 A periodic acid–Schiff stain performed on this ACC stains the mucin within true lumina bright pink and the basement membrane–like material produced by the myoepithelial cells pale pink.

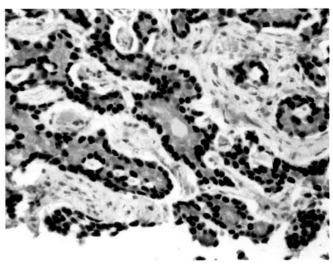

FIGURE 7.38 p63 immunohistochemical stain highlights the myoepithelial cells in this ACC. Note the absence of staining of luminal epithelial cells surrounding the true lumina.

differentiation despite the capacity for local invasion is consistent with the usual lack of distant metastasis.

Management

The preferred initial treatment of breast ACC is local excision to negative margins since this is a relatively indolent disease. However, it is important to emphasize that when excisional biopsy is performed as the primary initial surgical procedure, special attention must be given to the margins because these tumors grow in an infiltrative pattern. We advocate performing mastectomy and/or axillary node dissection only in patients with obviously large tumors and/or clinically involved axillary lymph nodes (85,87,89,102,106,107). Although the incidence of local recurrence increases with more conservative surgery (similar to other breast cancer histologies), distant metastasis after local failure is exceedingly rare with only 7 confirmed cases in the literature since 1970 (92,101,104,108,109). Patients who experience local failures can almost always be salvaged with more extensive surgical procedures. Because ACCs are estrogen receptor– and progesterone receptor–negative, there is no role for adjuvant hormonal therapy and chemotherapy is not advocated.

Key Points

- Adenoid cystic carcinoma of the breast accounts for about 0.1% of all invasive breast malignancies.
- Adenoid cystic carcinoma in the breast typically presents as a mobile, slowly growing mass in the region of the nipple or areola, which may be present for years before diagnosis.
- By definition, ACC contains a dual-cell population of epithelial and myoepithelial cells forming small, sharply defined glandular and pseudoglandular structures with true lumina filled with brightly eosinophilic mucin and pseudolumens filled with more basophilic basement membrane–like material.
- Strictly defined ACC are estrogen receptor– and progesterone receptor–negative. Overexpression of HER2/neu is also not seen.
- Unlike other sites, ACC in the breast has an excellent prognosis.
- The preferred initial treatment of breast ACC is local excision to negative margins since this is a relatively indolent disease.

■ LOW-GRADE SPINDLE CELL METAPLASTIC CARCINOMA

Pathologic Features

Metaplastic carcinomas of the breast are a heterogeneous group of cancers that collectively represent less than 1%

of all breast cancers. By definition, metaplastic carcinomas are of epithelial origin with intermixed nonepithelial elements including spindle cells, bone, cartilage, myxoid stroma, anaplastic stroma, and giant cells. The metaplastic spindle cells in metaplastic carcinomas can range from relatively bland to aggressive patterns resembling high-grade sarcoma. Low-grade spindle cell metaplastic carcinoma is a special variant of metaplastic carcinoma with relatively indolent growth which is capable of local recurrence but with no demonstrated distant spread or regional metastases (110). This contrasts sharply with the poor prognosis of cases with higher-grade features (26).

Average age at diagnosis of women diagnosed with low-grade spindle cell metaplastic carcinomas is 63 years (110). In the series of Page and Anderson (110), all women presented with a single palpable mass. Swelling and tenderness were present in a single patient.

Grossly, these tumors are firm and white, ranging in size from 1.2 to 7.0 cm in greatest extent (average size, 2.7 cm). The tumor borders may be circumscribed, nodular, and have irregular borders.

Histologically, spindle cell metaplastic carcinomas have a dominantly infiltrative growth pattern with cellular finger-like projections extending into adjacent mammary structures and fatty tissue reminiscent of fibromatosis. They are composed of bland-appearing, plump spindle cells arranged in interlacing short fascicles, often with a storiform pattern and usually without obvious epithelial differentiation on hematoxylin and eosin staining (110) (Figure 7.39). In some cases, the spindle cells merge with clusters of spindle cells, which take on fusiform or polygonal shapes with epithelioid nuclei that may cluster together (Figure 7.40A–B). Rarely, foci of glandular or squamous elements

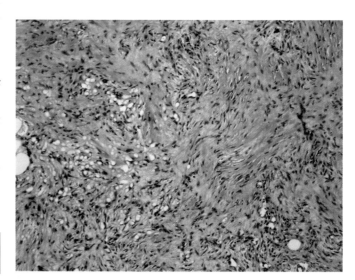

FIGURE 7.39 Low-grade spindle cell metaplastic carcinoma composed of bland-appearing spindle cells growing in short fascicles without obvious epithelial differentiation and a background of scattered mononuclear chronic inflammatory cells.

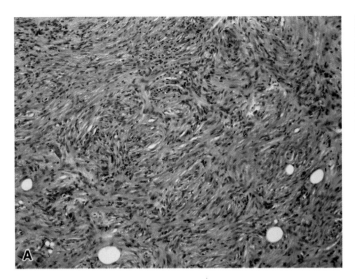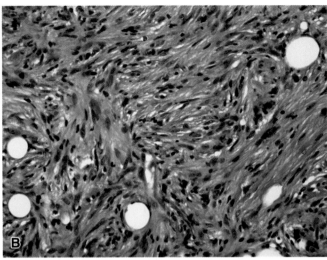

FIGURE 7.40 (A) Low-grade spindle cell metaplastic carcinoma with a vaguely storiform pattern and higher cellularity than Figure 7.39. (B) On higher power, the tumor cells in this case have a polygonal to epithelioid appearance with nesting of the nuclei.

may transition from the spindle cells, usually comprising less than 5% of the tumor. The cellularity of these lesions is variable, and often low, with low-grade nuclei and indistinct nucleoli. The nuclei are slender with tapered edges and finely dispersed chromatin. The cytoplasm is pale and eosinophilic.

Mitotic activity is low (range, none to 3 per 10 high-power fields). The stroma is mildly myxoid to edematous appearing, with a minimal to mild lymphoplasmacytic infiltrate that may focally resemble nodular fasciitis. Some cases also show varying degrees of fine stromal collagenization. Rarely, spindle cell metaplastic carcinomas may be seen arising from a number of fibrosclerotic breast lesions including papillomas, complex sclerosing lesions, and nipple duct adenomas (111).

The differential diagnosis for low-grade spindle cell metaplastic carcinoma includes higher-grade spindle cell carcinomas with increased spindle cell atypia and cellularity, low-grade spindle cell sarcoma, fibromatosis, and nodular fasciitis. Higher-grade spindle cell carcinomas demonstrate a higher density of keratin-positive cells, cellular atypia, and more obvious mitotic activity (regularly more than 4 per 10 high-power fields). Low-grade spindle cell sarcomas also show more cellularity and mild cytologic activity but lack evidence of keratin positivity. The fascicles of fibromatosis are long and sweeping in comparison to the short storiform fascicles of spindle cell metaplastic carcinoma. The spindle cells of nodular fasciitis are plumper, their nuclei contain prominent nucleoli, and they are arranged in short fascicles. Mitotic figures are also easily seen in nodular fasciitis and can be numerous. Foci of extravasated red blood cells may be a helpful clue to the diagnosis. Obvious nuclear pleomorphism and prominent mitotic figures including atypical mitoses are characteristic of low-grade spindle cell sarcoma.

Immunohistochemistry

Performance of immunohistochemistry with a battery of high- and low-molecular-weight cytokeratins is critical in confirming the diagnosis and may be helpful in evaluating margin status (110). In our practice, the strongest staining is typically obtained with p63 (Figure 7.41) and CK903 (Figure 7.42), followed by AE1/AE3, and orthokeratin.

Management

Excision to widely negative margins is critical to the successful treatment of spindle cell metaplastic carcinomas and prevention of local recurrence. Sentinel lymph node biopsy is unnecessary given the fact that low-grade spindle

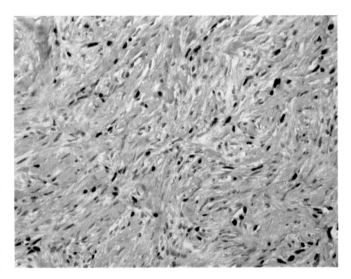

FIGURE 7.41 Immunohistochemical stain for p63 highlights the myoepithelial phenotype of spindle cell metaplastic carcinoma.

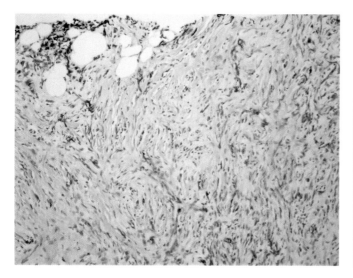

FIGURE 7.42 Immunohistochemical stain for CK903 is another helpful marker highlighting the myoepithelial phenotype of spindle cell metaplastic carcinoma.

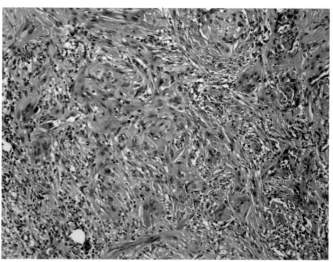

FIGURE 7.43 Low-grade adenosquamous carcinoma composed of cords and nests of bland-appearing infiltrative tumor with squamous differentiation.

cell metaplastic carcinoma essentially never metastasize to regional lymph nodes.

Key Points

- Low-grade spindle cell metaplastic carcinoma is a special variant of metaplastic carcinoma with relatively indolent growth which is capable of local recurrence but with no demonstrated distant spread or regional metastases.
- Low-grade spindle cell metaplastic carcinomas of the breast are very rare, representing less than 0.1% of all breast cancers.
- They are composed of bland-appearing, plump spindle cells arranged in interlacing short fascicles, often with a storiform pattern and usually without obvious epithelial differentiation on hematoxylin and eosin stain. The stroma is mildly myxoid to edematous with a mild lymphoplasmacytic infiltrate.
- Performance of immunohistochemistry with a battery of high- and low-molecular-weight cytokeratins is critical in confirming the diagnosis and may be helpful in evaluating margin status.
- Excision to widely negative margins is critical to the successful treatment of spindle cell metaplastic carcinomas and prevention of local recurrence. Sentinel node biopsy is unnecessary.

■ LOW-GRADE ADENOSQUAMOUS CARCINOMA

Pathologic Features

Low-grade adenosquamous carcinoma is a special variant of metaplastic carcinoma, which is low grade and has an excellent prognosis (112) but is not to be confused with

adenosquamous carcinoma, which is typically high grade with a poor prognosis. Grossly, these tumors are small, averaging 2.4 cm (range, 0.5–8.6) (112–114), firm, and yellow-tan with indistinct margins. Histologically, adenosquamous carcinomas are composed of a mixture of low-grade, well-formed glandular elements and angulated tumor cords with an immature squamous metaplasia-like phenotype that may predominate in some cases (Figures 7.43 and 7.44). The background stroma has a similar appearance to low-grade spindle cell metaplastic carcinoma with a fibromatosis-like appearance and an associated mononuclear inflammatory cell infiltrate but may be sclerotic. These tumors may arise in association with a

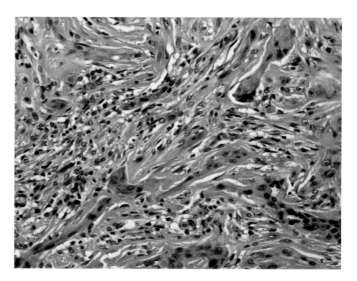

FIGURE 7.44 Low-grade adenosquamous carcinoma showing elongated islands of tumor with a bland squamoid appearance and abundant eosinophilic cytoplasm which blend imperceptibly with the desmoplastic stroma. Note the mild chronic inflammatory background.

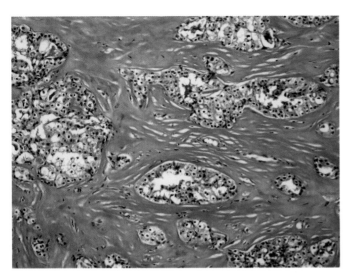

FIGURE 7.45 Secretory carcinoma composed of lobules of tumor cells with abundant cytoplasmic secretory material in the characteristic densely sclerotic stroma.

benign sclerosing lesion, such as a sclerosing papilloma or a complex sclerosing lesion (111–112).

The differential diagnosis for low-grade adenosquamous carcinoma includes syringomatous adenoma of the nipple, tubular carcinoma, and reactive squamous metaplasia.

Immunohistochemistry

Low-grade adenosquamous carcinomas are estrogen receptor– and progesterone receptor–negative and do not show evidence of HER2 overexpression or amplification.

Management

Excision to negative margins is critical to the successful treatment of low-grade adenosquamous carcinomas and prevention of local recurrence. Sentinel lymph node biopsy is unnecessary given the fact that a low-grade spindle cell metaplastic tumor essentially never metastasize to regional lymph nodes.

Key Points

- Low-grade adenosquamous carcinoma is another rare variant of metaplastic carcinoma, which is very low grade and has an excellent prognosis.
- Histologically, they are composed of a mixture of low-grade, well-formed glandular elements and angulated tumor cords with an immature squamous metaplasia-like phenotype.
- The background stroma has a similar appearance to low-grade spindle cell metaplastic carcinoma with a fibromatosis-like appearance and an associated mononuclear inflammatory infiltrate.

- These tumors may arise in association with a benign sclerosing lesion, such as a sclerosing papilloma or a complex sclerosing lesion.
- Low-grade adenosquamous carcinomas are estrogen receptor– and progesterone receptor–negative and do not show evidence of HER2 overexpression or amplification.
- Excision to negative margins is adequate treatment to prevent local recurrence. Sentinel lymph node biopsy is unnecessary.

■ SECRETORY CARCINOMA

Secretory carcinoma, first termed *juvenile carcinoma* by McDivitt and Stewart (115), as the original cases were identified in children, may also occur in adults (115–118). It is the main type of carcinoma diagnosed in the first 2 decades, and in this age group, it has been reported in males (117) and in females. This tumor usually presents as an asymptomatic mass under the nipple. Grossly, these tumors are 1.0 to 2.5 cm in greatest dimension and gray-white and firm on cut section. They are circumscribed and distinct from the nipple. Histologically, lobules of tumor are separated by prominant bands of often densely sclerotic collagen (Figure 7.45). A microcystic appearance is imparted histologically as a result of numerous intercellular lumina containing extracellular secretions (Figure 7.46). Individual tumor cells show only mild to moderate cytologic atypia. The tumor cell cytoplasm may be clear as a result of cytoplasmic vacuolization or finely granular. The secretory material both within tumor cells and within the intercellular lumina stains positively for periodic acid–Schiff (diastase resistant) and Alcian blue (14). Although

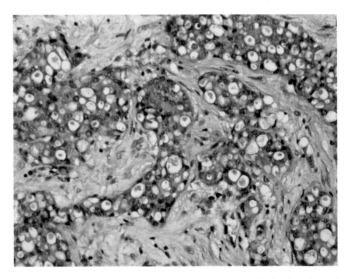

FIGURE 7.46 Secretory carcinoma with grade 2 epithelioid nuclei and large inter- and intracytoplasmic lumina filled with secretory material.

most cases will have a well-delineated border often with a layer of connectve tissue between the neoplasm and the surrounding connective tissue (14), occasional cases will show invasion into the surrounding tissue. Therefore, careful examination of the margins is especially critical.

Recently, a t(12;15)(p12;q26.1) translocation was identfied in 12 of 13 cases of secretory carcinoma tested (119). Three of these patents were younger than 20 years old. This translocation has been previously identified in congenital fibrosarcoma, mesoblastic nephroma, and a case report of acute myelod leukemia (117,120–122). The resulting ETV6-NTRK3 fusion gene encodes a chimeric tyrosine kinase with potent transforming activity in fbroblasts (123–124). Because secretory carcinoma is a histologically distinct lesion, it is unclear whether there will be a role for translocation studies in diagnosis of this lesion; however, it is remarkable in that the occurrence of such translocations as the sole cytogenetic abnormality in epithelial tumors is extremely rare.

Secretory carcinoma has an indolent behavior and an excellent prognosis in women younger than 20 years (118,123–127). Only 2 of the 22 originally reported cases recurred locally and were successfully managed surgically (115,117–118,126,128–135). Only 3 of these cases had involved axillary nodes, and none had distant metastases. When secretory carcinoma occurs in adults, the prognosis is less favorable (116,118,136). Local recurrences are probably related to inadequate excision. Metastatic lesions and death from disseminated tumor have only been reported in women more than 20 years old (116,118).

Immunohistochemistry

Secretory carcinoma is negative for estrogen receptor expression in the few reported cases in the literature. Strong positivity for alpha-lactalbumin, S100 protein, and carcino embryonic antigen (CEA) have been documented.

Management

Breast-conserving therapy, which preserves cosmesis and lactational ability, should be the goal of treatment in children and adolescents unless the tumor is large or has clinically involved axillary lymph nodes. Consideration may be given for a sentinel node biopsy in older women. There is no role for radiation in children.

Key Points

- Although secretory carcinoma is rare, it is the most common type of mammary carcinoma diagnosed in the first 2 decades and may also occur in older women.

- This tumor usually presents as an asymptomatic mass under the nipple.
- Secretory carcinoma is composed of lobules of tumor cells containing abundant cytoplasmic secretory material in a background of densely sclerotic stroma.
- Secretory carcinoma has indolent behavior and an excellent prognosis in women younger than 20 years old; however, when secretory carcinoma occurs in adults, the prognosis is less favorable.
- Breast-conserving therapy, which preserves cosmesis and lactational ability, should be the goal of treatment in children and adolescents unless the tumor is large or has clinically involved axillary lymph nodes.

■ REFERENCES

1. Patchefsky AS, Shaber GS, Schwartz GF, Feig SA, Nerlinger RE. The pathology of breast cancer detected by mass population screening. *Cancer.* 1977;40:1659–1670.

2. Carstens PH. Tubular carcinoma of the breast. A study of frequency. *Am J Clin Pathol.* 1978;70:204–210.

3. Carstens PH, Greenberg RA, Francis D, Lyon H. Tubular carcinoma of the breast. A long term follow-up. *Histopathology.* 1985;9:271–280.

4. Cooper HS, Patchefsky AS, Krall RA. Tubular carcinoma of the breast. *Cancer.* 1978;42:2334–2342.

5. McDivitt RW, Boyce W, Gersell D. Tubular carcinoma of the breast. Clinical and pathological observations concerning 135 cases. *Am J Surg Pathol.* 1982;6:401–411.

6. Anderson TJ, Alexander FE, Forrest PM. The natural history of breast carcinoma: what have we learned from screening? *Cancer.* 2000;88:1758–1759.

7. Anderson TJ, Lamb J, Alexander F, et al. Comparative pathology of prevalent and incident cancers detected by breast screening. Edinburgh Breast Screening Project. *Lancet.* 1986;1:519–523.

8. Anderson TJ, Lamb J, Donnan P, et al. Comparative pathology of breast cancer in a randomised trial of screening. *Br J Cancer.* 1991;64:108–113.

9. Anderson TJ, Waller M, Ellis IO, Bobrow L, Moss S. Influence of annual mammography from age 40 on breast cancer pathology. *Hum Pathol.* 2004;35:1252–1259.

10. Feig SA, Shaber GS, Patchefsky A, et al. Analysis of clinically occult and mammographically occult breast tumors. *AJR Am J Roentgenol.* 1977;128:403–408.

11. Rajakariar R, Walker RA. Pathological and biological features of mammographically detected invasive breast carcinomas. *Br J Cancer.* 1995;71:150–154.

12. Elson BC, Helvie MA, Frank TS, Wilson TE, Adler DD. Tubular carcinoma of the breast: mode of presentation, mammographic appearance, and frequency of nodal metastases. *AJR Am J Roentgenol.* 1993;161:1173–1176.

13. Oberman HA, Fidler WJ Jr. Tubular carcinoma of the breast. *Am J Surg Pathol.* 1979;3:387–395.

14. Page DL, Anderson TJ. *Diagnostic Histopathology of the Breast.* Edinburgh: Churchill Livingstone; 1987.

15. Tavassoli F. Infiltrating carcinomas, common and familiar special types. In: Tavassoli F, ed. *Pathology of the Breast.* Norwalk: Appleton & Lange; 1992: 293–294.

16. Leibman AJ, Lewis M, Kruse B. Tubular carcinoma of the breast: mammographic appearance. *AJR Am J Roentgenol.* 1993;160:263–265.

17. Tavassoli F, Devilee P, eds. *Tumors of the Breast and Female Genital Organs.* 1st ed. Lyon: IRC Press; 2003.

18. Kitchen PR, Smith TH, Henderson MA, et al. Tubular carcinoma of the breast: prognosis and response to adjuvant systemic therapy. *ANZ J Surg.* 2001;71: 27–31.

19. Cabral AH, Recine M, Paramo JC, McPhee MM, Poppiti R, Mesko TW. Tubular carcinoma of the breast: an institutional experience and review of the literature. *Breast J.* 2003;9:298–301.

20. Diab SG, Clark GM, Osborne CK, Libby A, Allred DC, Elledge RM. Tumor characteristics and clinical outcome of tubular and mucinous breast carcinomas. *J Clin Oncol.* 1999;17:1442–1448.

21. Elston CW, Ellis IO. *The Breast.* 3rd ed. London: Churchill Livingstone; 1998.

22. Papadatos G, Rangan AM, Psarianos T, Ung O, Taylor R, Boyages J. Probability of axillary node involvement in patients with tubular carcinoma of the breast. *Br J Surg.* 2001;88:860–864.

23. Leonard CE, Howell K, Shapiro H, Ponce J, Kercher J. Excision only for tubular carcinoma of the breast. *Breast J.* 2005;11:129–133.

24. Livi L, Paiar F, Meldolesi E, et al. Tubular carcinoma of the breast: outcome and loco-regional recurrence in 307 patients. *Eur J Surg Oncol.* 2005;31:9–12.

25. Thurman SA, Schnitt SJ, Connolly JL, et al. Outcome after breast-conserving therapy for patients with stage I or II mucinous, medullary, or tubular breast carcinoma. *Int J Radiat Oncol Biol Phys.* 2004;59: 152–159.

26. Ellis IO, Schnitt SJ, Sastre-Garau X. Invasive breast carcinoma. In: Tavassoli FA, Devilee P, eds. *Tumours of the Breast and Female Genital Organs.* Lyon: IARC Press; 2003:13–59.

27. Page DL, Dixon JM, Anderson TJ, Lee D, Stewart HJ. Invasive cribriform carcinoma of the breast. *Histopathology.* 1983;7:525–536.

28. Venable JG, Schwartz AM, Silverberg SG. Infiltrating cribriform carcinoma of the breast: a distinctive clinicopathologic entity. *Hum Pathol.* 1990;21:333–338.

29. Wheeler JE, Enterline HT. Lobular carcinoma of the breast in situ and infiltrating. *Pathol Annu.* 1976;11:161–188.

30. Bharat A, Gao F, Margenthaler JA. Tumor characteristics and patient outcomes are similar between invasive lobular and mixed invasive ductal/lobular breast cancers but differ from pure invasive ductal breast cancers. *Am J Surg.* 2009;198:516–519.

31. Orvieto E, Maiorano E, Bottiglieri L, et al. Clinicopathologic characteristics of invasive lobular carcinoma of the breast: results of an analysis of 530 cases from a single institution. *Cancer.* 2008;113:1511–1520.

32. Wasif N, Maggard MA, Ko CY, Giuliano AE. Invasive lobular vs. ductal breast cancer: a stage-matched comparison of outcomes. *Ann Surg Oncol.* 2010;17:1862–1869.

33. Dian D, Herold H, Mylonas I, et al. Survival analysis between patients with invasive ductal and invasive lobular breast cancer. *Arch Gynecol Obstet.* 2009;279:23–28.

34. Rakha EA, El-Sayed ME, Menon S, Green AR, Lee AH, Ellis IO. Histologic grading is an independent prognostic factor in invasive lobular carcinoma of the breast. *Breast Cancer Res Treat.* 2008;111:121–127.

35. Rakha EA, Ellis IO. Lobular breast carcinoma and its variants. *Semin Diagn Pathol.* 2010;27:49–61.

36. Adams AL, Li Y, Pfeifer JD, Hameed O. Nuclear grade and survival in invasive lobular carcinoma: a case series with long-term follow-up. *Breast J.* 2010;16: 445–447.

37. Viale G, Rotmensz N, Maisonneuve P, et al. Lack of prognostic significance of "classic" lobular breast carcinoma: a matched, single institution series. *Breast Cancer Res Treat.* 2009;117:211–214.

38. Mhuircheartaigh JN, Curran C, Hennessy E, Kerin MJ. Prospective matched-pair comparison of outcome after treatment for lobular and ductal breast carcinoma. *Br J Surg.* 2008;95:827–833.

39. Dixon JM, Page DL, Anderson TJ, et al. Long-term survivors after breast cancer. *Br J Surg.* 1985;72: 445–448.

40. Dixon JM, Anderson TJ, Page DL, Lee D, Duffy SW. Infiltrating lobular carcinoma of the breast. *Histopathology.* 1982;6:149–161.

41. Fechner RE. Histologic variants of infiltrating lobular carcinoma of the breast. *Hum Pathol.* 1975;6:373–378.

42. Martinez V, Azzopardi JG. Invasive lobular carcinoma of the breast: incidence and variants. *Histopathology.* 1979;3:467–488.

43. Shousha S, Backhous CM, Alaghband-Zadeh J, Burn I. Alveolar variant of invasive lobular carcinoma of

the breast. A tumor rich in estrogen receptors. *Am J Clin Pathol.* 1986;85:1–5.

44. Eusebi V, Magalhaes F, Azzopardi JG. Pleomorphic lobular carcinoma of the breast: an aggressive tumor showing apocrine differentiation. *Hum Pathol.* 1992;23:655–662.

45. Weidner N, Semple JP. Pleomorphic variant of invasive lobular carcinoma of the breast. *Hum Pathol.* 1992;23:1167–1171.

46. DiCostanzo D, Rosen PP, Gareen I, Franklin S, Lesser M. Prognosis in infiltrating lobular carcinoma. An analysis of "classical" and variant tumors. *Am J Surg Pathol.* 1990;14:12–23.

47. du Toit RS, Locker AP, Ellis IO, Elston CW, Nicholson RI, Blamey RW. Invasive lobular carcinomas of the breast—the prognosis of histopathological subtypes. *Br J Cancer.* 1989;60:605–609.

48. Chen CL, Weiss NS, Newcomb P, Barlow W, White E. Hormone replacement therapy in relation to breast cancer. *JAMA.* 2002;287:734–741.

49. Eheman CR, Shaw KM, Ryerson AB, Miller JW, Ajani UA, White MC. The changing incidence of in situ and invasive ductal and lobular breast carcinomas: United States, 1999–2004. *Cancer Epidemiol Biomarkers Prev.* 2009;18:1763–1769.

50. Peiro G, Bornstein BA, Connolly JL, et al. The influence of infiltrating lobular carcinoma on the outcome of patients treated with breast-conserving surgery and radiation therapy. *Breast Cancer Res Treat.* 2000;59:49–54.

51. Sastre-Garau X, Jouve M, Asselain B, et al. Infiltrating lobular carcinoma of the breast. Clinicopathologic analysis of 975 cases with reference to data on conservative therapy and metastatic patterns. *Cancer.* 1996;77:113–120.

52. Azzopardi JG, Ahmed A, Millis RR. Problems in breast pathology. *Major Probl Pathol.* 1979;11:i–xvi, 1–466.

53. Fisher ER, Gregorio RM, Redmond C, Fisher B. Tubulolobular invasive breast cancer: a variant of lobular invasive cancer. *Hum Pathol.* 1977;8:679–683.

54. Bentz JS, Yassa N, Clayton F. Pleomorphic lobular carcinoma of the breast: clinicopathologic features of 12 cases. *Mod Pathol.* 1998;11:814–822.

55. Middleton LP, Palacios DM, Bryant BR, Krebs P, Otis CN, Merino MJ. Pleomorphic lobular carcinoma: morphology, immunohistochemistry, and molecular analysis. *Am J Surg Pathol.* 2000;24:1650–1656.

56. Reis-Filho JS, Simpson PT, Jones C, et al. Pleomorphic lobular carcinoma of the breast: role of comprehensive molecular pathology in characterization of an entity. *J Pathol.* 2005;207:1–13.

57. Simpson PT, Reis-Filho JS, Lambros MB, et al. Molecular profiling pleomorphic lobular carcinomas of the breast: evidence for a common molecular genetic pathway with classic lobular carcinomas. *J Pathol.* 2008;215:231–244.

58. Berx G, Cleton-Jansen AM, Strumane K, et al. E-cadherin is inactivated in a majority of invasive human lobular breast cancers by truncation mutations throughout its extracellular domain. *Oncogene.* 1996;13:1919–1925.

59. Moll R, Mitze M, Frixen UH, Birchmeier W. Differential loss of E-cadherin expression in infiltrating ductal and lobular breast carcinomas. *Am J Pathol.* 1993;143:1731–1742.

60. Nishizaki T, Chew K, Chu L, et al. Genetic alterations in lobular breast cancer by comparative genomic hybridization. *Int J Cancer.* 1997;74:513–517.

61. Palacios J, Benito N, Pizarro A, et al. Anomalous expression of P-cadherin in breast carcinoma. Correlation with E-cadherin expression and pathological features. *Am J Pathol.* 1995;146: 605–612.

62. Rasbridge SA, Gillett CE, Sampson SA, Walsh FS, Millis RR. Epithelial (E-) and placental (P-) cadherin cell adhesion molecule expression in breast carcinoma. *J Pathol.* 1993;169:245–250.

63. Acs G, Lawton TJ, Rebbeck TR, LiVolsi VA, Zhang PJ. Differential expression of E-cadherin in lobular and ductal neoplasms of the breast and its biologic and diagnostic implications. *Am J Clin Pathol.* 2001;115:85–98.

64. Porter PL, Garcia R, Moe R, Corwin DJ, Gown AM. C-erbB-2 oncogene protein in in situ and invasive lobular breast neoplasia. *Cancer.* 1991;68:331–334.

65. Ridolfi RL, Rosen PP, Port A, Kinne D, Mike V. Medullary carcinoma of the breast: a clinicopathologic study with 10 year follow-up. *Cancer.* 1977;40:1365–1385.

66. Armes JE, Egan AJ, Southey MC, et al. The histologic phenotypes of breast carcinoma occurring before age 40 years in women with and without BRCA1 or BRCA2 germline mutations: a population-based study. *Cancer.* 1998;83:2335–2345.

67. Honrado E, Benitez J, Palacios J. The pathology of hereditary breast cancer. *Hered Cancer Clin Pract.* 2004;2:131–138.

68. Honrado E, Benitez J, Palacios J. The molecular pathology of hereditary breast cancer: genetic testing and therapeutic implications. *Mod Pathol.* 2005;18: 1305–1320.

69. Honrado E, Benitez J, Palacios J. Histopathology of BRCA1- and BRCA2-associated breast cancer. *Crit Rev Oncol Hematol.* 2006;59:27–39.

70. Lakhani SR, Jacquemier J, Sloane JP, et al. Multifactorial analysis of differences between sporadic breast cancers and cancers involving BRCA1 and BRCA2 mutations. *J Natl Cancer Inst.* 1998;90: 1138–1145.

71. Turner NC, Reis-Filho JS. Basal-like breast cancer and the BRCA1 phenotype. *Oncogene.* 2006;25:5846–5853.

72. Ellis IO, Galea M, Broughton N, Locker A, Blamey RW, Elston CW. Pathological prognostic factors in breast cancer. II. Histological type. Relationship with survival in a large study with long-term follow-up. *Histopathology.* 1992;20:479–489.

73. Ferguson DJ, Anderson TJ, Wells CA, Battersby S. An ultrastructural study of mucoid carcinoma of the breast: variability of cytoplasmic features. *Histopathology.* 1986;10:1219–1230.

74. Wilson TE, Helvie MA, Oberman HA, Joynt LK. Pure and mixed mucinous carcinoma of the breast: pathologic basis for differences in mammographic appearance. *AJR Am J Roentgenol.* 1995;165:285–289.

75. Adair F, Berg J, Joubert L, Robbins GF. Long-term follow up of breast cancer patients: the 30-year report. *Cancer.* 1974;33:1145–1150.

76. Hamele-Bena D, Cranor ML, Rosen PP. Mammary mucocele-like lesions. Benign and malignant. *Am J Surg Pathol.* 1996;20:1081–1085.

77. Ro JY, Sneige N, Sahin AA, Silva EG, del Junco GW, Ayala AG. Mucocelelike tumor of the breast associated with atypical ductal hyperplasia or mucinous carcinoma. A clinicopathologic study of seven cases. *Arch Pathol Lab Med.* 1991;115:137–140.

78. Rosen PP. Mucocele-like tumors of the breast. *Am J Surg Pathol.* 1986;10:464–469.

79. Page DL, Anderson TJ. How should we categorize breast cancer. *Breast.* 1993;2:217–219.

80. Pereira H, Pinder SE, Sibbering DM, et al. Pathological prognostic factors in breast cancer. IV: Should you be a typer or a grader? A comparative study of two histological prognostic features in operable breast carcinoma. *Histopathology.* 1995;27:219–226.

81. Prioleau PG, Santa Cruz DJ, Buettner JB, Bauer WC. Sweat gland differentiation in mammary adenoid cystic carcinoma. *Cancer.* 1979;43:1752–1760.

82. Simpson JF, Page DL. Prognostic value of histopathology in the breast. *Semin Oncol.* 1992;19:254–262.

83. Hjorth S, Magnusson PH, Blomquist P. Adenoid cystic carcinoma of the breast. Report of a case in a male and review of the literature. *Acta Chir Scand.* 1977;143:155–158.

84. Lusted D. Structural and growth patterns of adenoid cystic carcinoma of breast. *Am J Clin Pathol.* 1970;54:419–425.

85. Cavanzo FJ, Taylor HB. Adenoid cystic carcinoma of the breast. An analysis of 21 cases. *Cancer.* 1969;24:740–745.

86. Galloway JR, Woolner LB, Clagett OT. Adenoid cystic carcinoma of the breast. *Surg Gynecol Obstet.* 1966;122:1289–1294.

87. Anthony PP, James PD. Adenoid cystic carcinoma of the breast: prevalence, diagnostic criteria, and histogenesis. *J Clin Pathol.* 1975;28:647–655.

88. Friedman BA, Oberman HA. Adenoid cystic carcinoma of the breast. *Am J Clin Pathol.* 1970;54:1–14.

89. Qizilbash AH, Patterson MC, Oliveira KF. Adenoid cystic carcinoma of the breast. Light and electron microscopy and a brief review of the literature. *Arch Pathol Lab Med.* 1977;101:302–306.

90. Jaworski RC, Kneale KL, Smith RC. Adenoid cystic carcinoma of the breast. *Postgrad Med J.* 1983;59:48–51.

91. Leeming R, Jenkins M, Mendelsohn G. Adenoid cystic carcinoma of the breast. *Arch Surg.* 1992;127:233–235.

92. Wells CA, Nicoll S, Ferguson DJ. Adenoid cystic carcinoma of the breast: a case with axillary lymph node metastasis. *Histopathology.* 1986;10:415–424.

93. Shin SJ, Rosen PP. Solid variant of mammary adenoid cystic carcinoma with basaloid features: a study of nine cases. *Am J Surg Pathol.* 2002;26:413–420.

94. Acs G, Simpson JF, Bleiweiss IJ, et al. Microglandular adenosis with transition into adenoid cystic carcinoma of the breast. *Am J Surg Pathol.* 2003;27:1052–1060.

95. Kleer CG, Oberman HA. Adenoid cystic carcinoma of the breast: value of histologic grading and proliferative activity. *Am J Surg Pathol.* 1998;22:569–575.

96. Clement PB, Young RH, Azzopardi JG. Collagenous spherulosis of the breast. *Am J Surg Pathol.* 1987;11:411–417.

97. Simpson JF, Page DL. Status of breast cancer prognostication based on histopathologic data. *Am J Clin Pathol.* 1994;102:S3–S8.

98. Koss LG, Brannan CD, Ashikari R. Histologic and ultrastructural features of adenoid cystic carcinoma of the breast. *Cancer.* 1970;26:1271–1279.

99. Kasami M, Olson SJ, Simpson JF, Page DL. Maintenance of polarity and a dual cell population in adenoid cystic carcinoma of the breast: an immunohistochemical study. *Histopathology.* 1998;32:232–238.

100. Mastropasqua MG, Maiorano E, Pruneri G, et al. Immunoreactivity for c-kit and p63 as an adjunct in the diagnosis of adenoid cystic carcinoma of the breast. *Mod Pathol.* 2005;18:1277–1282.

101. Ro JY, Silva EG, Gallager HS. Adenoid cystic carcinoma of the breast. *Hum Pathol.* 1987;18:1276–1281.

102. Zaloudek C, Oertel YC, Orenstein JM. Adenoid cystic carcinoma of the breast. *Am J Clin Pathol.* 1984;81:297–307.

103. Pastolero G, Hanna W, Zbieranowski I, Kahn HJ. Proliferative activity and p53 expression in

adenoid cystic carcinoma of the breast. *Mod Pathol.* 1996;9:215–219.

104. Trendell-Smith NJ, Peston D, Shousha S. Adenoid cystic carcinoma of the breast: a tumour commonly devoid of oestrogen receptors and related proteins. *Histopathology* 1999;35:241–248.

105. Sheen-Chen SM, Eng HL, Chen WJ, Cheng YF, Ko SF. Adenoid cystic carcinoma of the breast: truly uncommon or easily overlooked? *Anticancer Res.* 2005;25:455–458.

106. Peters GN, Wolff M. Adenoid cystic carcinoma of the breast. Report of 11 new cases: review of the literature and discussion of biological behavior. *Cancer.* 1983;52:680–686.

107. Sumpio BE, Jennings TA, Merino MJ, Sullivan PD. Adenoid cystic carcinoma of the breast. Data from the Connecticut Tumor Registry and a review of the literature. *Ann Surg.* 1987;205:295–301.

108. Herzberg AJ, Bossen EH, Walther PJ. Adenoid cystic carcinoma of the breast metastatic to the kidney. A clinically symptomatic lesion requiring surgical management. *Cancer.* 1991;68:1015–1020.

109. Koller M, Ram Z, Findler G, Lipshitz M. Brain metastasis: a rare manifestation of adenoid cystic carcinoma of the breast. *Surg Neurol.* 1986;26:470–472.

110. Gobbi H, Simpson JF, Borowsky A, Jensen RA, Page DL. Metaplastic breast tumors with a dominant fibromatosis-like phenotype have a high risk of local recurrence. *Cancer.* 1999;85:2170–2182.

111. Gobbi H, Simpson JF, Jensen RA, Olson SJ, Page DL. Metaplastic spindle cell breast tumors arising within papillomas, complex sclerosing lesions, and nipple adenomas. *Mod Pathol.* 2003;16:893–901.

112. Van Hoeven KH, Drudis T, Cranor ML, Erlandson RA, Rosen PP. Low-grade adenosquamous carcinoma of the breast. A clinocopathologic study of 32 cases with ultrastructural analysis. *Am J Surg Pathol.* 1993;17:248–258.

113. Drudis T, Arroyo C, Van Hoeven K, Cordon-Cardo C, Rosen PP. The pathology of low-grade adenosquamous carcinoma of the breast. An immunohistochemical study. *Pathol Annu.* 1994;29(Pt 2):181–197.

114. Rosen PP, Ernsberger D. Low-grade adenosquamous carcinoma. A variant of metaplastic mammary carcinoma. *Am J Surg Pathol.* 1987;11:351–358.

115. McDivitt RW, Stewart FW. Breast carcinoma in children. *JAMA.* 1966;195:388–390.

116. Rosen PP, Cranor ML. Secretory carcinoma of the breast. *Arch Pathol Lab Med.* 1991;115:141–144.

117. Serour F, Gilad A, Kopolovic J, Krispin M. Secretory breast cancer in childhood and adolescence: report of a case and review of the literature. *Med Pediatr Oncol.* 1992;20:341–344.

118. Tavassoli FA, Norris HJ. Secretory carcinoma of the breast. *Cancer.* 1980;45:2404–2413.

119. Tognon C, Knezevich SR, Huntsman D, et al. Expression of the ETV6-NTRK3 gene fusion as a primary event in human secretory breast carcinoma. *Cancer Cell.* 2002;2:367–376.

120. Eguchi M, Eguchi-Ishimae M, Tojo A, et al. Fusion of ETV6 to neurotrophin-3 receptor TRKC in acute myeloid leukemia with t(12;15)(p13;q25). *Blood.* 1999;93:1355–1363.

121. Knezevich SR, Garnett MJ, Pysher TJ, Beckwith JB, Grundy PE, Sorensen PH. ETV6-NTRK3 gene fusions and trisomy 11 establish a histogenetic link between mesoblastic nephroma and congenital fibrosarcoma. *Cancer Res.* 1998;58:5046–5048.

122. Knezevich SR, McFadden DE, Tao W, Lim JF, Sorensen PH. A novel ETV6-NTRK3 gene fusion in congenital fibrosarcoma. *Nat Genet.* 1998;18:184–187.

123. Liu Q, Schwaller J, Kutok J, et al. Signal transduction and transforming properties of the TEL-TRKC fusions associated with t(12;15)(p13;q25) in congenital fibrosarcoma and acute myelogenous leukemia. *EMBO J.* 2000;19:1827–1838.

124. Wai DH, Knezevich SR, Lucas T, Jansen B, Kay RJ, Sorensen PH. The ETV6-NTRK3 gene fusion encodes a chimeric protein tyrosine kinase that transforms NIH3T3 cells. *Oncogene.* 2000;19:906–915.

125. Farrow JH, Ashikari H. Breast lesions in young girls. *Surg Clin North Am.* 1969;49:261–269.

126. Oberman HA, Stephens PJ. Carcinoma of the breast in childhood. *Cancer.* 1972;30:470–474.

127. Tanimura A, Konaka K. Carcinoma of the breast in a 5 years old girl. *Acta Pathol Jpn.* 1980;30:157–160.

128. Ferguson TB Jr, McCarty KS Jr, Filston HC. Juvenile secretory carcinoma and juvenile papillomatosis: diagnosis and treatment. *J Pediatr Surg.* 1987;22:637–639.

129. Heydenrych JJ, Villet WT, von der Heyden U. Carcinoma of the breast in children: a case report and review of the literature. *S Afr Med J.* 1980;57:1005–1008.

130. Rosen PP, Cantrell B, Mullen DL, DePalo A. Juvenile papillomatosis (Swiss cheese disease) of the breast. *Am J Surg Pathol.* 1980;4:3–12.

131. Simpson JS, Barson AJ. Breast tumours in infants and children: a 40-year review of cases at a children's hospital. *Can Med Assoc J.* 1969;101:100–102.

132. Byrne MP, Fahey MM, Gooselaw JG. Breast cancer with axillary metastasis in an eight and one-half-year-old girl. *Cancer.* 1973;31:726–728.

133. Karl SR, Ballantine TV, Zaino R. Juvenile secretory carcinoma of the breast. *J Pediatr Surg.* 1985;20:368–371.

134. Masse SR, Rioux A, Beauchesne C. Juvenile carcinoma of the breast. *Hum Pathol.* 1981;12:1044–1046.

135. Rosen PP, Lyngholm B, Kinne DW, Beattie EJ Jr. Juvenile papillomatosis of the breast and family history of breast carcinoma. *Cancer.* 1982;49: 2591–2595.

136. Krausz T, Jenkins D, Grontoft O, Pollock DJ, Azzopardi JG. Secretory carcinoma of the breast in adults: emphasis on late recurrence and metastasis. *Histopathology.* 1989;14:25–36.

8

Mesenchymal Lesions of the Breast

MELINDA E. SANDERS

JOHN S. J. BROOKS

JUAN P. PALAZZO

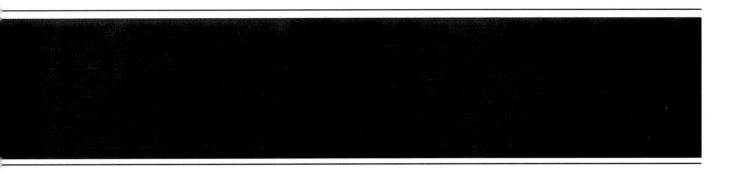

There are a number of benign and malignant mesenchymal lesions in the breast that can present difficult diagnostic dilemmas to the surgical pathologist because their differential diagnoses may overlap. This chapter covers a multitude of benign and malignant stromal and mixed stromal and epithelial lesions and discusses their diagnostic features and differential diagnoses.

■ BENIGN NONNEOPLASTIC STROMAL LESIONS

Pseudoangiomatous Stromal Hyperplasia

Pathologic Features

Pseudoangiomatous stromal hyperplasia (PASH) is a hormone-dependent stromal change of the breast characterized by a proliferation of myofibroblasts that resembles a vascular lesion due to the presence of small slit-like spaces (1–3). It affects predominantly, but not exclusively, premenopausal women and can be seen in men in association with gynecomastia. It is often an incidental finding but may present as a radiographic or palpable mass in young patients. Pseudoangiomatous stromal hyperplasia can be associated with other lesions, including fibroadenomas and phyllodes tumors.

The classic PASH lesion consists of a proliferation of slit-shaped spaces without red blood cells in a dense, keloid-like stroma (Figure 8.1). Some of the spaces are lined by a single layer of spindle-shaped myofibroblasts resembling endothelial cells (Figure 8.2). The stromal cellularity varies from hypocellular in the classic lesion to myofibroblastoma-like where the myofibroblasts form short fascicles. This latter appearance has been called fascicular PASH. Pseudoangiomatous stromal hyperplasia has ill-defined margins, and it blends with the surrounding breast stroma. Mitotic figures, nuclear atypia, necrosis, and calcifications should not be present in PASH.

The main differential diagnostic consideration for PASH is a vascular lesion, such as well-differentiated angiosarcoma. Other considerations include well-differentiated fibro-

sarcoma variants and biphasic tumors that show a dense cellular stroma as one of the components. Pseudoangiomatous stromal hyperplasia does not show the infiltrating and anastomosing vascular spaces of angiosarcoma. The myofibroblasts that line the slit-like spaces of PASH lack the atypia seen in the endothelial cells of angiosarcoma and are negative for endothelial markers by immunohistochemistry. Low-grade fibrosarcomas are composed of a monotonous proliferation of spindle cells that infiltrate the breast parenchyma and adipose tissue. In contrast to PASH, their nuclei are larger and atypical and show mitotic figures.

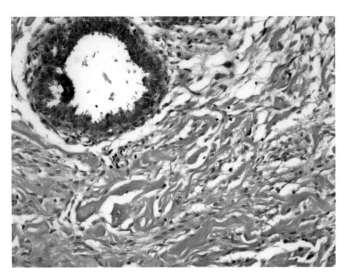

FIGURE 8.1 Pseudoangiomatous stromal hyperplasia showing a proliferation of slit-shaped spaces within a keloid stroma.

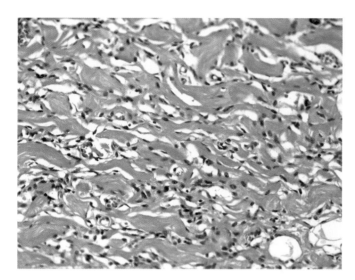

FIGURE 8.2 The pseudovascular spaces of PASH lack red blood cells are lined by benign myofibroblastic cells, and lack atypia and mitotic activity.

Immunohistochemistry

The cells lining the pseudovascular spaces of PASH are positive for vimentin and CD34 and negative for factor VIII, CD31, estrogen receptor, and epithelial markers. Other markers that can be positive in the spindle cells are progesterone receptor, smooth muscle actin, calponin, desmin, and BCL2.

Management

Pseudoangiomatous stromal hyperplasia does not need to be excised once other lesions have been excluded by morphology or with the help of immunohistochemical markers.

Reactive Spindle Cell Nodule After Biopsy or Fine-Needle Aspiration

Pathologic Features

After fine-needle aspiration or core biopsy of the breast, the stroma may become quite cellular with proliferation of spindled and epithelioid fibroblasts with large atypical nuclei forming a reactive spindle cell nodule. These changes are typically present 2 weeks after the procedure. A history of a previous procedure (core biopsy or fine-needle aspiration) is critical to correctly identify these benign lesions and differentiate them from other neoplastic spindle cell lesions. A careful search for the focal presence of hemosiderin, acute and chronic inflammation, fat necrosis, and foreign body giant cell reaction are also important clues to the diagnosis when present (4–5).

Reactive spindle cell nodules have been described with greater frequency in patients with papillary and sclerosing lesions but may be seen after biopsy of any breast lesion. They are nonencapsulated and composed of plump spindle cells arranged in a storiform pattern. Cellularity

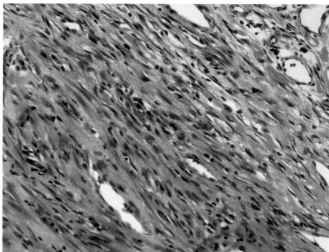

FIGURE 8.3 Reactive spindle cell nodule showing a dense cellular proliferation of spindle and epithelioid cells.

varies from hypocellular to hypercellular. Entrapment of the surrounding breast parenchyma is a typical feature. The fibroblastic cells have mild to moderate atypia, but mitotic activity is low. Chronic inflammation and hemosiderin-laden macrophages are typically present (Figures 8.3 and 8.4). The differential diagnosis includes metaplastic carcinoma, inflammatory pseudotumor, myofibroblastoma, nodular fasciitis, and fibromatosis. Metaplastic carcinomas often show areas of typical carcinoma, infiltrative margins, and cytokeratin expression.

Immunohistochemistry

The proliferating cells in reactive spindle cell nodules express muscle markers and vimentin but are negative for epithelial markers. In contrast, p63 and other keratins such as CK5/6 and CK903 are expressed in metaplastic carcinomas. β-Catenin is positive in fibromatosis and

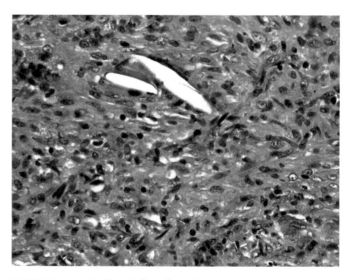

FIGURE 8.4 In this spindle cell nodule, there are macrophages and chronic inflammatory cells.

negative in metaplastic carcinoma and reactive spindle cell nodules.

Management

Reactive spindle cell nodules involute spontaneously, and there is no need for reexcision.

Nodular Fasciitis

Pathologic Features

Nodular fasciitis is a reactive condition that can affect the subcutaneous tissue of the skin and the breast parenchyma (6). Patients typically report a history of rapid growth and tenderness, which tends to regress spontaneously after weeks or months. Histologically, nodular fasciitis lacks a capsule but is well circumscribed. It is characterized by a proliferation of spindle cell myofibroblasts arranged in short fascicles embedded in a collagenous and myxoid stroma. Mitotic figures are usually present, but necrosis or significant cellular atypia is absent. Initially, lesions are more cellular and become with time hypocellular, and the cells are immersed in a keloid-like hyalinized stroma. Extravasated red blood cells and focal lymphocytic infiltrates are frequently present (Figure 8.5).

The main differential diagnosis of nodular fasciitis (NF) is myxoma, metaplastic carcinoma, fibromatosis, and sarcomas of the breast. Myxomas have relatively well-circumscribed margins, and the spindle cells are seen immersed in a myxoid stroma. The vascular pattern is not prominent, and the cells of myxoma lack atypical features. Fibromatosis shows infiltrative margins involving breast and soft tissues and is composed of a monotonous population of spindle cells. Both sarcomas and carcinomas show areas with more atypical cells, necrosis, atypical mitoses, and carcinomas express cytokeratins.

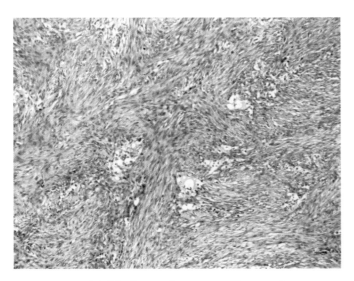

FIGURE 8.5 Nodular fasciitis showing a proliferation of monotonous spindle cells with microcysts and extravasated red blood cells.

Immunohistochemistry

The cells of NF express the muscle markers actin and desmin. Immunohistochemical markers are helpful to distinguish NF from metaplastic carcinoma by the lack of expression of epithelial markers in NF.

Management

There is no need to recommend reexcision of NF if the diagnosis can be rendered in core biopsy material and other entities are excluded.

■ BENIGN NEOPLASTIC STROMAL LESIONS

Fibromatosis

Pathologic Features

Clinically, fibromatosis presents as a firm, discrete mass that may distort the overlying skin or involve the chest wall. This infiltrative process can be locally aggressive, simulating carcinoma clinically and mammographically. Fibromatosis is usually sporadic but may be rarely associated with familial adenomatous polyposis or Gardner syndrome or as a component of hereditary desmoid syndrome (6–8).

Most examples of fibromatosis are gray-white and fibrous with ill-defined margins, ranging in size from 1 to greater than 10 cm. Rare cases may show some circumscription. Histologically, fibromatosis is composed of bland spindle cells with oval to spindled nuclei and poorly defined cell borders. The cells assemble in long, broad fascicles that infiltrate the surrounding stroma and may be accompanied by varying degrees of collagenization, which when particularly abundant may impart a keloid-like appearance (Figure 8.6A–C). Benign lobular units and ducts are often entrapped in the tumor. Myxoid foci, calcifications, and lymphoid aggregates may also be present. The cellularity of fibromatosis may vary, with the more cellular regions typically present at the periphery. Mitoses, when present, are usually in these peripheral cellular areas and number less than 3 per 10 high-power fields (HPF). Fibromatosis tends to be more cellular and mitotically active in children and in women of child-bearing age than in older women (9).

The most important consideration in the differential diagnosis for fibromatosis is the fibromatosis-like metaplastic carcinoma. The presence of scattered epithelioid cells, squamoid morules, slight myxoid character to the stroma, and scattered to rare mononuclear inflammatory cells are subtle clues to this diagnosis. The use of a battery of immunohistochemical stains for cytokeratins should correctly identify the carcinoma component

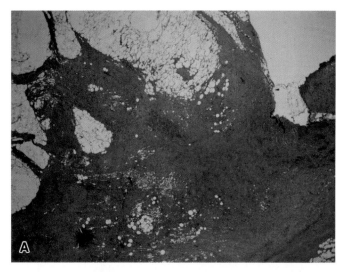

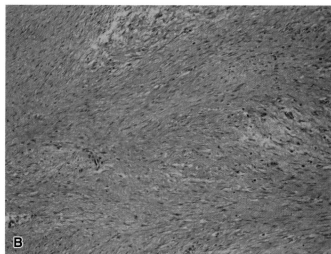

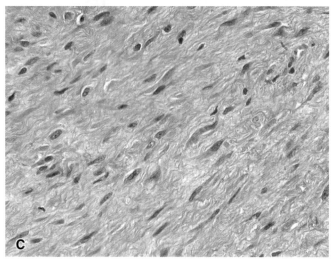

FIGURE 8.6 (A) Fibromatosis at low power is characterized by long sweeping fascicles and infiltrative margins. (B) Fibromatosis is composed of a monotonous population of elongated bland spindle cells with oval to spindled nuclei and poorly defined cell borders. (C) Fibromatosis at high power shows bland nuclei and a dense collagenous, often with keloid-like stroma. Note the lack of nuclear atypia.

of this lesion. In our practice, we find p63 to be the most informative of the keratins followed by CK903 and orthokeratin. Cytokeratin AE1/3 is often the least informative.

The differential diagnosis also includes a scar from a prior procedure or trauma. Accompanying features such as fat necrosis, foreign body giant cell reaction, and hemosiderin deposition are typically present in association with a scar. In patients undergoing reexcision or a recurrence, distinction of fibromatosis from scar at the margins may be very difficult. Staining of the margin sections with β-catenin may be useful in such cases but should be interpreted with caution. Lesser considerations are nodular fasciitis and spindle cell sarcoma. In contrast to fibromatosis, the spindle cells of nodular fasciitis are plumper, their nuclei contain prominent nucleoli, and they are arranged in short fascicles. Mitotic figures are easily seen and can be numerous. The foci of extravasated red blood cells and histiocytic giant cells may be helpful clues to the diagnosis. Spindle cell sarcomas are typically more cellular than fibromatosis, demonstrating obvious nuclear pleomorphism and prominent mitotic figures including atypical mitoses.

Immunohistochemistry

Fibromatosis typically demonstrates cytoplasmic staining for actin and nuclear staining for β-catenin in 80% of the cases (10) (Figure 8.7). Desmin and S-100 positivity may be detected in a minority of cells. Fibromatosis is negative for cytokeratins, BCL-2, CD34, estrogen, progesterone, and androgen receptors (9).

Management

If anatomically feasible, wide local excision to obtain negative margins should be undertaken to minimize the risk of local recurrence (7,8).

Myofibroblastoma

Pathologic Features

Myofibroblastomas are benign, slowly growing myofibroblastic proliferations that occur in equal frequency among men and women (11). Mammographically and clinically, they may be mistaken for fibroadenomas because they are

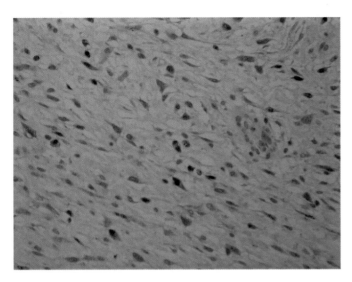

FIGURE 8.7 Immunohistochemical stain for β-catenin showing strong nuclear staining.

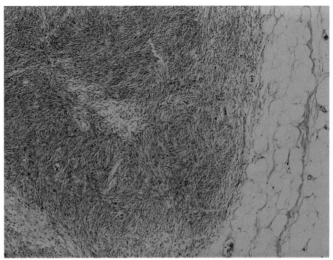

FIGURE 8.8 Myofibroblastoma showing a well-circumscribed proliferation of short fascicles of spindle cells separated by dense collagenous stroma.

circumscribed and mobile. There are no reports of association with microcalcifications. Grossly, myofibroblastomas are rubbery and firm, pink to white-tan, and often with a whorled cut surface similar to a uterine leiomyoma. The described size range is less than 1 to 13 cm (6,11). Histologically, myofibroblastomas are well circumscribed but nonencapsulated. In occasional cases, a portion of the margin may be irregular but should not be infiltrative.

Myofibroblastomas are composed of short fascicles of uniform spindle cells with bland oval nuclei and ill-defined cell borders that are interspersed with hyalinized collagen. The eosinophilic collagen component may be equally proportionate to the spindle cell component or highly abundant with limited numbers of spindle cells (Figures 8.8 and 8.9). Occasionally, the spindle cells have an epithelioid appearance simulating infiltrating lobular carcinoma. Scattered mast cells are usually present. Mitoses are rare, and necrosis is absent. The lesion also

contains a mature lipomatous component that can range from a few adipocytes to a predominantly fatty lesion (12). The morphologic similarity to spindle cell lipoma and a report of shared genetic abnormalities including partial monosomy of 13q and partial monosomy of 16q (13) suggest that the two entities represent a spectrum of the same lesion. Cases where the lipomatous component predominates have been termed lipomatous myofibroblastoma by some authors (12).

Important considerations in the differential diagnosis for myofibroblastoma include fibromatosis, nodular fasciitis, lobular carcinoma, and spindle cell metaplastic carcinoma. In contrast to the long sweeping fascicles of fibromatosis, the fascicles of myofibroblastoma are short. The spindle cells are similarly bland, but fibromatosis lacks the interspersed eosinophilic collagen bundles of myofibroblastoma. The characteristic spindle cells of nodular fasciitis with vesicular nuclei and prominent nucleoli contrast with the bland spindle cells of myofibroblastoma. In myofibroblastoma, extravasated erythrocytes are not seen, but this finding is common in nodular fasciitis. Mitoses are rare if observed in myofibroblastoma, whereas they are common and may be numerous in nodular fasciitis. Myofibroblastomas with epithelioid features can be mistaken for infiltrating lobular carcinoma. Immunohistochemical staining with a pan keratin marker should resolve this diagnosis and should either precede or accompany estrogen and progesterone receptor studies, as both of the latter may be positive in myofibroblastomas. When the differential diagnosis includes a metaplastic spindle cell carcinoma, the performance of immunohistochemistry for several high- and low-molecular-weight keratin stains is mandatory and should highlight the carcinoma cells, which can be subtle. The scattered epithelioid cells and squamoid nests that may be seen in spindle cell

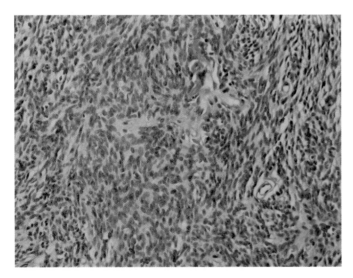

FIGURE 8.9 Higher-power magnification of myofibroblastoma showing the cellular stroma and epithelioid myofibroblasts.

metaplastic carcinomas are absent in myofibroblastoma. Pseudoangiomatous stromal hyperplasia and fibroadenomas may have myofibroblastoma-like areas that are of no clinical significance. In rare fibroadenomas, such areas may be prominent.

Immunohistochemistry

The spindle cells of myofibroblastoma are positive for vimentin, desmin, CD34, and BCL-2 and variably positive for smooth muscle actin. Estrogen receptor, progesterone receptor, and androgen receptor positivity can be seen, but tumor cells should always be negative for keratin.

Management

Adequate treatment for these benign lesions is local excision.

Solitary Fibrous Tumor

Pathologic Features

Solitary fibrous tumor in the breast typically presents as a single well-circumscribed, indolently growing nodule in an elderly patient (14,15). Tumor sizes have ranged from 6 to 30 mm. Grossly, solitary fibrous tumors are unencapsulated but well-circumscribed firm nodules with a smooth external surface. Histologically, they are similar to solitary fibrous tumors seen elsewhere, characterized by a random arrangement ("patternless" pattern) of uniform, nonatypical, round to ovoid spindled tumor cells with little cytoplasm, indistinct borders, and vesicular nuclei with dispersed chromatin and inconspicuous nucleoli (16–18) (Figures 8.10 and 8.11). Hypercellular areas containing these cells are randomly admixed with thick eosinophilic bands of keloid-like collagen. Mast cells may

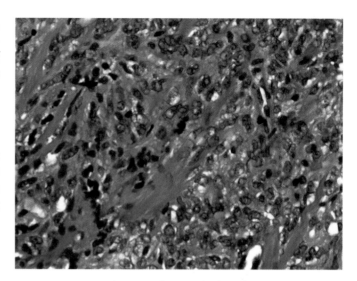

FIGURE 8.11 Higher magnification of solitary fibrous tumor showing lack of atypia and patternless growth.

be abundant. Vessels with thick and hyalinized walls are frequently present, which may have a "staghorn" appearance. Additional findings include myxomatous stroma and chronic inflammation.

Fortunately, most solitary fibrous tumors in the breast are benign. Mitoses are typically rare, uncommonly exceeding 3 per 10 HPF. Malignant solitary fibrous tumors are typically hypercellular lesions with moderate to marked cellular atypia at least focally, necrosis, obvious mitotic activity (≥4 mitoses per 10 HPF), and/or infiltrative margins.

The differential diagnosis for solitary fibrous tumor includes other spindle cell lesions of the breast such as myofibroblastoma, PASH, post-biopsy spindle cell nodules, metaplastic carcinoma, synovial sarcoma, and low-grade fibromyxoid sarcoma.

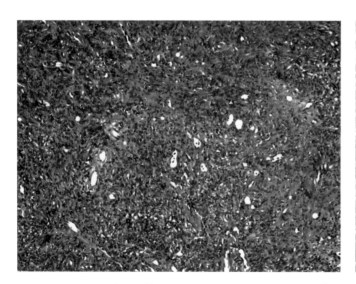

FIGURE 8.10 Solitary fibrous tumor with hypercellular areas of round cells between bands of keloid-like collagen.

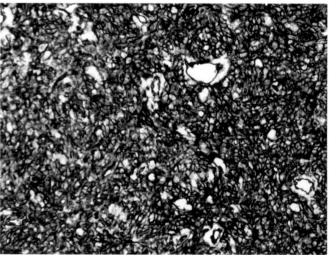

FIGURE 8.12 Immunohistochemistry showing strong CD34 positivity in most cells in solitary fibrous tumor.

Immunohistochemistry

The tumor cells in solitary fibrous tumor are typically strongly and diffusely positive for CD34 (90%–95% of cases) (14,16–18) and CD99 (70% of cases) (Figure 8.12). Tumor cells show variable positivity in 20% to 35% of cases for BCL-2 (15,19) and epithelial membrane antigen. A subset of cases are positive for estrogen and progesterone receptors (19,20). Solitary fibrous tumors are typically negative for actin, desmin, and smooth muscle actin; however, focal reactivity for S-100, cytokeratin, and/or desmin has been reported.

Management

Although most cases of solitary fibrous tumor are benign, the behavior of solitary fibrous tumor can be unpredictable with approximately 10% to 15% demonstrating malignant behavior. Thus, solitary fibrous tumor is best treated by complete surgical excision.

Other Benign Soft Tissue Tumors

The breast can uncommonly be the primary site of benign tumors such as leiomyoma, nerve sheath tumors, and myxomas. All these tumors are histologically identical to their counterparts elsewhere. They tend to be well circumscribed, encapsulated, and lack cytologic atypia. Immunohistochemical stains can be very useful to definitively identify these tumors. Leiomyomas can occur in the breast, almost exclusively arising in the nipple region. Leiomyomas express smooth muscle actin and desmin, whereas nerve sheath tumors express S-100 protein and neurofilament (21). Neurofibromas and schwannomas are both S-100–positive; however, neurofibromas are more often neurofilament-positive than schwannomas. Myxomas consist of round-, spindle-, and stellate-shaped cells embedded in an abundant myxoid matrix with inconspicuous supporting vascularity (Figure 8.13). These cells express vimentin and calponin but are negative for muscle and myofibroblastic markers (22).

■ MASS-FORMING CHRONIC FIBROINFLAMMATORY PROLIFERATIONS IN THE BREAST

This is an uncommon group of lesions that can be thought of collectively as "inflammatory pseudotumors" of the breast characterized by proliferation of fibroblasts and myofibroblasts accompanied by a prominent chronic inflammatory infiltrate. These encompass a wide spectrum of reactive, possibly autoimmune, and neoplastic conditions published as case reports and small case series diagnosed as diabetic mastopathy, IgG4-related sclerosing mastitis, and inflammatory myofibroblastic tumor (IMT). At present, the relationship between these entities, if any, is unclear; therefore, the most appropriate classification system and nomenclature for these lesions should be considered a work in progress.

Diabetic Mastopathy/Sclerosing Lymphocytic Lobulitis

Diabetic mastopathy, also known as sclerosing lymphocytic lobulitis and lymphocytic mastopathy, is a distinctive clinicopathologic entity with a strong association with autoimmune disease, likely representing an immune reaction to abnormal matrix production (23). These patients typically have painless, palpable ill-defined, or nodular breast masses that are predominantly subareolar (24). They are usually unilateral but may be bilateral and have been described in male breasts (24). The condition was

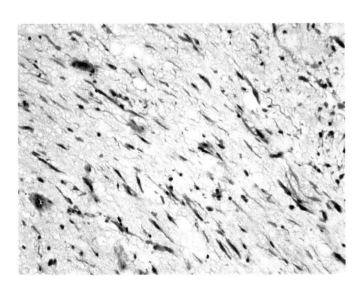

FIGURE 8.13 Breast myxoma showing a myxoid matrix with spindle and stellate cells and inconspicuous vessels.

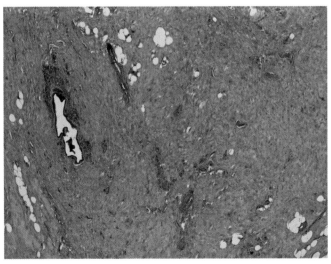

FIGURE 8.14 Sclerosing lymphocytic lobulitis with perilobular and periductal lymphocytic infiltrates and dense fibrosis.

first reported by Soler and Khardori (25) in 1984 in a group of 12 women with long-standing type 1 diabetes mellitus with secondary complications and shortly after designated diabetic mastopathy (26). The defining criteria for diabetic mastopathy as proposed by Tomaszewski et al. (23) are dense fibrosis associated with (1) lymphocytic lobulitis and ductitis, (2) lymphocytic perivasculitis, and (3) epithelioid fibroblasts, with the presence of epithelioid fibroblasts being the most sensitive and specific feature (Figures 8.14 and 8.15). However, the specificity of these features has been questioned because identical findings have now been reported in a few patients with type 2 diabetes and nondiabetic patients without evidence of other autoimmune diseases (24). Patients with Hashimoto thyroiditis (23,25,27), Graves disease (28), Sjogren syndrome (29), or a combination of goiter and diabetes (25) have also been reported to have histologic features of diabetic mastopathy, giving further support to the concept of an underlying autoimmune etiology. The chronic inflammatory infiltrate is composed of predominantly B cells that are polyclonal (29) and may include follicles with germinal centers.

In nondiabetic patients, the appearance of diabetic mastopathy may precede the onset of clinical diabetes or another autoimmune process. Once the diagnosis is established, no further treatment is necessary. For excised lesions, recurrences are common and can be ipsilateral, bilateral, or contralateral on repeated occasions (24). It may be that the more generic term *sclerosing lymphocytic lobulitis* is the better name for this entity given its documented association with nondiabetic conditions.

IgG4-Related Sclerosing Mastitis

Immunoglobulin (IgG) 4–related sclerosing disease is characterized by mass-forming lesions in various organs composed

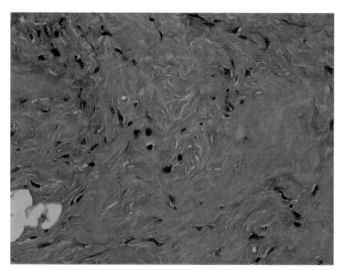

FIGURE 8.15 Higher magnification showing epithelioid fibroblasts embedded in the dense stroma.

of dense lymphoplasmacytic infiltrates and stromal sclerosis, elevated serum IgG4 titer, and increased tissue IgG4 plasma cells (30). To date, only 4 cases of IgG4-related sclerosing disease have been reported in the breast (31). All patients were Asian women, with ages ranging from 37 to 54, who presented with painless masses in both breasts. Histologically, the breast masses contained dense lymphoplasmacytic infiltrates, prominent stromal sclerosis, and loss of breast lobules. Plasma cells represented a significant proportion of the chronic inflammatory infiltrate and showed polytypic staining for Ig. IgG4+ cells ranged from 272 to 495 per HPF. These lesions differ from diabetic mastopathy in that the fibrosis usually predominates over the lymphocytic infiltration, which is characteristically limited to a narrow zone around lobular units, ducts, and vessels, and also, plasma cells are scanty. The differential diagnosis would also include lymphoma, which should be excluded based on appropriate immunohistochemical stains. Once the diagnosis was established in the reported patients, no recurrences occurred after excision of the mass. Thus, this entity appears to have a benign clinical course.

Inflammatory Myofibroblastic Tumor

Inflammatory myofibroblastic tumor has been reported in pulmonary and many extrapulmonary sites (32,33), including the breast (33–38). Although initially thought to be an aberrant inflammatory response, as our understanding of this entity has evolved, IMT is now classified as an intermediate, rarely metastasizing neoplasm (39). Fortunately, most affected individuals regardless of the primary site have had favorable clinical outcomes.

Histologically, IMT at other sites has 3 patterns: (1) myxoid, vascular, and inflammatory areas resembling nodular fasciitis; (2) compact spindle cells with intermingled inflammatory cells (lymphocytes, plasma cells, and eosinophils) resembling fibrous histiocytoma; and (3) dense plate-like collagen resembling a desmoid or scar (33). Immunohistochemically, the spindle cells are strongly positive for vimentin and variably positive for smooth muscle actin, muscle-specific actin, and desmin consistent with myofibroblasts (37,40,41). Recently, anaplastic lymphoma kinase (ALK) expression, resulting from translocations involving 2p23, has been demonstrated in 60% to 75% of IMT in the bladder (42,43) and other sites (44). A 9p deletion has also been reported in 3 cases of IMT, including one in the breast (36).

In the breast, reported cases of IMT are very rare with only 8 putative cases in the literature (33,34,36,38,45). These have been benign, nonmetastasizing proliferations of myofibroblasts with the potential for recurrence and persistent local growth. These cases have been reported to be multiple and bilateral (37) and recur several times locally (37,38), but there are no reports of malignant transformation. None of the cases in the breast have presented with constitutional symptoms, although the lesion in other sites has been associated with fever, malaise, and weight loss (32). The age at presentation among reported cases is 16 to 79 years. Grossly, these lesions are firm, pale, gray-white, ill-defined nodules (37). The average tumor size reported in the breast is 3.1 cm (range, 1.5–8.0 cm). Most lesions in the breast have infiltrative margins, although one case reportedly had well-circumscribed margins (45). Histologically and immunohistochemically, the lesions are reportedly similar to other sites; however, ALK-1 expression has not been demonstrated (36,37). In the breast, the cytology and histology have always been benign despite the fact that clinically and on imaging, it can resemble carcinoma (37). The differential diagnoses at this site include IgG4-related sclerosing disease (31), low-grade spindle cell sarcoma, fibromatosis, and nodular fasciitis. Given the lack of ALK-1 staining and constitutional symptoms in any of the reported cases calls the diagnosis of IMT at this site into question. The best designation for these lesions in the breast may be forthcoming (personal communication with Cheryl M. Coffin, MD).

■ FIBROEPITHELIAL LESIONS OF THE BREAST

Fibroadenoma

Pathologic Features

Fibroadenoma is a benign tumor composed of mesenchymal (stromal) and epithelial elements, likely resulting from a hyperplasia of the lobular unit with the fibrous elements usually predominating. Fibroadenoma occurs most commonly in women of child-bearing age, especially those younger than 30 years. They usually present as painless,

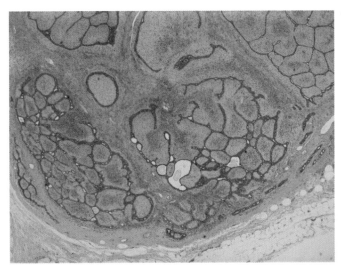

FIGURE 8.17 Fibroadenoma, intracanalicular type, stromal cell proliferation compresses the ducts that show a narrow lumen and cleft spaces.

firm, slowly growing, well-defined, mobile nodules. Symptoms may occur in the setting of rapid growth or infarction. In 15% to 20% of cases, fibroadenomas present as multiple nodules arising synchronously or asynchronously in the same or both breasts. The finding of multiple myxomatous fibroadenomas should raise the possibility of Carney syndrome (46,47).

Most fibroadenomas are 2 to 5 cm in greatest dimension. Grossly, they have a bulging, lobulated, gray-white cut surface with a few slit-like spaces. Myxoid areas may be evident. Histologically, the mixture of stromal and epithelial elements gives rise to a variety of growth patterns and varying degrees of cellularity, which have no significance clinically. The *pericanalicular* pattern results from the proliferation of stromal cells around glandular structures in a circumferential fashion and retains an acinar

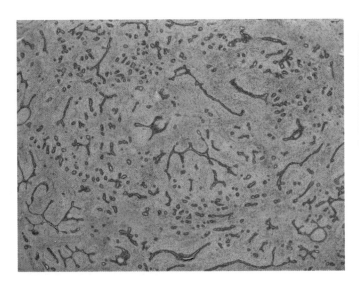

FIGURE 8.16 Fibroadenoma, pericanalicular type, in which the stromal cells proliferate around ducts with retention of the ducts and lobular units.

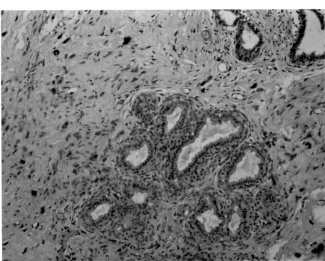

FIGURE 8.18 Fibroadenoma with bizzare multinucleated stromal giant cells.

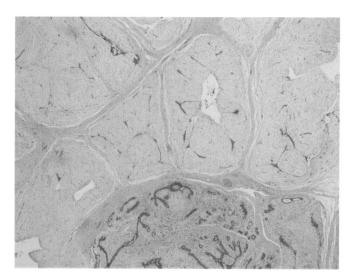

FIGURE 8.19 Fibroadenoma with extensive myxoid change of the stroma.

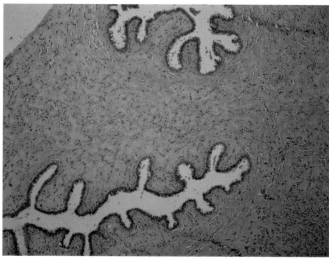

FIGURE 8.20 Pseudoangiomatous stromal hyperplasia in the stroma of a fibroadenoma.

arrangement of ducts and lobular units (Figure 8.16). The *intracanalicular* pattern is the result of compression of the ducts into clefts by the proliferating stromal cells (Figure 8.17). The stromal component may exhibit focal or diffuse hypercellularity, atypical multinucleated giant cells, extensive myxoid change (Figures 8.18 and 8.19), areas of PASH (Figure 8.20), myofibroblastic change (Figure 8.21) or hyalinization with dystrophic calcification, and rarely, ossification. Foci of lipomatous (Figure 8.22), smooth muscle, and osteochondroid metaplasia may rarely occur. Mitotic figures are uncommon.

The epithelial component may show varying degrees of epithelial hyperplasia, especially in adolescents, but it does not affect prognosis even in the presence of formal patterns of atypical hyperplasia when confined to the fibroadenoma (48). Extensive myoepithelial proliferation can be seen in some lesions and should not be confused with atypical hyperplasia.

Cellular fibroadenomas are characterized by increased stromal cellularity but do not demonstrate significant mitotic activity (usually <3 per 10 HPF) or stromal overgrowth (Figure 8.23). The cleft-like spaces, leaf-like projections, and periductal stromal cell condensation typical of phyllodes tumors are lacking. Although most fibroadenomas are well circumscribed and clearly delineated from the adjacent normal breast tissue, the occasional lesion will have borders that seem to merge with the surrounding breast tissue without a discrete margin. In the absence of stromal atypia or mitotic activity, such foci should not be of concern. The clinical entity "giant" or so-called juvenile fibroadenoma, typically accompanied by a history of rapid growth, may show focal areas with branching elongated clefts reminiscent of a benign phyllodes tumor. However, in the absence of a florid, true leaf-like growth pattern and/or moderately increased stromal cellularity accompanied by mitotic activity averaging 3

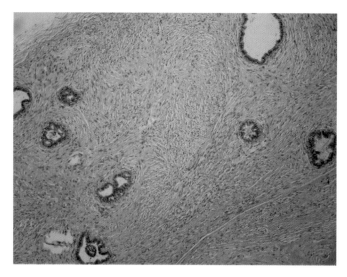

FIGURE 8.21 Fibroadenoma with benign myofibroblastic stroma.

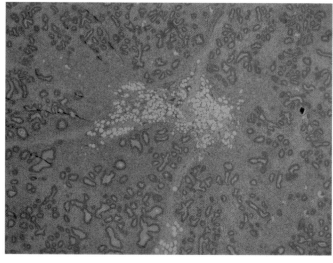

FIGURE 8.22 Lipomatous metaplasia in the stroma of a fibroadenoma.

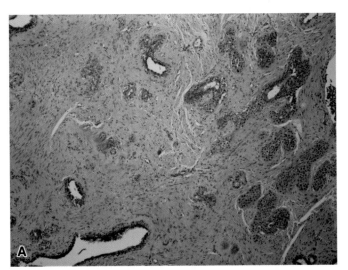

FIGURE 8.23 Cellular fibroadenoma demonstrating increased stromal cellularity without evidence of stromal overgrowth, atypia, or mitotic activity. Note the slight irregularity of the margin.

to 4 per 10 HPF, they should be designated as cellular fibroadenoma.

Prominent myoepithelial proliferation can be seen in some lesions and should not be confused with atypical hyperplasia. Immunohistochemical stains for smooth muscle actin and p63 are helpful in making this distinction. Foci of sclerosing adenosis, papillary apocrine change, and cysts greater than 3.0 mm are the features of a complex fibroadenoma, so named given the slight increase in the relative risk of carcinoma proposed to be associated with these features (49). Atypical ductal hyperplasia (ADH) and atypical lobular hyperplasia (ALH) are occasionally identified in a fibroadenoma (Figure 8.24A and B) but have not been found to increase the future risk of breast cancer unless they are also present outside the

fibroadenoma (48,49). Ductal carcinoma in situ is rarely found in association with fibroadenomas (50).

Management

Fibroadenomas can usually be managed by simple excision; however, in rare cases of multiple or giant fibroadenoma, a mastectomy may be required (51). If diagnosed on core biopsy or fine-needle aspiration, fibroadenomas may be followed clinically. After excision, the finding of an additional fibroadenoma may represent recurrence of an incompletely excised lesion or a metachronous lesion.

Tubular Variant and Nodular Gestational Hyperplasia

Pathologic Features

The tubular variant of fibroadenoma and clinically detectable nodules in the spectrum of nodular gestational hyperplasia aka "tubular adenomas" and "lactating adenomas" are best considered to be variants of fibroadenoma rather than actual "adenomas," as they are not truly neoplastic. Clinically and grossly, the tubular variant is well circumscribed, with a distinct interface with the normal breast and a homogeneous cut surface. They are white-tan and firm, whereas nodules in gestational hyperplasia are tan-yellow and somewhat softer. Histologically, tubular variants are composed of compactly arranged uniform tubules lined by a dual-cell population composed of an inner layer of cuboidal to columnar epithelial cells and an outer layer of myoepithelial cells with minimal amounts of specialized connective tissue between the tubules (Figure 8.25). Occasionally, mild fibrosis and patchy, sparse mononuclear cells may be seen. Foci resembling the tubular variant maybe seen within an otherwise classic fibroadenoma, a finding of no clinical significance.

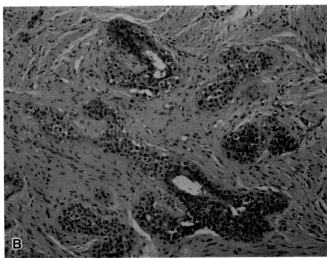

FIGURE 8.24 (A and B) Fibroadenoma with ALH. (B) Higher magnification of ALH with ductal involvement by cells of ALH.

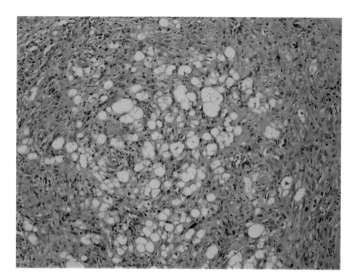

FIGURE 8.25 The tubular adenoma variant of fibroadenoma consists of a proliferation of benign tightly packed tubules similar to those in a normal lobular unit and has well-circumscribed margins.

Nodular gestational hyperplasia occurs during pregnancy or the postpartum period. Although the patient presentation suggests a discrete mass, the subsequent excision usually shows coalescence of several large lobular units forming a clinical mass. Prominent secretory activity is present throughout the breast tissue. Alternatively, the clinical mass may be a fibroadenoma with superimposed secretory change. Histologically, the lesions of nodular gestational hyperplasia form true acini with the alveolar pattern of the lactating breast. The luminal epithelial cells have large nuclei and abundant vacuolated cytoplasm (Figure 8.26). Tubular variants and foci within nodular gestational hyperplasia may infarct, especially during pregnancy (52,53) and should not be overdiagnosed as malignant based on the presence of necrosis.

Management

Excision is adequate therapy for tubular variants and discrete masses in nodular gestational hyperplasia but is not necessary. Negative margins are not required because these lesions are benign. If they are diagnosed on core biopsy or fine-needle aspiration, they may be followed clinically. Subsequent excision should be considered for a sudden rapid growth or symptomatic lesions.

Hamartoma

Pathologic Features

Hamartomas most commonly present in pre- and perimenopausal women as mobile nodules measuring 1 to 4 cm in size, similar to fibroadenomas. Radiographically, they form a distinctive, well-defined mass that may be centrally lucent. In fact, diagnosis of hamartoma should not be made in the absence of these characteristic findings. Grossly, they are gray-yellow, rubbery, and circumscribed. Histologically, hamartomas are composed of a disorganized combination of ductal and lobular structures, hyalinized stroma, and an adipose tissue component ranging from prominent to absent (Figure 8.27). Typically, the epithelial elements contain a single epithelial and myoepithelial cell layer. Epithelial hyperplasia is usually absent. The stromal component shows varying degrees of hyalinization haphazardly interposed among the epithelial elements. Foci of smooth muscle differentiation may be present, and when dominant, the lesions may be called a myoid hamartoma. Areas of PASH may also be present.

The differential diagnosis for mammary hamartoma includes fibroadenoma and benign phyllodes tumor. Both fibroadenomas and benign phyllodes tumors demonstrate a more regular relationship between the stromal and

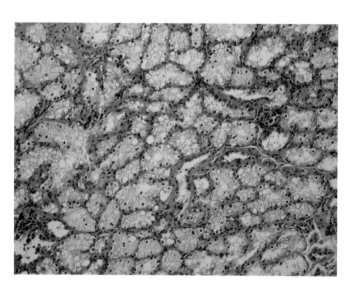

FIGURE 8.26 In nodular gestational hyperplasia, the tubules demonstrate prominant secretory change characterized by clear vacuolated cytoplasm.

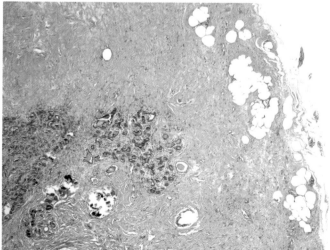

FIGURE 8.27 Hamartoma showing a disorganized proliferation of ductal and lobular units, hyalinized stroma, and adipose tissue.

epithelial elements compared with hamartomas. In addition, benign phyllodes tumors contain cleft-like spaces, and the stroma is more cellular.

Management

Hamartomas are benign, and simple excision is adequate. Similar to fibroadenomas, negative margins are not required.

Phyllodes Tumors

Pathologic Features

Phyllodes tumors account for less than 1% of breast tumors. They most commonly occur in middle-aged women with an average age at presentation of 40 to 50 years, which is about 15 to 20 years later than fibroadenomas. In Asian countries, phyllodes tumors occur at a younger age, averaging 25 to 30 years (54).

The usual presentation is a unilateral, firm, painless breast mass that is not adhesed to the skin. The average tumor size is 4 to 5 cm, and these lesions may have a history of rapid growth (55–57). Multifocal or bilateral lesions are rare. Very large tumors measuring 10 to 20 cm, which stretch the skin and distend the superficial veins, have been reported. Size does not appear to be a reliable criterion of biological behavior, although in a series reporting metastases, the average tumor size was greater (58). Spontaneous infarction may present clinically as bloody nipple discharge (59,60). Imaging studies usually demonstrate a rounded, sharply defined mass containing clefts and sometimes coarse calcifications.

Grossly, phyllodes tumors are bulging, well-circumscribed masses with a tan to pink-gray cut surface that may be mucoid. An alternating pattern of whorled leaf-like projection residing in curved clefts is usually visible in larger lesions, but smaller lesions often have a homogeneous

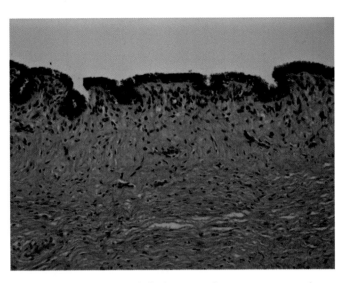

FIGURE 8.29 Benign phyllodes tumor demonstrating stromal condensation around the epithelial component.

appearance similar to fibroadenoma. The cystic areas are usually filled with serous or occasionally serosanguinous fluid (61). Because of their clearly defined margins, they can often be shelled out surgically (62). Hemorrhage or necrosis may be visible in large lesions.

Histologically, phyllodes tumors are circumscribed biphasic tumors characterized by a double-layered epithelial component forming alternating leaf-like projections and clefts surrounded by a cellular stromal component (Figure 8.28). Phyllodes tumors are thought to be derived from intralobular or periductal stroma. Some may develop from preexisting fibroadenomas. They are true neoplasms. Phyllodes tumors have been divided into 3 categories (benign, borderline, and malignant) based on a combination of their degree of cellular atypia and stromal overgrowth, the presence and extent of areas of sarcoma, mitotic activity, and relative circumscription versus growth into surrounding breast parenchyma (63). The luminal epithelial component may show usual-type or florid hyperplasia and occasionally areas of adenosis, apocrine, or squamous metaplasia (61). Malignant transformation of the epithelial component is exceptionally rare (64,65).

Fortunately, most cases are benign, especially in young women. Most are circumscribed and show a noninfiltrative interface with normal breast tissue, limited if any stromal overgrowth or sarcomatous foci, and absence of necrosis (66). Recent studies indicate that the major determinant of local recurrence in lesions classified as both benign and malignant is the presence of positive margins suggesting that the histologic features are in fact of lesser importance. In fact, the overwhelming majority of tumors classified as malignant never metastasize (58,67,68). The use of the older generic terms *cystosarcoma phyllodes* or *periductal sarcoma* for these lesions is not advocated because these names are nonspecific and convey the idea that all such

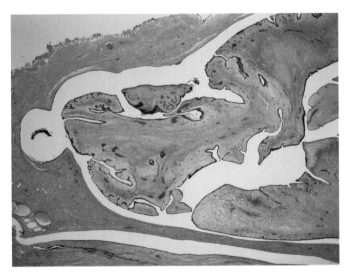

FIGURE 8.28 Low-magnification appearance of benign phyllodes tumor showing cleft-like projections surrounded by a cellular stroma.

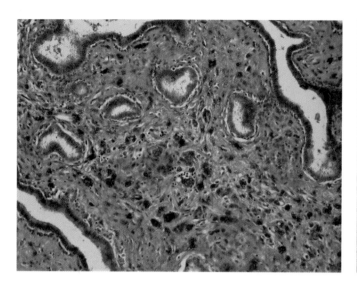

FIGURE 8.30 Benign phyllodes tumor with bizarre stromal giant cells should not raise concern in the absence of other cellular features of characteristic of malignancy.

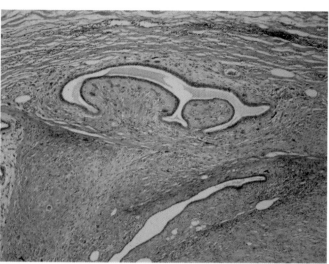

FIGURE 8.32 Malignant phyllodes tumor with stromal overgrowth, cellular stroma, and pleomorphic cells.

lesions are metastatic-capable sarcomas, whereas, in fact, only a very small percentage of lesions are truly malignant.

The stromal component in *benign phyllodes* tumors shows a monomorphic spindle cell population of moderate cellularity, mild pleomorphism, few to no mitoses (<5 per 10 HPF) and no evidence of stromal overgrowth. The margins are usually circumscribed. The stromal cellularity is regularly variable and generally highest closest to the epithelial component (Figure 8.29). The proportional stromal-epithelial relationship is maintained without overgrowth as defined by the absence of the epithelial component in one low-power ×4 field (69). Areas of sparse stromal cellularity, myxoid change, or sclerosis may also be seen. Scattered bizarre stromal giant cells in an otherwise benign phyllodes tumor should not raise concern (70) (Figure 8.30). Lipomatous, cartilaginous, and osseous metaplasia have all been described (71,72). At least

70% of all phyllodes tumor fall into the benign category (67).

Borderline phyllodes tumors are characterized by moderate to high stromal cellularity with moderate cellular pleomorphism and frequent mitoses (5–9 per 10 HPF), a heterogeneous stromal distribution without frank sarcomatous stromal overgrowth, and dominantly pushing borders (Figure 8.31A and B). Limited areas of infiltration into surrounding breast parenchyma are permissible as long as the lesion otherwise displays borderline features. Areas of low-grade sarcoma when present are limited (<5 mm) and centrally located in the lesion as opposed to peripheral with invasion of the surrounding breast tissue as is seen in malignant lesions. The most common sarcomatous pattern is fibrosarcoma followed by areas of well-differentiated liposarcoma (69). Approximately, 12.5% of phyllodes tumors fall in this category (67).

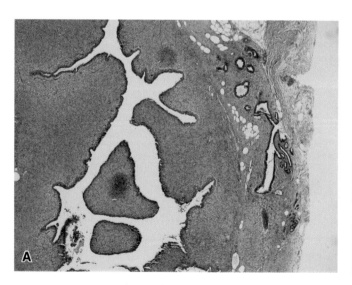

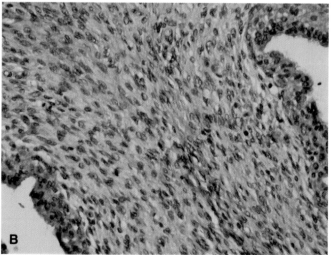

FIGURE 8.31 (A and B) Borderline phyllodes tumor with pushing borders, stromal expansion, and high cellularity. (B) Borderline phyllodes tumor showing a cellular stroma, moderate atypia, and mitotic figures.

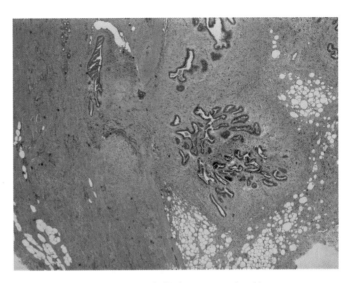

FIGURE 8.33 Marked nuclear atypia and cellularity with frequent mitotic figures in malignant phyllodes tumor.

FIGURE 8.34 Malignant phyllodes tumor with infiltrative margins.

Tumors classified as *malignant phyllodes* contain frank areas of intermediate- to high-grade sarcoma, which usually dominate the histologic picture. The stromal cellularity and degree of cellular pleomorphism are marked (Figure 8.32), usually with stromal overgrowth by the sarcomatous elements, high mitotic rate (10 or more mitosis per 10 HPF), and necrosis (Figure 8.33). There is usually some degree of infiltration of the surrounding breast parenchyma (Figure 8.34). Fibrosarcoma and/or liposarcoma are the most common sarcomatous elements (Figure 8.35); however, areas of chondrosarcoma, osteosarcoma, and rarely, rhabdomyosarcoma may also be present (71,73–76). Foci of metaplastic ossification or cartilage should not be overinterpreted as osteosarcoma or chondrosarcoma. Although, 15% or more of phyllodes tumors could fall into the malignant category (67) based on the above criteria, the fact remains that 2% (58,68) to none (67) of those lesions classified as malignant in studies

with clear case definition have resulted in distant metastasis and death. In the recent studies by Tan, Mofat, and Chen (58,67), the major determinant of local recurrence in lesions classified as both benign and malignant was the presence of positive margins suggesting that the histologic features are in fact of lesser importance.

The differential diagnosis for phyllodes tumors is cellular fibroadenoma at the benign end of the spectrum, and metaplastic carcinomas and primary sarcomas at the other. Benign phyllodes tumors can be distinguished from cellular fibroadenomas by the presence of a leaf-like growth pattern throughout the majority of the lesion and a more cellular stroma composed of monomorphic spindle cells. Mitotic figures, when present, should be confined to the periductal stroma in the cellular fibroadenoma, whereas in benign phyllodes, they will be more randomly distributed within the stroma. Stromal cellularity in fibroadenomas will also be more constant and will not vary in relation to the

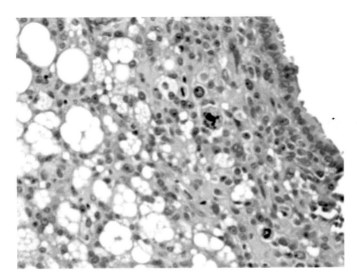

FIGURE 8.35 Liposarcomatous elements in the stroma of a malignant phyllodes tumor.

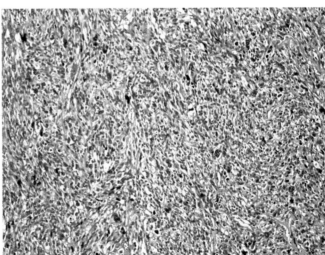

FIGURE 8.36 Primary leiomyosarcoma of the breast showing marked nuclear atypia of the spindle cells.

distance from the epithelial component. In metaplastic carcinomas, the malignant epithelial component often merges imperceptively with the stromal component, requiring immunohistochemical stains for cytokeratins for certain identification. In phyllodes tumors, the epithelial component remains discrete from the stromal component and is benign. Pure primary sarcomas are rare and should only be diagnosed after thorough sampling of the lesion fails to demonstrate any evidence of a phyllodes tumor component. It should also be remembered that phyllodes tumors may recur as pure sarcoma. Thus, in cases of pure sarcoma, a history of a previous phyllodes tumor should be pursued.

Management

Wide excision with clear surgical margins is the preferable initial treatment including malignant lesions (68), and routine axillary dissection is not recommended. Local recurrence can occur for both benign and malignant lesions and is likely a result of incomplete initial excision with the rate of local recurrence related to the width of the excision margins (67,77–79). The histologic features of recurrent lesions are usually similar to the original tumor but may progress to a worse lesion (78,80). The average interval between the diagnosis of primary benign and recurrent benign phyllodes is 2 years, although several years may pass before relapse. A relatively small number of patients with malignant phyllodes will develop hematogenous metastases (58,66,80–82), with the most common sites being the lung and skeleton. Most recurrences of malignant lesions will also occur within 2 years. Axillary lymph node metastases are rare but have been reported in 10% to 15% of cases with systemic metastases (67–83).

Other Primary Mammary Sarcomas

Primary sarcomas of the breast, excluding angiosarcoma (see subsequent section), are exceedingly rare (84,85). Their microscopic features are identical to their extrammary counterparts, and many may originate from the chest wall and infiltrate the breast parenchyma, especially those arising subsequent to radiation therapy. Primary liposarcoma (86), followed by fibrosarcoma, is the most common; however, osteosarcoma, chondrosarcoma, leiomyosarcoma (Figure 8.36), rhabdomyosarcoma, malignant peripheral nerve sheath tumor, and pleomorphic undifferentiated sarcoma have all been reported in the breast (84,85,87). Postradiation sarcomas of the breast are high-grade tumors with marked nuclear atypia, atypical mitotic figures, and myxoid stromal changes. These tumors develop in the breast several years after the radiation therapy (Figure 8.37). Before concluding that one is dealing with a pure sarcoma, it is critical to exclude the possibility that the sarcomatous elements are part of a malignant phyllodes tumor or a metaplastic carcinoma.

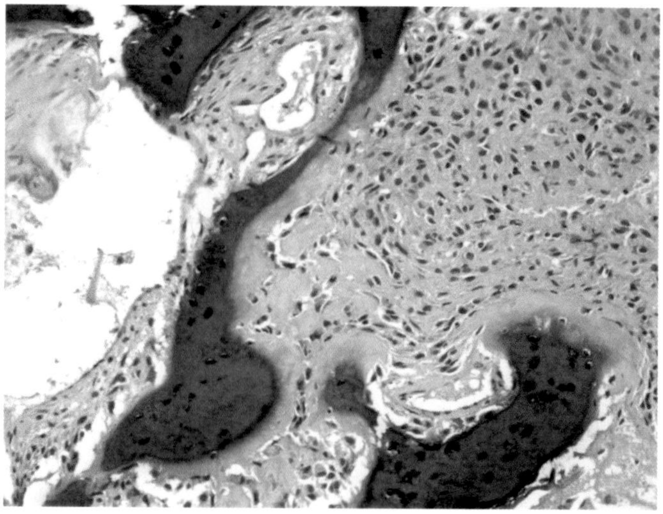

FIGURE 8.37 Postradiation sarcoma with bone formation.

Extensive sampling of the specimen should be undertaken to search for more typical areas of phyllodes tumor or carcinoma. The presence of coexistent ductal carcinoma in situ can also be an important clue to a metaplastic carcinoma. Performance of immunohistochemistry utilizing a battery of high- and low-molecular-weight cytokeratins including p63 can be valuable in excluding a metaplastic carcinoma. The possibility of metastasis should always be considered when a "pure" sarcoma is encountered. The epithelial component and relative circumscription of phyllodes tumors, as well as areas of more typical carcinoma, should help to differentiate them from sarcomas.

Immunohistochemistry

The diagnosis of breast sarcoma should be based on morphologic grounds. Sarcomas can have overlapping immunohistochemical profiles. Metaplastic carcinomas express p63 and other cytokeratins that are almost always negative in sarcomas. The stromal component of phyllodes tumors can express markers that overlap with those seen in sarcomas.

Management

All sarcomas of the breast should be excised with the primary goal of achieving negative margins. The overall prognosis of breast sarcomas is similar to that of subcutaneous sarcomas, but survival is poor for some tumors, such as rhabdomyosarcoma and osteosarcoma.

■ VASCULAR LESIONS

All vascular tumors seen in the skin and soft tissues may occur in the breast. Fortunately, most can be readily characterized histologically as benign or malignant.

Benign Vascular Lesions

Pathologic Features

Collectively, benign vascular lesions are well circumscribed and lack the endothelial hyperplasia, atypia, and inter-anastomosing vascular channels of angiosarcoma. Variants of hemangioma recognized in the breast include perilobular, capillary, cavernous, and venous hemangiomas, as well as angiomatosis. There is no evidence to suggest that any of these hemangiomas develop into angiosarcomas.

The *perilobular hemangioma* is the most common vascular lesion seen in the breast, with a reported frequency of 1% to 12% (88). They are capillary hemangiomas that are incidental microscopic findings. Histologically, they are composed of a proliferation of well-circumscribed, thin-walled, capillary spaces lined by attenuated to barely visible, nonatypical endothelial cells with small nuclei (Figure 8.38). Mitotic activity is absent. They may involve the intralobular and the extralobular stromas.

The remaining categories of hemangioma are large enough to be detected clinically or mammographically. *Capillary hemangiomas* are characterized by a well-circumscribed proliferation of small-sized vascular spaces with a lobular appearance, which can resemble a pyogenic granuloma (Figure 8.39). The endothelial cells lining these spaces are flat to slightly cuboidal without evidence of atypia (89). In *cavernous hemangiomas*, the vascular spaces are larger, cystically dilated, and filled with red blood cells (Figure 8.40). The spaces are lined by non-atypical endothelial cells (89). *Venous hemangiomas* are uncommon and characterized by large venous channels with variably thickened muscular walls and lined by flat endothelial cells without atypia (90).

Angiomatosis is an uncommon lesion composed of a proliferation of cystically dilated vascular spaces filled with red blood cells. Mammographically, they may

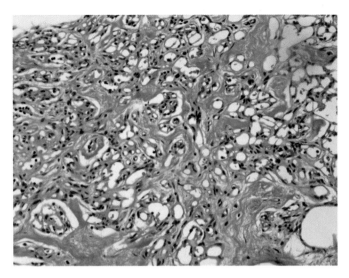

FIGURE 8.39 Capillary hemangioma with a proliferation of small vessels lacking nuclear atypia or anastomosing spaces.

simulate a tumor. The nonanastomosing, cystic spaces grow in between the breast epithelial elements without infiltration of the surrounding tissue and may involve large areas of the breast (91) (Figure 8.41). The spaces are lined by flat endothelial cells without atypia, and pericytes are present. There is no mitotic activity. Distinction from low-grade angiosarcoma may be difficult; however, angiomatosis lacks the anastomosing spaces, the prominent nuclei, and the infiltrative pattern present in angiosarcomas. Immunohistochemical stains may be helpful in this differential since the pericytes are smooth muscle actin–positive, whereas most angiosarcomas lack this marker.

Angiolipomas are more often seen in the skin than in the breast parenchyma. They are often painful and may be multiple. They are relatively well-circumscribed lesions composed of an admixture of mature adipose and benign capillary hemangioma components. The presence of hyaline

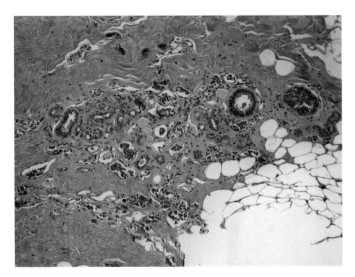

FIGURE 8.38 Perilobular hemangioma showing a well-circumscribed proliferation of capillary vessels, without atypia.

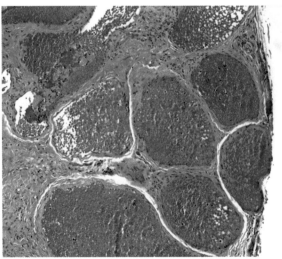

FIGURE 8.40 Cavernous hemangioma showing large cystic vascular spaces lined by nonatypical endothelial cells.

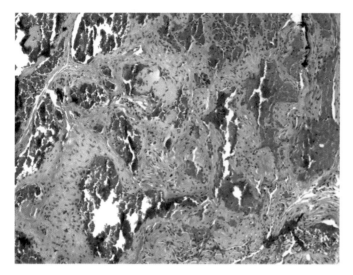

FIGURE 8.41 Angiomatosis consisting of nonanastomosing vascular spaces lined by bland endothelial cells and lacking an invasive pattern.

microthrombi is characteristic. Angiolipomas lack the infiltrate pattern and atypia of angiosarcoma.

Papillary endothelial hyperplasia represents an exuberant organization and recanalization of a thrombus. Its appearance in the breast is identical to that in other sites. It is exclusively an intravascular process characterized by hyaline papillary stalks lined by attenuated endothelial cells, lacking necrosis or atypia (92) (Figure 8.42). These lesions are typically small, usually less than 2 cm in diameter, and well circumscribed. The presence of anastomosing spaces may simulate a well-differentiated angiosarcoma (92); however, recognition of the lack of endothelial cell atypia, necrosis, and mitotic activity usually makes the distinction straightforward.

Immunohistochemistry

In most cases, the diagnosis of benign vascular tumors of the breast should be achievable based on microscopic findings alone. All benign vascular lesions express endothelial cell markers (CD31, CD34, factor VIII, and Fli-1) (93). The use of cell cycle markers such as Ki67 may help to highlight proliferative activity in borderline vascular lesions (94).

Management

In most cases, benign vascular lesions do not require reexcision. When the diagnosis is made in core biopsy and the entire lesion cannot be fully visualized, reexcision should be recommended to exclude a more aggressive lesion. In contrast, complete excision is recommended for angiomatosis, as it has a potential for local recurrence.

Angiosarcoma

Pathologic Features

Angiosarcoma is the most common primary sarcoma of the breast and yet accounts for less than 0.05% of malignant breast lesions. Angiosarcoma can occur in the parenchyma of the breast or the skin, sporadically or after radiotherapy (95–98). When subsequent to radiotherapy, they more frequently involve the skin rather than the mammary parenchyma (99). The time frame between development of subsequent angiosarcoma and radiotherapy can be less than 5 years, but most cases are detected at least 5 years after treatment. Frequently, these are multifocal high-grade tumors. In the past, when radical mastectomy was common practice, angiosarcoma was occasionally seen in the setting of chronic lymphedema of the arm (Stewart-Treves syndrome) (100).

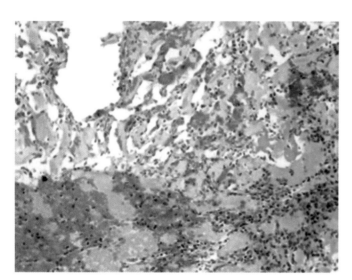

FIGURE 8.42 Papillary endothelial hyperplasia composed of vascular spaces lined by benign-appearing endothelial cells that surround hyalinized cores.

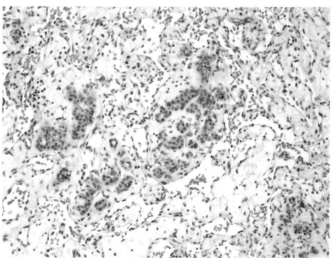

FIGURE 8.43 Well-differentiated angiosarcoma infiltrating the surrounding tissue and showing anastomosing vascular spaces.

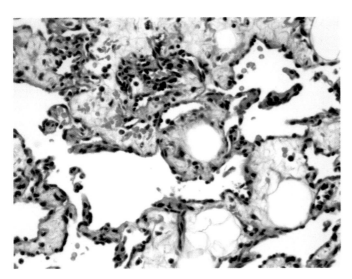

FIGURE 8.44 The endothelial cells lining this angiosarcoma show prominent and hyperchromatic nuclei.

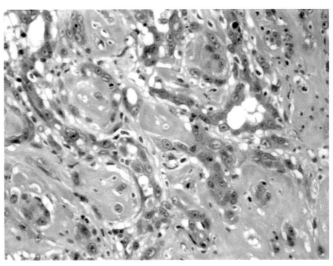

FIGURE 8.45 In addition to the infiltrating anastomosing vascular spaces, this angiosarcomas shows prominent vesicular nuclei and mitotic figures.

Angiosarcomas of the breast typically present as a painless mass, ranging in size from than 1.0 cm to greater than 15 cm. The skin lesions are characterized by a blue-purple color. Histologically, angiosarcomas are characterized by anastomosing vascular channels that infiltrate the dermis in cutaneous tumors and adipose tissue in the breast proper. Angiosarcoma may be categorized as low intermediate or high grade based on presence or absence of specific histologic features (101).

In low-grade angiosarcomas, the vascular spaces are well defined and lined by cells with prominent nuclei (Figures 8.43 and 8.44). Endothelial tufting is minimal, and papillary formations are absent. Solid and spindle cell foci, blood lakes, and necrosis are absent. Mitoses are rare to absent. Intermediate-grade angiosarcoma shows increased cellularity, endothelial tufting, focal presence of papillary

formations, rare if any spindle cell foci, and the absence of blood lakes and necrosis. The papillary areas are typically characterized by obvious mitotic activity. High-grade angiosarcomas are characterized by prominent endothelial cell tufting, papillary formations with obviously malignant endothelial cells, and numerous mitoses (Figures 8.45 and 8.46). Solid and spindle cell foci, blood lakes, and necrosis are almost always present. Occasional high-grade angiosarcomas have an epithelioid appearance that resembles a carcinoma. The histologic grade can be variable within a given lesion. Most postradiation therapy angiosarcomas have at least focal intermediate or high-grade areas cytologically.

Earlier studies have shown a relationship between grade and outcome (102), whereas a more recent study by Nascimento et al (103) with more precise case definition suggests angiosarcomas of the breast behave poorly

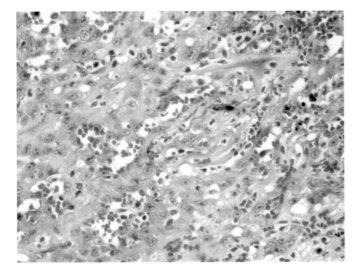

FIGURE 8.46 This high-grade angiosarcoma is characterized by spindle and epithelioid cells. The search for more typical areas and the use of immunostains can be helpful to confirm the diagnosis.

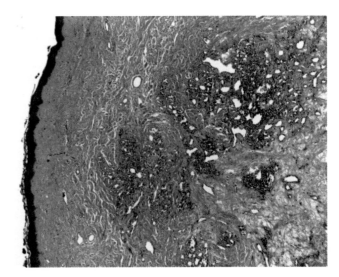

FIGURE 8.47 This atypical vascular lesion of the skin of the breast is relatively well circumscribed with nonanastomosing vascular spaces and lacks atypical endothelial cells.

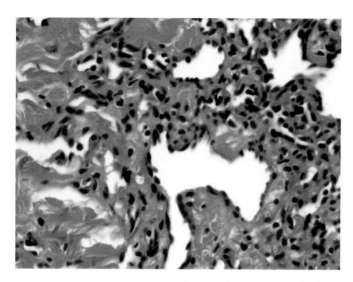

FIGURE 8.48 Atypical vascular lesion with endothelial cells showing moderate nuclear atypia without mitotic figures.

regardless of grade, with 60% of patients developing distant metastases at a mean follow-up time of 49 months. The differential diagnosis for low-grade mammary angiosarcomas includes hemangioma, PASH, papillary endothelial hyperplasia, and atypical vascular lesions. High-grade angiosarcomas, especially epithelioid angiosarcoma, may be confused with carcinomas. However, most carcinomas can be differentiated by the presence of more typical epithelial components, such as carcinoma in situ or invasive tumor at least focally, and by the immunohistochemical profile.

Immunohistochemistry

In difficult cases, immunohistochemistry for endothelial markers including factor VIII–related antigen, CD31, CD34, D2-40, and Fli-1 (93) can be performed. High-grade angiosarcomas can be more difficult to diagnose because they may not diffusely express endothelial cell markers, may be focally cytokeratin-positive, and may lack vasoformative areas.

Management

Angiosarcomas require complete excision and are usually treated with mastectomy. Involvement of axillary lymph nodes is rare. Their management can be further complicated by multifocality in some cases. When metastasis occurs, the most common sites are lungs, liver, contralateral breast, skin, soft tissue, and bone.

Atypical Vascular Lesions

These lesions have been described in the skin of the breast after radiation therapy for breast cancer and occasionally after conservative surgery only (104–109). The typical presentation for these lesions is a small, red, brown or pink papule or plaque on the skin. In general, they are smaller than angiosarcomas, tend to be relatively circumscribed, and involve the dermis or subcutis of the breast. Histologically, they consist of dilated anastomosing vascular spaces, often with a complex branching pattern, lined by plump endothelial cells and separated by small bundles of dermal collagen (Figures 8.47 and 8.48). However, in contrast to well-differentiated angiosarcoma, the endothelial cells lack prominent nucleoli, significant atypia, multilayering, and papillary tufting. A chronic inflammatory infiltrate is often present. Red blood cells are usually not found in the vascular spaces, and their extravasation into the surrounding tissue is not present. Necrosis is absent. Two microscopic patterns have been described, the more common being the lymphatic type, which shows a resemblance to lymphangioma. The less common variant is the vascular type that forms capillary-like spaces and shows compact vascular spaces and spindle cells. Papillary endothelial hyperplasia and fibrin thrombi may be present centrally. Most of these lesions pursue a benign clinical course, with a few cases reportedly recurring locally or progressing to angiosarcoma (104,105,110).

Immunohistochemistry

Immunohistochemistry is not helpful to differentiate between atypical lesions and angiosarcomas since they both express endothelial cell markers.

Management

Similar to angiosarcomas, atypical vascular lesions should be excised with the aim of obtaining negative margins.

■ KEY POINTS

- Many of the mesenchymal lesions of the breast show the same morphologic features as their soft tissue counterparts.
- Reactive mesenchymal conditions may show atypical morphologic features similar to more aggressive lesions.
- Correlation with imaging findings to determine their size and extension is important in the evaluation of these breast lesions.
- Proper evaluation of the margins is crucial for the diagnosis as well as for prognostic and therapeutic purposes.
- Vascular lesions of the breast can show a morphologic spectrum, and the more atypical components may not be present in smaller samples.
- Immunohistochemical stains play a significant role in the diagnosis of mesenchymal lesions; however, they need to be interpreted in conjunction with the morphologic findings.

■ REFERENCES

1. AbdullGaffar B. Pseudoangiomatous stromal hyperplasia of the breast. *Arch Pathol Lab Med.* 2009;133:1335–1338.
2. Ferreira M, Albarracin CT, Resetkova E. Pseudoangiomatous stromal hyperplasia tumor: a clinical, radiologic and pathologic study of 26 cases. *Mod Pathol.* 2008; 21:201–207.
3. Powell CM, Cranor ML, Rosen PP. Pseudoangiomatous stromal hyperplasia (PASH). A mammary stromal tumor with myofibroblastic differentiation. *Am J Surg Pathol.* 1995;19:270–277.
4. Gobbi H, Tse G, Page DL, Olson SJ, Jensen RA, Simpson JF. Reactive spindle cell nodules of the breast after core biopsy or fine-needle aspiration. *Am J Clin Pathol.* 2000; 113:288–294.
5. Lee KC, Chan JK, Ho LC. Histologic changes in the breast after fine-needle aspiration. *Am J Surg Pathol.* 1994;18:1039–1047.
6. McMenamin ME, DeSchryver K, Fletcher CD. Fibrous lesions of the breast: a review. *Int J Surg Pathol.* 2000;8:99–108.
7. Rosen PP, Ernsberger D. Mammary fibromatosis. A benign spindle-cell tumor with significant risk for local recurrence. *Cancer.* 1989;63:1363–1369.
8. Wargotz ES, Norris HJ, Austin RM, Enzinger FM. Fibromatosis of the breast. A clinical and pathological study of 28 cases. *Am J Surg Pathol.* 1987;11:38–45.
9. Devouassoux-Shisheboran M, Schammel MD, Man YG, Tavassoli FA. Fibromatosis of the breast: age-correlated morphofunctional features of 33 cases. *Arch Pathol Lab Med.* 2000;124:276–280.
10. Carlson JW, Fletcher CD. Immunohistochemistry for beta-catenin in the differential diagnosis of spindle cell lesions: analysis of a series and review of the literature. *Histopathology.* 2007;51:509–514.
11. Nucci MR, Fletcher CDM. Myofibroblastoma of the breast: a distinctive benign stromal tumor. *Pathology Case Reviews.* 1999;4:214–219.
12. Magro G, Michal M, Vasquez E, Bisceglia M. Lipomatous myofibroblastoma: a potential diagnostic pitfall in the spectrum of the spindle cell lesions of the breast. *Virchows Arch.* 2000;437:540–544.
13. Pauwels P, Sciot R, Croiset F, Rutten H, Van den Berghe H, Dal Cin P. Myofibroblastoma of the breast: genetic link with spindle cell lipoma. *J Pathol.* 2000;191:282–285.
14. Salomao DR, Crotty TB, Nascimento AG. Myofibroblastoma and solitary fibrous tumour of the breast: histopathologic and immunohistochemical studies. *Breast.* 2001;10:49–54.
15. Falconieri G, Lamovec J, Mirra M, Pizzolitto S. Solitary fibrous tumor of the mammary gland: a potential pitfall in breast pathology. *Ann Diagn Pathol.* 2004;8:121–125.
16. Damiani S, Miettinen M, Peterse JL, Eusebi V. Solitary fibrous tumour (myofibroblastoma) of the breast. *Virchows Arch.* 1994;425:89–92.
17. Khalifa MA, Montgomery EA, Azumi N, et al. Solitary fibrous tumors: a series of lesions, some in unusual sites. *South Med J.* 1997;90:793–799.
18. Magro G. Mammary myofibroblastoma: a tumor with a wide morphologic spectrum. *Arch Pathol Lab Med.* 2008;132:1813–1820.
19. Magro G, Bisceglia M, Michal M, Eusebi V. Spindle cell lipoma-like tumor, solitary fibrous tumor and myofibroblastoma of the breast: a clinico-pathological analysis of 13 cases in favor of a unifying histogenetic concept. *Virchows Arch.* 2002;440:249–260.
20. Meguerditchian AN, Malik DA, Hicks DG, Kulkarni S. Solitary fibrous tumor of the breast and mammary myofibroblastoma: the same lesion? *Breast J.* 2008;14:287–292.
21. Jones MW, Norris HJ, Wargotz ES. Smooth muscle and nerve sheath tumors of the breast. A clinicopathologic study of 45 cases. *Int J Surg Pathol.* 1994;2:85–92.
22. Magro G, Cavanaugh B, Palazzo J. Clinico-pathological features of breast myxoma: report of a case with histogenetic considerations. *Virchows Arch.* 2010;456:581–586.
23. Tomaszewski JE, Brooks JS, Hicks D, Livolsi VA. Diabetic mastopathy: a distinctive clinicopathologic entity. *Hum Pathol.* 1992;23:780–786.
24. Ely KA, Tse G, Simpson JF, Clarfeld R, Page DL. Diabetic mastopathy. A clinicopathologic review. *Am J Clin Pathol.* 2000;113:541–545.
25. Soler NG, Khardori R. Fibrous disease of the breast, thyroiditis, and cheiroarthropathy in type I diabetes mellitus. *Lancet.* 1984;1:193–195.
26. Byrd BF Jr, Hartmann WH, Graham LS, Hogle HH. Mastopathy in insulin-dependent diabetics. *Ann Surg.* 1987;205:529–532.
27. Lammie GA, Bobrow LG, Staunton MD, Levison DA, Page G, Millis RR. Sclerosing lymphocytic lobulitis of the breast—evidence for an autoimmune pathogenesis. *Histopathology.* 1991;19:13–20.
28. Dubenko M, Breining D, Surks MI. Sclerosing lymphocytic lobulitis of the breast in a patient with Graves' disease. *Thyroid.* 2003;13:309–311.
29. Schwartz IS, Strauchen JA. Lymphocytic mastopathy. An autoimmune disease of the breast? *Am J Clin Pathol.* 1990;93:725–730.
30. Kamisawa T, Okamoto A. IgG-related sclerosing disease. *World J Gastroenterol.* 2008;14:3948–3955.
31. Cheuk W, Chan AC, Lam WL, et al. IgG4-related sclerosing mastitis: description of a new member of the IgG4-related sclerosing diseases. *Am J Surg Pathol.* 2009;33:1058–1064.
32. Coffin CM, Humphrey PA, Dehner LP. Extrapulmonary inflammatory myofibroblastic tumor: a clinical and pathological survey. *Semin Diagn Pathol.* 1998;15:85–101.
33. Coffin CM, Watterson J, Priest JR, Dehner LP. Extrapulmonary inflammatory myofibroblastic tumor (inflammatory pseudotumor). A clinicopathologic and immunohistochemical study of 84 cases. *Am J Surg Pathol.* 1995;19:859–872.
34. Chetty R, Govender D. Inflammatory pseudotumor of the breast. *Pathology.* 1997;29:270–271.
35. Pettinato G, Manivel JC, Kelly DR, Wold LE, Dehner LP. Lesions of the breast in children exclusive of typical fibroadenoma and gynecomastia. A clinicopathologic study of 113 cases. *Pathol Annu.* 1989;24(pt 2):296–328.
36. Sastre-Garau X, Couturier J, Derre J, Aurias A, Klijanienko J, Lagace R. Inflammatory myofibroblastic tumour (inflammatory pseudotumour) of the breast. Clinicopathological and genetic analysis of a case with evidence for clonality. *J Pathol.* 2002;196:97–102.
37. Zardawi IM, Clark D, Williamsz G. Inflammatory myofibroblastic tumor of the breast. A case report. *Acta Cytol.* 2003;47:1077–1081.

38. Yip CH, Wong KT, Samuel D. Bilateral plasma cell granuloma (inflammatory pseudotumour) of the breast. *Aust N Z J Surg.* 1997;67:300–302.

39. Coffin CM, Fletcher JA. Inflammatory myofibroblastic tumour. In: Fletcher CD, Unni KK, Mertens F, eds. *World Health Organization Classification of Tumours Pathology and Genetics of Tumours of Soft Tissue and Bone.* Lyon: IARC Press; 2002:91–93.

40. Coffin CM, Dehner LP, Meis-Kindblom JM. Inflammatory myofibroblastic tumor, inflammatory fibrosarcoma, and related lesions: an historical review with differential diagnostic considerations. *Semin Diagn Pathol.* 1998;15:102–110.

41. Biselli R, Boldrini R, Ferlini C, Boglino C, Inserra A, Bosman C. Myofibroblastic tumours: neoplasias with divergent behaviour. Ultrastructural and flow cytometric analysis. *Pathol Res Pract.* 1999;195:619–632.

42. Freeman A, Geddes N, Munson P, et al. Anaplastic lymphoma kinase (ALK 1) staining and molecular analysis in inflammatory myofibroblastic tumours of the bladder: a preliminary clinicopathological study of nine cases and review of the literature. *Mod Pathol.* 2004;17:765–771.

43. Tsuzuki T, Magi-Galluzzi C, Epstein JI. ALK-1 expression in inflammatory myofibroblastic tumor of the urinary bladder. *Am J Surg Pathol.* 2004;28:1609–1614.

44. Cook JR, Dehner LP, Collins MH, et al. Anaplastic lymphoma kinase (ALK) expression in the inflammatory myofibroblastic tumor: a comparative immunohistochemical study. *Am J Surg Pathol.* 2001;25:1364–1371.

45. Pettinato G, Manivel JC, Insabato L, De Chiara A, Petrella G. Plasma cell granuloma (inflammatory pseudotumor) of the breast. *Am J Clin Pathol.* 1988;90:627–632.

46. Carney JA, Toorkey BC. Myxoid fibroadenoma and allied conditions (myxomatosis) of the breast. A heritable disorder with special associations including cardiac and cutaneous myxomas. *Am J Surg Pathol.* 1991;15:713–721.

47. Courcoutsakis NA, Chow CK, Shawker TH, Carney JA, Stratakis CA. Syndrome of spotty skin pigmentation, myxomas, endocrine overactivity, and schwannomas (Carney complex): breast imaging findings. *Radiology.* 1997;205:221–227.

48. Carter BA, Page DL, Schuyler P, et al. No elevation in long-term breast carcinoma risk for women with fibroadenomas that contain atypical hyperplasia. *Cancer.* 2001;92:30–36.

49. Dupont WD, Page DL, Parl FF, et al. Long-term risk of breast cancer in women with fibroadenoma. *N Engl J Med.* 1994;331:10–15.

50. Diaz NM, Palmer JO, McDivitt RW. Carcinoma arising within fibroadenomas of the breast. A clinicopathologic study of 105 patients. *Am J Clin Pathol.* 1991;95:614–622.

51. Silfen R, Skoll PJ, Hudson DA. Florid juvenile (cellular) fibroadenomatosis in the adolescent: a case for subcutaneous mastectomy? *Aesthetic Plast Surg.* 1999;23:413–415.

52. Behrndt VS, Barbakoff D, Askin FB, Brem RF. Infarcted lactating adenoma presenting as a rapidly enlarging breast mass. *AJR Am J Roentgenol.* 1999;173:933–935.

53. Rickert RR, Rajan S. Localized breast infarcts associated with pregnancy. *Arch Pathol.* 1974;97:159–161.

54. Chua CL, Thomas A, Ng BK. Cystosarcoma phyllodes—Asian variations. *Aust N Z J Surg.* 1988;58:301–305.

55. Bernstein L, Deapen D, Ross RK. The descriptive epidemiology of malignant cystosarcoma phyllodes tumors of the breast. *Cancer.* 1993;71:3020–3024.

56. Keelan PA, Myers JL, Wold LE, Katzmann JA, Gibney DJ. Phyllodes tumor: clinicopathologic review of 60 patients and flow cytometric analysis in 30 patients. *Hum Pathol.* 1992;23:1048–1054.

57. Mollitt DL, Golladay ES, Gloster ES, Jimenez JF. Cystosarcoma phyllodes in the adolescent female. *J Pediatr Surg.* 1987;22:907–910.

58. Tan PH, Jayabaskar T, Chuah KL, et al. Phyllodes tumors of the breast: the role of pathologic parameters. *Am J Clin Pathol.* 2005;123:529–540.

59. Martino A, Zamparelli M, Santinelli A, Cobellis G, Rossi L, Amici G. Unusual clinical presentation of a rare case of phyllodes tumor of the breast in an adolescent girl. *J Pediatr Surg.* 2001;36:941–943.

60. Tagaya N, Kodaira H, Kogure H, Shimizu K. A case of phyllodes tumor with bloody nipple discharge in juvenile patient. *Breast Cancer.* 1999;6:207–210.

61. Page DL, Anderson TJ. *Diagnostic Histopathology of the Breast.* Edinburgh: Churchill Livingstone; 1987.

62. Coffin CM. The breast. In: Stocker JT, Dehner LP, eds. *Pediatric Pathology.* 2nd ed. Philadelphia: Lippincott, Williams & Wilkins; 2001:993–1015.

63. Bellocq JP, Magro G. Fibroepithelial tumors. In: Tavassoli FA, Devilee P, eds. *Tumors of the Breast and Genital Organs.* Lyon: IARC Press; 2003:100–103.

64. Grove A, Deibjerg Kristensen L. Intraductal carcinoma within a phyllodes tumor of the breast: a case report. *Tumori.* 1986;72:187–190.

65. Ozzello L, Gump FE. The management of patients with carcinomas in fibroadenomatous tumors of the breast. *Surg Gynecol Obstet.* 1985;160:99–104.

66. Rajan PB, Cranor ML, Rosen PP. Cystosarcoma phyllodes in adolescent girls and young women: a study of 45 patients. *Am J Surg Pathol.* 1998;22:64–69.

67. Moffat CJ, Pinder SE, Dixon AR, Elston CW, Blamey RW, Ellis IO. Phyllodes tumours of the breast: a clinicopathological review of thirty-two cases. *Histopathology.* 1995;27:205–218.

68. Chen WH, Cheng SP, Tzen CY, et al. Surgical treatment of phyllodes tumors of the breast: retrospective review of 172 cases. *J Surg Oncol.* 2005;91:185–194.

69. Ward RM, Evans HL. Cystosarcoma phyllodes. A clinicopathologic study of 26 cases. *Cancer.* 1986;58:2282–2289.

70. Powell CM, Cranor ML, Rosen PP. Multinucleated stromal giant cells in mammary fibroepithelial neoplasms. A study of 11 patients. *Arch Pathol Lab Med.* 1994;118:912–916.

71. Norris HJ, Taylor HB. Relationship of histologic features to behavior of cystosarcoma phyllodes. Analysis of ninety-four cases. *Cancer.* 1967;20:2090–2099.

72. Smith BH, Taylor HB. The occurrence of bone and cartilage in mammary tumors. *Am J Clin Pathol.* 1969;51:610–618.

73. Cohn-Cedermark G, Rutqvist LE, Rosendahl I, Silfversward C. Prognostic factors in cystosarcoma phyllodes. A clinicopathologic study of 77 patients. *Cancer.* 1991;68:2017–2022.

74. Hawkins RE, Schofield JB, Fisher C, Wiltshaw E, McKinna JA. The clinical and histologic criteria that predict metastases from cystosarcoma phyllodes. *Cancer.* 1992;69:141–147.

75. Pietruszka M, Barnes L. Cystosarcoma phyllodes: a clinicopathologic analysis of 42 cases. *Cancer.* 1978;41: 1974–1983.

76. Qizilbash AH. Cystosarcoma phyllodes with liposarcomatous stroma. *Am J Clin Pathol.* 1976;65:321–327.

77. Barth RJ Jr. Histologic features predict local recurrence after breast conserving therapy of phyllodes tumors. *Breast Cancer Res Treat.* 1999;57:291–295.

78. Chua CL, Thomas A. Cystosarcoma phyllodes tumors. *Surg Gynecol Obstet.* 1988;166:302–306.

79. Chua CL, Thomas A, Ng BK. Cystosarcoma phyllodes: a review of surgical options. *Surgery.* 1989;105:141–147.

80. Grimes MM. Cystosarcoma phyllodes of the breast: histologic features, flow cytometric analysis, and clinical correlations. *Mod Pathol.* 1992;5:232–239.

81. Leveque J, Meunier B, Wattier E, Burtin F, Grall JY, Kerisit J. Malignant cystosarcomas phyllodes of the breast in adolescent females. *Eur J Obstet Gynecol Reprod Biol.* 1994;54:197–203.

82. Turalba CI, el-Mahdi AM, Ladaga L. Fatal metastatic cystosarcoma phyllodes in an adolescent female: case report and review of treatment approaches. *J Surg Oncol.* 1986;33: 176–181.

83. Tavassoli F. *Pathology of the Breast.* 2nd ed. Stamford: Appleton & Lange; 1999.

84. Adem C, Reynolds C, Ingle JN, Nascimento AG. Primary breast sarcoma: clinicopathologic series from the Mayo Clinic and review of the literature. *Br J Cancer.* 2004;91:237–241.

85. Callery CD, Rosen PP, Kinne DW. Sarcoma of the breast. A study of 32 patients with reappraisal of classification and therapy. *Ann Surg.* 1985;201:527–532.

86. Austin RM, Dupree WB. Liposarcoma of the breast: a clinicopathologic study of 20 cases. *Hum Pathol.* 1986;17:906–913.

87. Silver SA, Tavassoli, FA. Primary osteogenic sarcoma of the breast: a clinicopathologic analysis of 50 cases. *Hum Pathol.* 1998;17:906–913.

88. Rosen PP, Ridolfi RL. The perilobular hemangioma. A benign microscopic vascular lesion of the breast. *Am J Clin Pathol.* 1977;68:21–23.

89. Jozefczyk MA, Rosen PP. Vascular tumors of the breast. II. Perilobular hemangiomas and hemangiomas. *Am J Surg Pathol.* 1985;9:491–503.

90. Rosen PP, Jozefczyk MA, Boram LH. Vascular tumors of the breast. IV. The venous hemangioma. *Am J Surg Pathol.* 1985;9:659–665.

91. Rosen PP. Vascular tumors of the breast. III. Angiomatosis. *Am J Surg Pathol.* 1985;9:652–658.

92. Branton PA, Lininger R, Tavassoli FA. Papillary endothelial hyperplasia of the breast: the great impostor for angiosarcoma: a clinicopathologic review of 17 cases. *Int J Surg Pathol.* 2003;11:83–87.

93. Folpe AL, Chand EM, Goldblum JR, Weiss SW. Expression of Fli-1, a nuclear transcription factor, distinguishes vascular neoplasms from potential mimics. *Am J Surg Pathol.* 2001;25:1061–1066.

94. Shin SJ, Lesser M, Rosen PP. Hemangiomas and angiocomas of the breast: diagnostic utility of cell cycle markers with emphasis on Ki-67. *Arch Pathol Lab Med.* 2007;131: 538–544.

95. Monroe AT, Feigenberg SJ, Mendenhall NP. Angiosarcoma after breast-conserving therapy. *Cancer.* 2003;97:1832–1840.

96. Vorburger SA, Xing Y, Hunt KK, et al. Angiosarcoma of the breast. *Cancer.* 2005;104:2682–2688.

97. Billings SD, McKenney JK, Folpe AL, Hardacre MC, Weiss SW. Cutaneous angiosarcoma following breast-conserving surgery and radiation: an analysis of 27 cases. *Am J Surg Pathol.* 2004;28:781–788.

98. Lucas DR. Angiosarcoma, radiation-associated angiosarcoma, and atypical vascular lesion. *Arch Pathol Lab Med.* 2009;133:1804–1809.

99. Schnitt SJ. Angiosarcoma of the mammary skin following conservative surgery and radiation therapy for breast cancer. *Pathology Case Reviews.* 1999;4:194–198.

100. Heitmann C, Ingianni G. Stewart-Treves syndrome: lymphangiosarcoma following mastectomy. *Ann Plast Surg.* 2000;44:72–75.

101. Donnell RM, Rosen PP, Lieberman PH, et al. Angiosarcoma and other vascular tumors of the breast. *Am J Surg Pathol.* 1981;5:629–642.

102. Rosen PP, Kimmel M, Ernsberger D. Mammary angiosarcoma. The prognostic significance of tumor differentiation. *Cancer.* 1988;62:2145–2151.

103. Nascimento AF, Raut CP, Fletcher CDM. Primary angiosarcoma of the breast: clinicopathologic analysis of 49 cases, suggesting that grade is not prognostic. *Am J Surg Pathol.* 2008;32:1896–1904.

104. Brenn T, Fletcher CD. Radiation-associated cutaneous atypical vascular lesions and angiosarcoma: clinicopathologic analysis of 42 cases. *Am J Surg Pathol.* 2005;29:983–996.

105. Fineberg S, Rosen PP. Cutaneous angiosarcoma and atypical vascular lesions of the skin and breast after radiation therapy for breast carcinoma. *Am J Clin Pathol.* 1994;102:757–763.

106. Requena L, Kutzner H, Mentzel T, Duran R, Rodriguez-Peralto JL. Benign vascular proliferations in irradiated skin. *Am J Surg Pathol.* 2002;26:328–337.

107. Brenn T, Fletcher CD. Postradiation vascular proliferations: an increasing problem. *Histopathology.* 2006;48:106–114.

108. Hoda S, Cranor M, Rosen PP. Hemangiomas of the breast with atypical histological features further analysis of histological subtypes confirming their benign character. *Am J Surg Pathol.* 1992;16:553–560.

109. Patton KT, Deyrup AT, Weiss SW. Atypical vascular lesions after surgery and radiation of the breast: a clinicopathologic study of 32 cases analyzing histologic heterogeneity and association with angiosarcoma. *Am J Surg Pathol.* 2008;32:943–950.

110. Gengler C, Coindre JM, Leroux A, et al. Vascular proliferations of the skin after radiation therapy for breast cancer: clinicopathologic analysis of a series in favor of a benign process: a study from the French Sarcoma Group. *Cancer.* 2007;109:1584–1598.

9

Lymphomas of the Breast

JUDITH A. FERRY

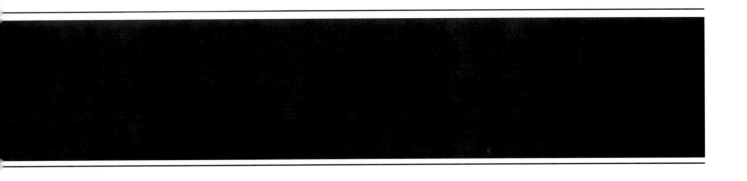

■ PRIMARY LYMPHOMAS OF THE BREAST

Primary lymphoma of the breast is usually defined as lymphoma involving one or both breasts with or without ipsilateral axillary lymph node involvement, without evidence of disease elsewhere at presentation, in a patient without a prior history of lymphoma (1). The breast is a very uncommon primary site for a lymphoma, possibly correlating with the very sparse endogenous lymphoid tissue in this site. Primary lymphoma of the breast accounts for 0.1% to 0.15% (2–5) of all malignant neoplasms of the breast, for 0.34% to 0.85% (3–4,6–7) of all non-Hodgkin lymphomas, and for less than 2% of all extranodal non-Hodgkin lymphomas (3).

Clinical Features

Most patients are middle-aged to elderly women, although occasionally, young women, and, rarely, adolescents are affected (1–2,8–10), with a median age in the sixth or seventh decade in most series (4–7,11–20). Approximately 2% of patients with primary breast lymphoma are men (4–7,12–20). Occasionally, the disease affects pregnant or lactating women. Rarely, patients have had prior carcinoma of the breast (1).

Almost all patients present with a palpable breast mass with or without ipsilateral axillary lymphadenopathy (4,6,13,15,18,19). The lesions are typically painless, but in a few cases, they are painful (18,21). In a few cases, patients are asymptomatic, and the lymphoma is detected by mammography (4,9–11). Constitutional symptoms are very uncommon (6,11,13,15,17,22). Most present with unilateral disease, but occasionally, primary lymphoma of the breast is bilateral (1–2,5,7,14,15,17,20,22). A few patients have a history of autoimmune disease, diabetes mellitus, or mastitis (3–5,13). Several HIV-positive patients have developed lymphoma presenting with involvement of the breast (23). On physical examination, patients usually have discrete, mobile masses. The overlying skin is involved infrequently; it may be thickened (18), erythematous, or inflamed (2,24), mimicking inflammatory carcinoma.

Mammographic Features

Although most breast lymphomas are not initially detected by mammography, they do have characteristic radiographic features. The most common finding is a solitary lesion with irregular or indistinct borders, in most cases lacking microcalcifications. In some cases, the lymphoma has a rounded border, potentially mimicking a benign condition. Less commonly, primary lymphoma of the breast manifests as multiple lesions or as diffuse, unilateral, or bilateral enlargement of the breast (13,18,19).

Pathologic Features

In most series, diffuse large B-cell lymphoma is the most common type, accounting for approximately 60% of cases of all primary breast lymphomas overall (2,4–6, 11,15,16,19,25–26). The remainder are mostly extranodal marginal zone lymphoma (mucosa-associated lymphoid tissue [MALT] lymphoma) or follicular lymphoma. However, recent studies suggest that low-grade B-cell lymphomas may be more prevalent than previously recognized, with marginal zone lymphoma being more common, followed by follicular lymphoma (5,10). Marginal zone lymphoma accounts for approximately 20% of all primary breast lymphomas, but the proportion varies widely among different series (2–6,9,11,15,16,19,25). Approximately 6% of primary breast lymphomas are follicular lymphomas. It is possible that a larger number of low-grade lymphomas are being detected because of the wider use of routine mammography that identifies asymptomatic lesions (10), and because with the wider recognition of marginal zone lymphomas and greater variety of immunostains for paraffin sections and ready availability of polymerase chain reaction (PCR) to evaluate clonality, pathologists are now better able to recognize and

■ **Table 9.1** Primary lymphoma of the breast: clinical and pathologic features

Type of Lymphoma	Patients	Pattern	Composition	Immunophenotype	Outcome
DLBCL	Adults, women >> men, broad age range, few pregnant	Diffuse	Large lymphoid cells, usually centroblasts or immunoblasts	CD20+, CD10 usually negative, bcl6+/−, bcl2 and MUM1/IRF4 usually positive, Ki67 high; non-GC > GC	Aggressive; most common sites of relapse are CNS and opposite breast; good outcomes in some with chemo +/− RT.
Extranodal MZL (MALT lymphoma)	Middle-aged and older adults; women >> men	Diffuse, vaguely nodular	Marginal zone cells, plasma cells+/−, reactive follicles+/−. LELs may not be found	CD20+, CD5−, CD10−, CD23−, CD43+/−, bcl2+/−, cyclin D1−, cIg+/−	Good prognosis. Localized extranodal relapses may occur. Few have transformation to DLBCL. Few die of lymphoma.
Follicular lymphoma (FL)	Middle-aged and older women	Follicular +/− diffuse areas	Centrocytes (small cleaved cells) usually predominate; variable number of centroblasts	CD20+, CD10+, CD5−, CD23−, CD43−, bcl2+, cyclin D1−, sIg+	Prognosis less good than MZL. Behavior similar to nodal FL.
Burkitt lymphoma	Young to middle-aged, few older women, some pregnant or lactating	Diffuse	Medium-sized uniform round cells, many mitoses, tingible body macrophages	CD20+, CD10+, bcl6+, bcl2−, sIgM+, Ki67 ~100%	Very aggressive; lymphoma is often widespread at presentation.
Anaplastic large cell lymphoma associated with implant	Women with saline or silicone implants, cosmetic or post mastectomy; often years after implant; seroma more common than discrete mass	Diffuse; neoplastic cells may be present focally	Large atypical cells with oval or indented nuclei associated with inflammation and fibrosis	CD45+, CD30+, ALK−, T-cell associated antigens+/−, EMA usually +, EBV−, HHV8−	Very good prognosis.

DLBCL indicates diffuse large B-cell lymphoma; MZL, marginal zone lymphoma; CNS, central nervous system; non-GC, nongerminal center immunophenotype; GC, germinal center immunophenotype; RT, radiation therapy; LELs, lymphoepithelial lesions; cIg, monotypic cytoplasmic immunoglobulin; sIg, monotypic surface immunoglobulin.

diagnose these lymphomas. Burkitt lymphoma and T-cell lymphomas are rare (Table 9.1) (10,19).

Very rare cases of B-lymphoblastic lymphoma (19) and T-lymphoblastic lymphoma (4) apparently arising in the breast are reported. Classical Hodgkin lymphoma rarely presents with involvement of the breast; however, usually, there is concurrent lymph node involvement, suggesting that the breast involvement is secondary (19).

Although breast lymphomas may appear circumscribed on gross examination, microscopic examination often reveals some invasion into surrounding tissues at the periphery of the lesion (9). The neoplastic cells infiltrate around and within mammary ducts and lobules, sometimes with obliteration of these structures. Histologic changes of lymphocytic mastitis have been reported in association with rare cases of primary breast lymphoma (27).

Diffuse Large B-Cell Lymphoma

Diffuse large B-cell lymphoma primary in the breast affects adults over a broad age range, occasionally including young adults. Women are affected much more often than men, and occasionally, patients present during pregnancy. These lymphomas are larger on average than carcinomas of the breast, with a median size of 4 to 5 cm (7,13,15,17,20). The lesions may be discrete, hard, rubbery (14), soft, or fleshy (2); they are sometimes rapidly enlarging (1,14,24).

The lymphomas are composed of a diffuse infiltrate of large lymphoid cells, usually centroblasts, immunoblasts, or a combination of these cell types. Centroblasts are large lymphoid cells with round to oval nuclei, vesicular chromatin, nucleoli (typically several per cell) that are most often present along the nuclear membrane, and scant cytoplasm that is deep blue on a Giemsa stain. Immunoblasts are also large, transformed lymphoid cells with vesicular chromatin, but they have a single, centrally placed nucleolus and somewhat more abundant cytoplasm than centroblasts. In most cases of diffuse large B-cell lymphomas that have been subclassified, most are subclassified as centroblastic, whereas only a few are immunoblastic (2,16,19,28). Rare cases of diffuse large B-cell lymphoma, anaplastic variant, expressing CD30, are described (7). A few cases of diffuse large B-cell lymphoma have had a component of marginal zone lymphoma, consistent with histologic progression of the low-grade lymphoma (17,20). The lymphomas are CD45+ and CD20+, with rare CD5+ cases (20). CD10 is expressed in a small minority, bcl6 is expressed in approximately half of cases, bcl2 is expressed in most cases, and MUM1/IRF4 is expressed in nearly all cases (5,13,19,20,22). Most cases thus have a nongerminal center immunophenotype (CD10−, bcl6+/−, MUM1/IRF4+), whereas a minority has a germinal center phenotype (CD10+, bcl6+ or CD10−, bcl6+, MUM1/IRF4−) (19). The proliferation index as measured by mib1 is relatively high (60%-95%) (Figure 9.1) (20). Evaluation of the mutational status of the immunoglobulin heavy chain gene variable region reveals a frequency of mutation of 1% to 10%, usually without ongoing mutation. In conjunction with immunophenotypic features, these findings suggest that the neoplastic cells of most diffuse large B-cell lymphomas of the breast correspond to a postgerminal center stage of differentiation (20).

Staging and Prognostic Factors. In most studies of primary diffuse large B-cell lymphoma of the breast, cases have been included only when the lymphoma was confined to the breast (Ann Arbor stage I) or had spread to ipsilateral axillary lymph nodes (stage II). A designation of stage IV has been applied to those cases with bilateral mammary involvement (7,17). The relative proportion of stage I and II cases varies among series, but overall, most patients present with stage I disease. Most of the remainder have stage II disease. Stage IV (bilateral) disease is uncommon (6,12–14,16–17,20,25).

A number of factors may influence the prognosis. Mastectomy, however, does not improve survival; performing a large enough biopsy for optimal pathologic evaluation is the only surgery needed (13,15,17). There is no obvious difference in outcome between men and women (17). Diffuse large B-cell lymphomas arising as large cell transformation of marginal zone lymphoma and de novo diffuse large B-cell lymphoma appear to have a similar prognosis (17). Neither the size of the lesion nor stage (I vs II) has had a clear effect on prognosis in several studies (12,13,17). The immunophenotype of the tumor cells may affect outcome; patients with CD10+, bcl6+ lymphomas may fare better than those with CD10−, bcl6− lymphomas (13), and those with a nongerminal center immunophenotype may have a worse outcome than those with a germinal center immunophenotype (19).

Extranodal Marginal Zone Lymphoma of Mucosa-Associated Lymphoid Tissue (MALT Lymphoma)

Marginal zone lymphoma typically affects middle-aged and older adults. Almost all patients are women, but men are rarely affected (2–4,6,9,25). Their histologic features are similar to those of marginal zone lymphomas in other sites. The lymphoma has a diffuse to vaguely nodular pattern on low-power examination. The neoplastic cells are small to minimally enlarged cells with oval to slightly irregular nuclei with smooth chromatin, inconspicuous nucleoli, and variable quantity of pale cytoplasm (Figures 9.2 and 9.3). Interspersed reactive follicles are often identified (Figure 9.3B). They may be intact or they may be infiltrated and replaced to a variable extent by tumor cells (follicular colonization). A subset of cases shows plasmacytic differentiation; such cases show a variable number, often many, plasma cells and/or plasmacytoid cells (Figure 9.3C–E), sometimes containing Dutcher bodies, which are intranuclear protrusions of cytoplasm containing immunoglobulin. Sclerosis is usually inconspicuous. Well-developed lymphoepithelial lesions tend to be less conspicuous than in marginal zone lymphomas involving some other sites, although neoplastic cells may invade epithelial structures (4,9,19,28). Rarely, amyloid deposition in association with marginal zone lymphoma with plasmacytic differentiation has been found (2).

Immunophenotypic features are similar to those of marginal zone lymphoma in other sites. Tumor cells are CD45+, CD20+, CD5−, CD10−, CD23−, CD43+/−, cyclin D1−, with monotypic cytoplasmic immunoglobulin in cases with plasmacytic differentiation (Figures 9.2C and 9.3D–E) (5). Bcl2 is usually positive, but bcl2 expression may be lost, particularly in neoplastic cells that have infiltrated reactive follicles. The proliferation index as assessed

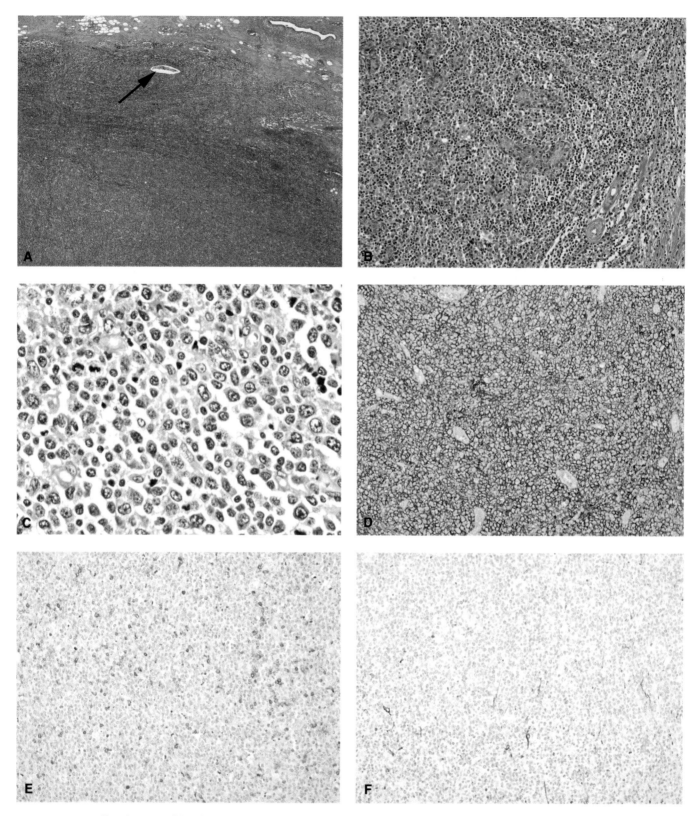

FIGURE 9.1 Diffuse large B-cell lymphoma arising in the breast. (A) Low power shows a large, densely cellular lesion replacing breast tissue. A small duct is present adjacent to the lymphoma (upper right corner of image). Another small duct has been engulfed by the lymphoma (arrow). (B) In this image, lymphoma invades around and distorts a lobule. (C) High power shows large lymphoid cells with vesicular nuclei, distinct nucleoli and scant cytoplasm. Mitoses are frequent. (D–I) Immunostains show that the atypical cells are diffusely positive for CD20 (D), with scattered admixed nonneoplastic T cells (E). The neoplastic B cells are negative for CD10 (F).

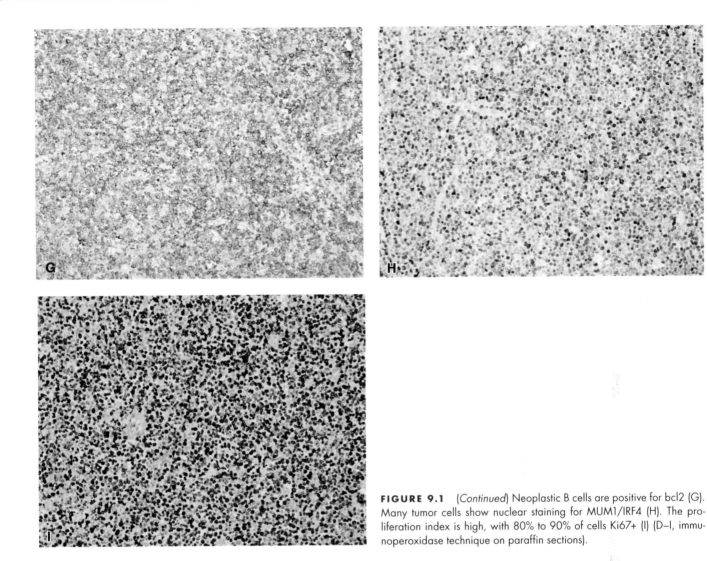

FIGURE 9.1 (*Continued*) Neoplastic B cells are positive for bcl2 (G). Many tumor cells show nuclear staining for MUM1/IRF4 (H). The proliferation index is high, with 80% to 90% of cells Ki67+ (I) (D–I, immunoperoxidase technique on paraffin sections).

by staining for Ki67 is low. If intact reactive follicles are present, their germinal centers are CD10+, bcl6+, bcl2–, with nearly all cells Ki67+. Even in cases in which reactive follicles are not readily identified on routine sections, immunostains for antibodies to follicular dendritic cells, such as CD21 and CD23, usually highlight irregular remnants of follicular dendritic meshworks.

Staging and Prognostic Factors. Most patients present with lymphoma confined to the breast (3–6,16,19). Patients typically remain well after treatment or develop relapses that are usually localized and extranodal in the ipsilateral or contralateral breast, subcutaneous tissue, larynx, chest wall, and other sites. Occasional patients develop lymph node involvement (2,3,25). Large cell transformation has been reported (2,9). Few patients die of lymphoma, sometimes after large cell transformation (9). Marginal zone lymphomas arising in the breast thus behave in a manner similar to that of marginal zone lymphomas in other sites (2,3,9,16).

Follicular Lymphoma

Follicular lymphoma primary in the breast predominantly affects middle-aged and older women (6,9,25). Histologic and immunophenotypic features are similar to those of nodal follicular lymphomas. The lymphomas are typically composed of crowded, poorly delineated follicles composed most often predominantly of centrocytes (small cleaved cells) with few to scattered admixed centroblasts (large noncleaved cells), with or without diffuse areas (Figure 9.4). Follicular lymphomas of all grades (1–3) have been reported (9,10,13,15). Cases with 0 to 5 centroblasts per average high-power field (hpf) in a count of 10 hpf are designated follicular lymphoma, grade 1 of 3. Those with 6 to 15 centroblasts per hpf are designated grade 2 of 3. In the 2008 *WHO Classification of Tumours of Haematopoietic and Lymphoid Tissues*, a change to the traditional grading scheme of follicular lymphoma has been introduced. Because there is no clear biologic difference between grade 1 and grade 2 follicular lymphoma, reporting the grade as "grade 1-2" for any follicular

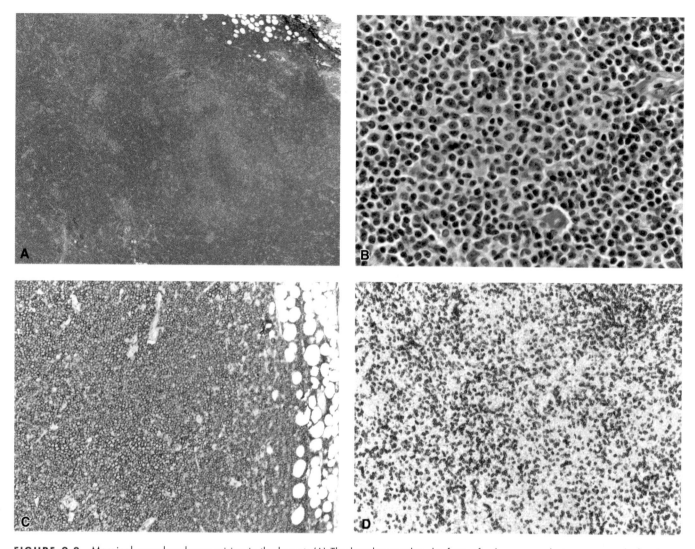

FIGURE 9.2 Marginal zone lymphoma arising in the breast. (A) The lymphoma takes the form of a large mass lesion composed of a dense proliferation of small dark lymphoid cells with ill-defined, slightly more palely stained areas, corresponding to cells with more abundant cytoplasm. (B) High-power examination shows small lymphocytes and minimally enlarged, slightly irregular cells with scant to moderate pale cytoplasm, consistent with marginal zone cells. Rare large cells are present. (C,D) Immunostains show that most cells are CD20+ B cells (C), although there are many admixed reactive CD3+ T cells (D) as well (immunoperoxidase technique on paraffin sections).

lymphoma with 0 to 15 centroblasts per average hpf is acceptable (29). Those with greater than 15 centroblasts per hpf with interspersed centrocytes are designated grade 3A, whereas those with solid aggregates of centroblasts are designated grade 3B. Single-cell epithelial infiltration has been described; this could suggest lymphoepithelial lesions and potentially lead to a mistaken impression of marginal zone lymphoma (5). Neoplastic follicles are typically composed of CD45+, CD20+, CD10+, CD5−, CD43−, bcl6+, bcl2+, cyclin D1−, monotypic surface immunoglobulin light chain+ B cells (5), although fresh tissue for flow cytometry is usually required to demonstrate the surface immunoglobulin. Patients present with disease involving the breast, sometimes accompanied by axillary nodal involvement and occasionally with widespread disease (4–6,9,16,25).

Burkitt Lymphoma

Burkitt lymphoma and lymphomas that have been classified as Burkitt-like lymphoma are mainly found in young to middle-aged women (4,15,16) who are sometimes pregnant or postpartum (see Lymphoma of the Breast in Pregnancy and Lactation) (4,15,16,30) and rarely in premenarchal girls (31). Some patients are from Africa (31,32). Burkitt lymphoma is typically composed of a diffuse proliferation of uniform, medium-sized cells with round nuclei, clumped chromatin, several nucleoli, and a modest amount of cytoplasm that is deeply basophilic on a Giemsa stain. The proliferation is highly cellular, with intervening stroma essentially absent. The mitotic rate is very high, and there is abundant apoptotic debris related to rapid turnover of neoplastic cells. Burkitt lymphoma has many interspersed pale tingible body macrophages

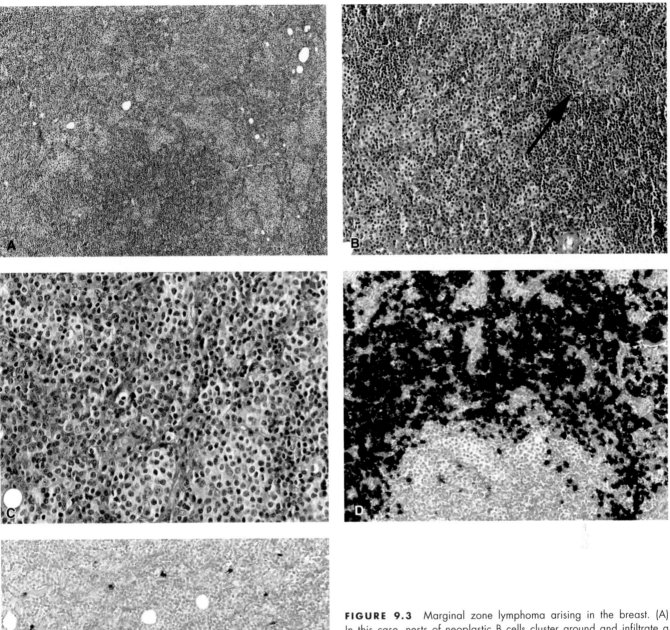

FIGURE 9.3 Marginal zone lymphoma arising in the breast. (A) In this case, nests of neoplastic B cells cluster around and infiltrate a lymphoid follicle at the bottom of the field. (B) Slightly higher power shows a reactive follicle with a small, discrete follicle center (arrow) surrounded by a mantle of small dark lymphocytes. The neoplastic marginal zone cells surrounding the follicle have abundant clear cytoplasm. (C) On high-power examination, many plasma cells can be seen scattered between clusters of clear cells. (D,E) In situ hybridization on paraffin sections shows intense positive staining of numerous plasma cells and plasmacytoid cells for κ immunoglobulin light chain (D), with only a few lambda light chain–positive plasma cells, consistent with a monotypic κ-positive population and demonstrating that the lymphoma has plasmacytic differentiation.

containing apoptotic debris in a background of deeply stained neoplastic cells creating the characteristic starry sky pattern (33).

Burkitt lymphoma also has a characteristic immunophenotype: neoplastic cells are uniformly CD20+, CD10+, bcl6+, bcl2−, monotypic surface immunoglobulin (IgM)+,

with virtually all cells positive for Ki67 (proliferation). As for other types of lymphoma, successful demonstration of surface immunoglobulin usually requires fresh tissue for flow cytometry. The underlying genetic event is a translocation involving *MYC* on chromosome 8 and *IGH* on chromosome 14. In a few cases, the rearrangement

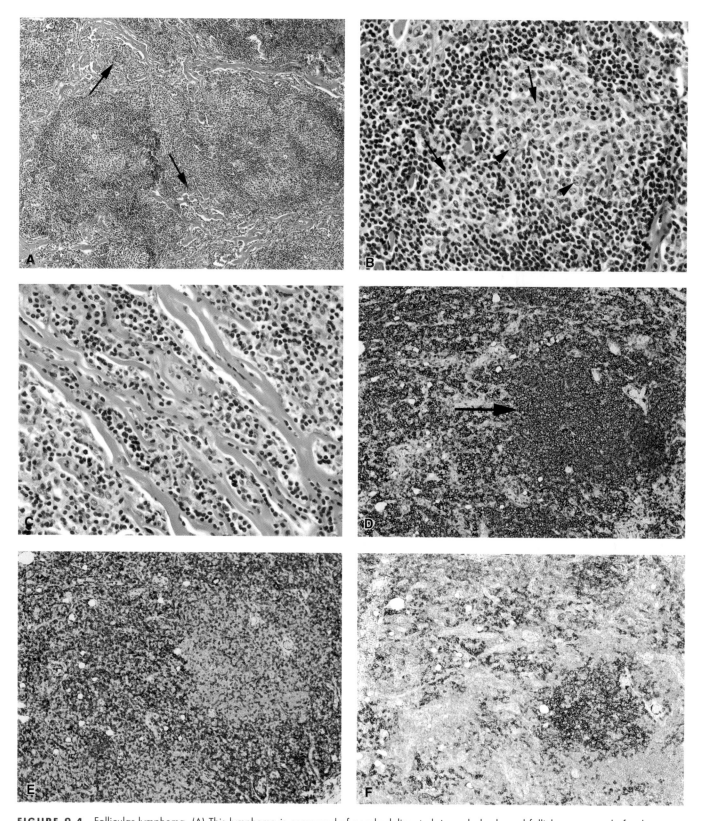

FIGURE 9.4 Follicular lymphoma. (A) This lymphoma is composed of poorly delineated, irregularly shaped follicles composed of pale aggregates of follicle center cells incompletely surrounded by small lymphocytes. Atypical cells are also present in a diffuse pattern outside follicles (arrows). This lymphoma is associated with prominent sclerosis, especially in diffuse areas. (B) High-power view of one follicle shows that it is composed of many small- to medium-sized, irregular centrocytes (arrows) and occasional large centroblasts (arrowheads). (C) The diffuse areas contain centrocytes and small dark lymphocytes that prove to be nonneoplastic T cells on immunostains. (D) Immunostains show that the lymphoma is composed of numerous CD20+ B cells in a follicle (arrow) and also outside follicles (D) with many admixed CD3+ T cells (E). B cells, both within and outside the follicle, are CD10+ (F) and coexpress bcl2 (G).

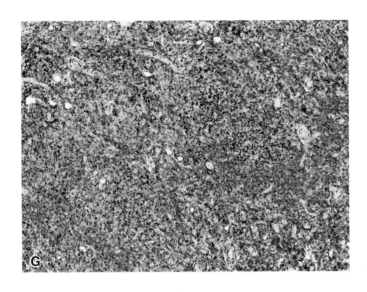

FIGURE 9.4 (*Continued*)

involves *MYC* and the gene for κ or λ light chain rather than the immunoglobulin heavy chain gene (33).

T-Cell Lymphomas

Primary breast lymphoma of T lineage is very uncommon, accounting for only about 2% to 3% of breast lymphomas (4,14,19). As for B-lineage breast lymphomas, patients usually present with unilateral, but occasionally bilateral, masses. ALK-negative anaplastic large cell lymphomas arising in association with breast implants are discussed separately below (see Breast Lymphoma in Association With Implants). Also reported are ALK+ anaplastic large cell lymphoma; peripheral T-cell lymphoma; NOS, including both CD4+ and CD8+ cases; T-lymphoblastic lymphoma (4,19,21,34–36); and subcutaneous panniculitis-like T-cell lymphoma (25). Based on the small number of cases and despite aggressive therapy in some cases, the prognosis appears poor overall. The behavior appears more aggressive than B-cell lymphomas arising in the breast. An exception to this is anaplastic large cell lymphoma arising in association with implants, which has a favorable prognosis (see below).

Breast Lymphoma in Pregnancy and Lactation

Women who are pregnant or breast-feeding rarely develop lymphoma presenting with involvement of the breast; lymphoma in this setting has distinctive features (1,6,17,19, 24,30,37–40). Patients typically present with rapidly enlarging breast masses that may be bilateral and extremely large. Most of the lymphomas are aggressive B-cell lymphomas classified as Burkitt lymphoma (or as small noncleaved cell lymphoma) (30,38–40) or diffuse large B-cell lymphoma (6,17,19), although pathologic features are often not described in detail and immunophenotyping studies are sometimes limited or are not performed at all. Most patients with aggressive B-cell lymphoma have died within a year of diagnosis; others are well on follow-up (1,19,40).

Although the explanation for the massive breast involvement and poor outcome in this setting is uncertain, a number of hypotheses have been suggested. Possible contributing factors include hypervascularity of the breast during pregnancy and lactation (38), changes in the immune system or decreased immune surveillance related to pregnancy (39), and homing of neoplastic cells to hormonally stimulated tissue (38). Another possible factor is delay in establishing a diagnosis or instituting therapy because the patient is pregnant (6).

Breast Lymphoma in Association With Implants

Rare patients with breast implants, including those used for both cosmetic purposes and reconstruction after mastectomy for carcinoma, have developed lymphoma of the breast (25,41–44). The interval from insertion of the implant to diagnosis of lymphoma has ranged from 3 to 16 years, with a median of about 7 to 8 years (25,41,45–47). Although lymphomas of a variety of types have involved the breast in this setting, most lymphomas arising in association with implants are ALK-negative anaplastic large cell lymphomas. Most patients with anaplastic large cell lymphoma present with swelling due to a seroma adjacent to the implant, sometimes accompanied by erythema, warmth or ulceration of the overlying skin, and tenderness or pain; a mass lesion is often absent (25,41–47).

The neoplastic cells are large, atypical, pleomorphic, and mitotically active; they have oval or indented nuclei, prominent nucleoli, and moderately abundant cytoplasm. The tumor is often accompanied by a mixed inflammatory infiltrate composed of lymphocytes, plasma cells, histiocytes, and sometimes granulocytes in a sclerotic background (Figure 9.5) (43,47). Neoplastic cells sometimes form a thin layer between the necrotic material adjacent to the implant and the surrounding fibrosis (42). Silicone from the implant may be identified adjacent to the infiltrate (47). The neoplastic cells are CD30+ (Figure 9.5D),

---

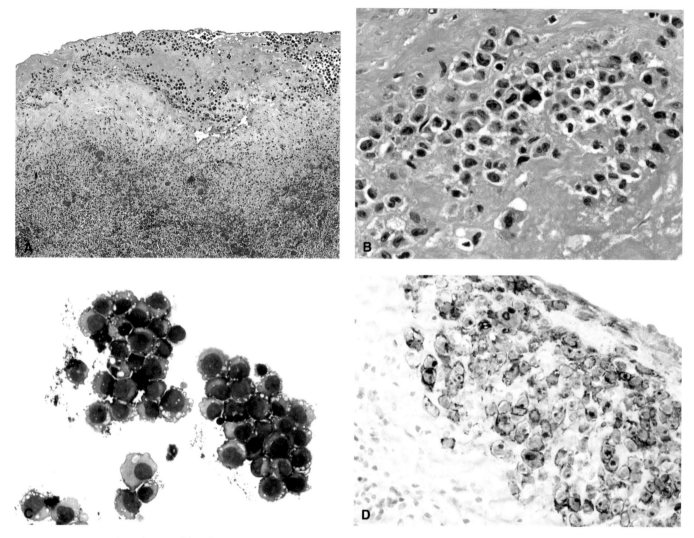

FIGURE 9.5 Anaplastic large cell lymphoma, ALK-negative, arising in association with an implant. (A) A section of the fibrous capsule shows a thin layer of large atypical cells near the surface (top of image); numerous chronic inflammatory cells are also present (bottom half of image). (B) High power shows large, atypical, discohesive cells with oval or bean-shaped nuclei, distinct nucleoli, and a moderate amount of eosinophilic cytoplasm in a fibrotic background. (C) Aspiration of the seroma present adjacent to the implant reveals large atypical lymphoid cells with relatively abundant, basophilic cytoplasm, often with vacuolization (Wright stain). (D) The large atypical cells are CD30+ (shown here) but were negative for ALK (immunoperoxidase technique on paraffin sections).

ALK−, CD45+ and often with coexpression of EMA and cytotoxic granule proteins such as granzyme B and TIA-1. T-cell antigens are variably expressed; there is frequently loss of one or more pan-T-cell antigens. Epstein-Barr virus (EBV) and human herpes virus 8 (HHV8) are absent (41–44,46,47). Clonal rearrangement of the T-cell receptor γ chain gene can usually be detected, but a clonal B-cell population is not found (41–42,47). The lymphoma is usually localized (41–42,45), and follow-up is uneventful in the most cases (41,45–47).

Differential Diagnosis

The diagnosis of lymphoma of the breast is almost never suspected preoperatively. The clinical impression is most often carcinoma, but depending on the findings on physical

examination and the mammographic features, the differential may also include fibroadenoma or phyllodes tumor (24). Establishing a diagnosis of lymphoma of the breast may present a variety of problems, particularly when the specimen submitted is small or a diagnosis is requested on frozen section. A stepwise approach to evaluating breast biopsies with lymphoid infiltrates is suggested below.

1. Determining the tissue involved: lymphoid infiltrate involving the breast versus lymph node.

   The first step in evaluating a specimen reported to be from the breast is determining whether it represents breast parenchyma or an intramammary or low axillary lymph node. This can be difficult, and on a small biopsy may be impossible. The area with the lymphoid proliferation should be evaluated for evidence of lymph nodal components, such as a discrete capsule or patent sinuses. If the lesion biopsied is determined to be a lymph node, the differential diagnosis then includes the wide variety of reactive and neoplastic lesions that may involve lymph nodes at any anatomic site. Finding the infiltrate in continuity with ducts or lobules without intervening lymph node structures supports breast parenchymal involvement. The discussion below focuses on breast parenchymal lymphoid infiltrates.

2. Evaluating the cellular composition

Most lymphoid infiltrates in the breast fall into 1 of 2 major categories: (1) diffuse infiltrates of obviously malignant lymphoid cells and (2) infiltrates composed predominantly of small lymphoid cells. In the first category, the differential diagnosis includes aggressive lymphoma and invasive carcinoma. Subclassification of the lymphoma may also pose diagnostic challenges. In the second category, the differential diagnosis includes low-grade lymphoma and a reactive, chronic inflammatory infiltrate.

A. Overtly malignant neoplasms
   i. Distinguishing lymphoma
      from carcinoma

Differentiating lymphoma from carcinoma can occasionally be difficult; neoplastic lymphoid cells can grow in a pattern mimicking carcinoma infiltrating in an Indian file pattern (13). In some instances, misdiagnosis of lymphoma as carcinoma has led to mastectomy and axillary lymph node dissection (22). Careful evaluation of the histologic features should suggest lymphoma. The presence of cohesive growth or lumen formation by the neoplastic cells and of ductal or lobular carcinoma in situ supports a diagnosis of carcinoma. Immunohistochemical evaluation using antibodies to cytokeratin and B- and T-cell–associated markers should establish a diagnosis.

Lymphoepithelioma-like carcinoma and medullary carcinoma present special problems in the differential diagnosis of lymphoma of the breast. Both of these carcinomas are associated with a dense lymphoid infiltrate; the tumor cells may be obscured by the lymphoid infiltrate or mistaken for large lymphoid cells. Lymphoepithelioma-like carcinoma takes the form of an ill-defined mass with infiltrative borders. Neoplastic epithelial cells are present as single cells, cords, nests, or sheets associated with a dense lymphoid infiltrate that sometimes contains reactive follicles (48). Medullary carcinoma characteristically produces a well-circumscribed mass composed of a high-grade carcinoma growing in a syncytial pattern; mitotic figures are numerous. The carcinoma is present in a background rich in

lymphoid cells (24). Careful examination of well-prepared slides is important in establishing a diagnosis. Lobular carcinoma in situ and atypical lobular hyperplasia have been described in association with lymphoepithelioma-like carcinoma. The presence of atypical epithelial structures may provide a clue to the diagnosis of carcinoma rather than lymphoma (48). Immunostains for cytokeratin and lymphocyte-associated antigens help to distinguish reactive lymphoid cells and neoplastic epithelial cells in cases of carcinoma. Lymphoepithelioma-like carcinoma arising in the breast is negative for EBV, so staining for EBV is not helpful; this is in contrast to the histologically similar undifferentiated nasopharyngeal carcinoma (48).

Establishing a diagnosis in cases of anaplastic large cell lymphoma, ALK–, arising in association with a breast implant may be problematic, with both carcinoma and nonneoplastic, reactive processes included in the differential diagnosis. The findings at presentation can lead to a clinical impression of inflammation, infection, or leaking implant. Neoplastic lymphoid cells may be mistaken for carcinoma, particularly in women with a prior diagnosis of breast carcinoma. Neoplastic cells may be present focally within the specimen and may be obscured by inflammation and fibrosis, so that they may be overlooked.

   ii. Subclassification of high-grade lymphomas

An important problem in the subclassification of diffuse aggressive breast lymphomas is distinguishing diffuse large B-cell lymphoma from Burkitt lymphoma. Diffuse large B-cell lymphoma is much more common, but Burkitt lymphoma, when properly treated, has a good prognosis; hence, the distinction is critical. Burkitt lymphoma, as noted above, is typically composed of a diffuse proliferation of medium-sized cells that are CD20+, CD10+, bcl6+, bcl2–, Ki67~100%. Diffuse large B-cell lymphomas are composed of cells that are overall larger and often more pleomorphic than those of Burkitt lymphoma. Their immunophenotype varies, with some cases having an immunophenotype similar to that of Burkitt lymphoma and others lacking CD10 or bcl6 and/or expressing bcl2. The distinction may be difficult in some cases. If fresh tissue is sent for cytogenetics, the results can be very helpful. Because this is often not available, fluorescence in situ hybridization on paraffin-embedded tissue for rearrangement of *MYC*, *BCL2*, and *BCL6* can be very helpful, as Burkitt lymphoma is characterized by *MYC* rearrangement but absence of translocations involving *BCL2* and *BCL6*, whereas diffuse large B-cell lymphomas may have *BCL2* or *BCL6* rearrangements. A minority of diffuse large

B-cell lymphomas have a *MYC* rearrangement, so the presence of this cytogenetic abnormality by itself does not establish a diagnosis of Burkitt lymphoma.

B. Predominantly small lymphoid cell infiltrate
    i. Low-grade lymphomas versus reactive lymphoid infiltrates

Reactive lymphoid infiltrates in the breast that are sufficiently dense that they may mimic lymphoma are uncommon. Diabetic mastopathy, however, can be associated with a prominent lymphoid infiltrate. Familiarity with its clinical and pathologic features will avoid its misinterpretation as a lymphoproliferative disorder. Diabetic mastopathy is an uncommon, fibroinflammatory process predominantly found in young or middle-aged, usually premenopausal, women, although older women and occasionally men may also be affected. Patients typically have long-standing type 1 diabetes mellitus, and a few have type 2 diabetes mellitus. This disorder is occasionally encountered in patients with other types of immunologic disorders or in individuals who are otherwise well; in such cases, the condition may be designated autoimmune mastopathy or lymphocytic mastitis. The typical presentation is with unilateral, or less often bilateral, firm to hard breast mass(es) (32,49–51) that may mimic carcinoma on physical examination. Microscopic examination reveals a perilobular, periductal, and/or perivascular infiltrate of small lymphocytes with a variable admixture of plasma cells (Figure 9.6). Lymphoid follicles with reactive follicle centers may be seen. Vascular invasion is sometimes identified. The infiltrate may be associated with lobular atrophy. Densely collagenized fibrous tissue,

sometimes reminiscent of keloidal fibrosis, is often prominent. In some cases, large, reactive, epithelioid fibroblasts can be identified in the fibrous tissue. Immunophenotyping reveals that lymphocytes are predominantly B cells with varying numbers of T cells. Lymphoepithelial lesions composed of B cells are found in some cases. No clonal B-cell population is identified using immunophenotyping or PCR (32,50,51). The discrete perilobular or periductal lymphoid aggregates, lack of cytologic atypia, absence of clonal B cells, and the distinctive sclerosis of diabetic mastopathy help to exclude lymphoma. Establishing a definite diagnosis may be difficult on a needle biopsy, as the characteristic histologic features may be difficult to appreciate on a small piece of tissue (51). Recurrences are reported in some cases (49) and thus are not necessarily indicative of malignancy. There is no known increased risk of malignancy in association with diabetic or lymphocytic mastopathy, but because lymphoma has rarely been reported in specimens showing this disorder (27), careful evaluation of the entire specimen is suggested to exclude areas of lymphoma.

Both extranodal marginal zone lymphoma and follicular lymphoma may enter the differential diagnosis of a chronic inflammatory, reactive lymphoid infiltrate. In the differential diagnosis of marginal zone lymphoma and a reactive process, large numbers of B cells with the morphology of marginal zone cells outside follicles, CD43 expression by B cells, and monotypic immunoglobulin expression by the lymphoid cells or by admixed plasma cells favor lymphoma. Florid follicular hyperplasia is not commonly found in the breast, but features that would favor a

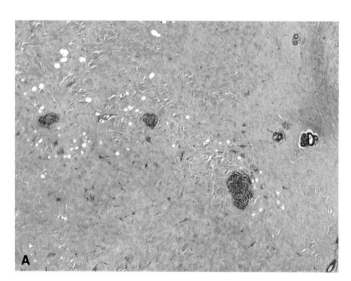
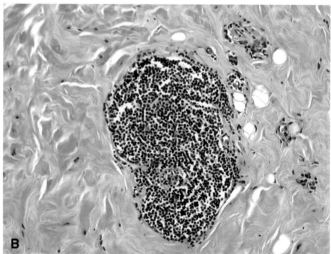

FIGURE 9.6 Diabetic mastopathy. (A) Low power shows extensive hypocellular sclerotic tissue with a few widely separated aggregates of lymphoid cells. (B) Higher power of one aggregate shows that it is composed of a uniform population of small lymphocytes; the aggregate appears to be centered on a small blood vessel.

low-grade follicular lymphoma over reactive follicular hyperplasia (in the breast and also in lymph nodes and other extranodal sites) include the presence of crowded follicles occupied by a monotonous population of lymphoid cells without polarization and with few mitoses or tingible body macrophages. Bcl2 expression by follicle center B cells confirms a diagnosis of follicular lymphoma. Follicular lymphoma is also more likely than follicular hyperplasia to have an interfollicular or occasionally diffuse component of atypical B cells that may express CD10 or bcl6. In some cases, a definite distinction between a low-grade lymphoma and a reactive lymphoid infiltrate cannot be made with certainty based on histologic and immunohistologic features. In such cases, a tissue may be submitted for molecular studies using PCR to investigate the presence of a clonal population.

ii. Subclassification of low-grade lymphomas

The 2 most common low-grade lymphomas that arise in the breast, that is, extranodal marginal zone lymphoma and follicular lymphoma, may occasionally be difficult to distinguish from one another in the breast and in other sites as well. In general, marginal zone lymphomas typically have a pattern that is predominantly diffuse, whereas follicular lymphomas usually have a follicular pattern, sometimes with diffuse areas. Marginal zone lymphomas often contain reactive follicles, which may be intact or which may be partially or completely replaced by neoplastic marginal zone cells (follicular colonization) resulting in an infiltrate that may in areas appear to have a follicular architecture, potentially mimicking follicular lymphoma. In favor of marginal zone lymphoma are the predominance of CD5–, CD10–, bcl6– marginal zone cells with cytologically bland, oval to slightly irregular nuclei and pale cytoplasm; remnants of follicle centers that appear reactive; and evidence of plasmacytic differentiation. Crowded, poorly delineated follicles composed predominantly of CD10+, bcl6+ centrocytes with more pronounced nuclear irregularity and scant cytoplasm favor follicular lymphoma (compare Figures 9.2 and 9.3 to Figure 9.4). Identification of lymphoepithelial lesions to support a diagnosis of marginal zone lymphoma over follicular lymphoma is not as useful in the breast as in some other extranodal sites because well-developed lymphoepithelial lesions may not be found in marginal zone lymphomas of the breast and because lymphocytic infiltration into the epithelium may be found in follicular lymphomas of the breast. Both of these lymphomas, as well as nearly all low-grade B-cell lymphomas and many normal lymphoid cells, are usually bcl2+. Bcl2 expression is mainly of use in the distinction between reactive and neoplastic follicles, not in distinguishing different types of lymphoma.

■ SECONDARY LYMPHOMAS OF THE BREAST

Secondary lymphoma of the breast includes cases of lymphoma with involvement of the breast in the setting of widespread disease, as well as those relapsing in the breast. Lymphoma is reported to be the most common type of malignancy to involve the breast secondarily (52). Secondary involvement of the breast by lymphoma appears to be more common than primary lymphoma of the breast (4,9,19,53). In nearly all cases, the neoplasms are B-cell lymphomas, among which the most common are diffuse large B-cell lymphoma, follicular lymphoma, and extranodal marginal zone lymphoma (4,9,19,25,26,53).

In general, the prognosis for patients with secondary lymphoma of the breast is inferior to that of primary lymphoma (26). Patients with marginal zone lymphoma may have isolated relapses in the breast and in other extranodal sites, with a favorable outcome, as is true of extranodal marginal zone lymphoma in general (9). However, some marginal zone lymphomas undergo histologic progression to diffuse large B-cell lymphoma; patients in whom this occurs may succumb to their disease (19).

■ CONCLUSIONS

Lymphomas of the breast are uncommon, but when they occur, they have characteristic features. Most are B-lineage lymphomas, including both high-grade and low-grade types. Among primary lymphomas of the breast, the most common pathologic types are diffuse large B-cell lymphoma, extranodal marginal zone lymphoma (MALT lymphoma), and follicular lymphoma. Cases of Burkitt lymphoma are rare but well described. T-cell lymphomas are very uncommon; the one type of T-cell lymphoma of the breast that emerges as a distinct clinicopathologic entity is ALK-negative anaplastic large cell lymphoma arising in association breast implants. The differential diagnosis of diffuse large B-cell lymphoma is mainly with poorly differentiated carcinoma. The differential diagnosis of marginal zone lymphoma and follicular lymphoma is mainly with chronic inflammatory processes; in some instances, these 2 types of lymphoma may be difficult to distinguish from one another. Because these breast lymphomas are rare, the possibility of lymphoma may not be considered initially, but establishing a precise diagnosis is critical, as the treatment and prognosis differ from those of other neoplasms involving the breast.

■ KEY POINTS

- Primary lymphoma of the breast is very uncommon; when it occurs, it has distinct clinical and pathologic features.
- Nearly all primary lymphomas of the breast are B-cell lymphomas; the most common types are diffuse large B-cell lymphoma, extranodal marginal zone lymphoma, and follicular lymphoma.
- T-cell lymphomas arising in the breast are extremely uncommon. Among T-lineage lymphomas, ALK-negative anaplastic large cell lymphoma arising in association with breast implants is a distinctive entity with a very good prognosis.
- Depending on the type of lymphoma, the differential diagnosis may include poorly differentiated carcinoma or chronic inflammatory processes.

■ REFERENCES

1. Wiseman C, Liao K. Primary lymphoma of the breast. *Cancer*. 1972;29:1705–1712.
2. Lamovec J, Jancar J. Primary malignant lymphoma of the breast—lymphoma of the mucosa-associated lymphoid tissue. *Cancer*. 1987;60:3033–3041.
3. Hugh J, Jackson F, Hanson J, Poppema S. Primary breast lymphoma—an immunohistologic study of 20 new cases. *Cancer*. 1990;66:2602–2611.
4. Domchek SM, Hecht JL, Fleming MD, Pinkus GS, Canellos GP. Lymphomas of the breast: primary and secondary involvement. *Cancer*. 2002;94:6–13.
5. Farinha P, Andre S, Cabecadas J, Soares J. High frequency of MALT lymphoma in a series of 14 cases of primary breast lymphoma. *Appl Immunohistochem Mol Morphol*. 2002;10:115–120.
6. Cabras MG, Amichetti M, Nagliati M, Orru P, Mamusa AM, Angelucci E. Primary non-Hodgkin's lymphoma of the breast: a report of 11 cases. *Haematologica*. 2004;89:1527–1528.
7. Vigliotti ML, Dell'olio M, La Sala A, Di Renzo N. Primary breast lymphoma: outcome of 7 patients and a review of the literature. *Leuk Lymphoma*. 2005;46:1321–1327.
8. Liu M, Hsieh C, Wang A, et al. Primary breast lymphoma: a pooled analysis of prognostic factors and survival in 93 cases. *Ann Saudi Med*. 2005;25:288–293.
9. Mattia A, Ferry J, Harris N. Breast lymphoma: a B-cell spectrum including the low grade B-cell lymphoma of mucosa associated lymphoid tissue. *Am J Surg Pathol*. 1993;17:574–587.
10. Wang LA, Harris NL, Ferry JA. Lymphoma of the breast and the role of mammography in the detection of low-grade lymphomas. *Mod Pathol*. 2004;17:276A.
11. Lyons J, Myles J, Pohlman B, Macklis R, Crowe J, Crownover R. Treatment and prognosis of primary breast lymphoma—a review of 13 cases. *Am J Clin Oncol*. 2000;23:334–336.
12. Aviles A, Delgado S, Nambo MJ, Neri N, Murillo E, Cleto S. Primary breast lymphoma: results of a controlled clinical trial. *Oncology*. 2005;69:256–260.
13. Fruchart C, Denoux Y, Chasle J, et al. High grade primary breast lymphoma: is it a different clinical entity? *Breast Cancer Res Treat*. 2005;93:191–198.
14. Uesato M, Miyazawa Y, Gunji Y, Ochiai T. Primary non-Hodgkin's lymphoma of the breast: report of a case with special reference to 380 cases in the Japanese literature. *Breast Cancer*. 2005;12:154–158.
15. Vignot S, Ledoussal V, Nodiot P, et al. Non-Hodgkin's lymphoma of the breast: a report of 19 cases and a review of the literature. *Clin Lymphoma*. 2005;6:37–42.
16. Ribrag V, Bibeau F, El Weshi A, et al. Primary breast lymphoma: a report of 20 cases. *Br J Haematol*. 2001;115:253–256.
17. Ryan G, Martinelli G, Kuper-Hommel M, et al. Primary diffuse large B-cell lymphoma of the breast: prognostic factors and outcomes of a study by the International Extranodal Lymphoma Study Group. *Ann Oncol*. 2008;19:233–241.
18. Sabate JM, Gomez A, Torrubia S, et al. Lymphoma of the breast: clinical and radiologic features with pathologic correlation in 28 patients. *Breast J*. 2002;8:294–304.
19. Talwalkar SS, Miranda RN, Valbuena JR, Routbort MJ, Martin AW, Medeiros LJ. Lymphomas involving the breast: a study of 106 cases comparing localized and disseminated neoplasms. *Am J Surg Pathol*. 2008;32:1299–1309.
20. Yoshida S, Nakamura N, Sasaki Y, et al. Primary breast diffuse large B-cell lymphoma shows a non-germinal center B-cell phenotype. *Mod Pathol*. 2005;18:398–405.
21. Kebudi A, Coban A, Yetkin G, et al. Primary T-lymphoma of the breast with bilateral involvement, unusual presentation. *Int J Clin Pract*. 2005:95–98.
22. Pisani F, Romano A, Anticoli Borza P, et al. Diffuse large B-cell lymphoma involving the breast. A report of four cases. *J Exp Clin Cancer Res*. 2006;25:277–281.
23. Chanan-Khan A, Holkova B, Goldenberg AS, Pavlick A, Demopoulos R, Takeshita K. Non-Hodgkin's lymphoma presenting as a breast mass in patients with HIV infection: a report of three cases. *Leuk Lymphoma*. 2005;46:1189–1193.
24. Jeon H, Akagi T, Hoshida Y, et al. Primary non-Hodgkin's malignant lymphoma of the breast. *Cancer*. 1992;70:2451–2459.
25. Gualco G, Bacchi CE. B-cell and T-cell lymphomas of the breast: clinical—pathological features of 53 cases. *Int J Surg Pathol*. 2008;16:407–413.
26. Lin YC, Tsai CH, Wu JS, et al. Clinicopathologic features and treatment outcome of non-Hodgkin lymphoma of the breast—a review of 42 primary and secondary cases in Taiwanese patients. *Leuk Lymphoma*. 2009;50:918–924.
27. Rooney N, Snead D, Goodman S, Webb A. Primary breast lymphoma with skin involvement arising in lymphocytic lobulitis. *Histopathology*. 1994;24:81–84.
28. Talwalkar SS, Valbuena JR, Abruzzo LV, et al. MALT1 gene rearrangements and NF-kB activation involving p65 and p50 are absent or rare in primary MALT lymphomas of the breast. *Mod Pathol*. 2006;19:1402–1408.
29. Harris N, Nathwani B, Swerdlow SH, et al. Follicular lymphoma In: Swerdlow S, Campo E, Harris N, et al, eds. *WHO Classification Tumours of Haematopoietic and Lymphoid Tissues*. 4th ed. Lyon: IARC; 2008:220–226.
30. Cordeiro A, Machado AI, Borges A, Alves MJ, Frade MJ. Burkitt's lymphoma related to Epstein-Barr virus

infection during pregnancy. *Arch Gynecol Obstet.* 2009;280:297–300.

31. Lingohr P, Eidt S, Rheinwalt KP. A 12-year-old girl presenting with bilateral gigantic Burkitt's lymphoma of the breast. *Arch Gynecol Obstet.* 2009;279:743–746.
32. Brogi E, Harris N. Lymphomas of the breast: pathology and clinical behavior. *Semin Oncol.* 1999;26:357–364.
33. Leoncini L, Raphael M, Stein H, Harris N, Jaffe E, Kluin P. Burkitt lymphoma In: Swerdlow S, Campo E, Harris N, et al, eds. *WHO Classification Tumours of Haematopoietic and Lymphoid Tissues.* 4th ed. Lyon: IARC; 2008:262–264.
34. Vakiani E, Savage DG, Pile-Spellman E, et al. T-cell lymphoblastic lymphoma presenting as bilateral multinodular breast masses: a case report and review of the literature. *Am J Hematol.* 2005;80:216–222.
35. Aguilera NS, Tavassoli FA, Chu WS, Abbondanzo SL. T-cell lymphoma presenting in the breast: a histologic, immunophenotypic and molecular genetic study of four cases. *Mod Pathol.* 2000;13:599–605.
36. Briggs JH, Algan O, Stea B. Primary T-cell lymphoma of the breast: a case report. *Cancer Invest.* 2003;21:68–72.
37. Burkitt D, Wright D. *Burkitt's Lymphoma.* 1st ed. Edinburgh and London: E and S Livingstone; 1970.
38. Armitage JO, Feagler JR, Skoog DP. Burkitt lymphoma during pregnancy with bilateral breast involvement. *JAMA.* 1977;237:151.
39. Durodola JI. Burkitt's lymphoma presenting during lactation. *Int J Gynaecol Obstet.* 1976;14:225–231.
40. Miyoshi I, Yamamoto K, Saito T, Taguchi H. Burkitt lymphoma of the breast. *Am J Hematol.* 2006;81:147–148.
41. Roden AC, Macon WR, Keeney GL, Myers JL, Feldman AL, Dogan A. Seroma-associated primary anaplastic large-cell lymphoma adjacent to breast implants: an indolent T-cell lymphoproliferative disorder. *Mod Pathol.* 2008;21:455–463.
42. Wong AK, Lopategui J, Clancy S, Kulber D, Bose S. Anaplastic large cell lymphoma associated with a breast implant capsule: a case report and review of the literature. *Am J Surg Pathol.* 2008;32:1265–1268.

43. Farkash E, Ferry J, Harris N, et al. Rare lymphoid malignancies of the breast: a report of two cases illustrating potential diagnostic pitfalls. *J Hematop.* 2009;2:237–244.
44. Miranda RN, Lin L, Talwalkar SS, Manning JT, Medeiros LJ. Anaplastic large cell lymphoma involving the breast: a clinicopathologic study of 6 cases and review of the literature. *Arch Pathol Lab Med.* 2009;133:1383–1390.
45. Newman MK, Zemmel NJ, Bandak AZ, Kaplan BJ. Primary breast lymphoma in a patient with silicone breast implants: a case report and review of the literature. *J Plast Reconstr Aesthet Surg.* 2008;61:822–825.
46. Olack B, Gupta R, Brooks GS. Anaplastic large cell lymphoma arising in a saline breast implant capsule after tissue expander breast reconstruction. *Ann Plast Surg.* 2007;59:56–57.
47. Sahoo S, Rosen PP, Feddersen RM, Viswanatha DS, Clark DA, Chadburn A. Anaplastic large cell lymphoma arising in a silicone breast implant capsule: a case report and review of the literature. *Arch Pathol Lab Med.* 2003;127:e115–e118.
48. Sanati S, Ayala AG, Middleton LP. Lymphoepithelioma-like carcinoma of the breast: report of a case mimicking lymphoma. *Ann Diagn Pathol.* 2004;8:309–315.
49. Ely KA, Tse G, Simpson JF, Clarfeld R, Page DL. Diabetic mastopathy. A clinicopathologic review. *Am J Clin Pathol.* 2000;113:541–545.
50. Valdez R, Thorson J, Finn WG, Schnitzer B, Kleer CG. Lymphocytic mastitis and diabetic mastopathy: a molecular, immunophenotypic, and clinicopathologic evaluation of 11 cases. *Mod Pathol.* 2003;16:223–228.
51. Oba M, Sasaki M, Ii T, et al. A case of lymphocytic mastopathy requiring differential diagnosis from primary breast lymphoma. *Breast Cancer.* 2009;16:141–146.
52. Vizcaino I, Torregrosa A, Higueras V, et al. Metastasis to the breast from extramammary malignancies: a report of four cases and a review of literature. *Eur Radiol.* 2001;11:1659–1665.
53. Duncan VE, Reddy VV, Jhala NC, Chhieng DC, Jhala DN. Non-Hodgkin's lymphoma of the breast: a review of 18 primary and secondary cases. *Ann Diagn Pathol.* 2006;10:144–148.

10

Immunohistochemistry in Breast Pathology

FELIPE C. GEYER

MAGALI LACROIX-TRIKI

JORGE S. REIS-FILHO

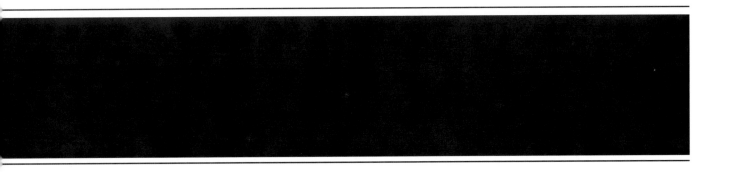

Immunohistochemistry (IHC) is an ancillary technique widely used in daily clinical practice to assist in the histological diagnosis of breast lesions and in the management of patients with breast cancer. Apart from its usefulness in a diagnostic setting for determining invasion and for the differential diagnosis between distinct entities (1), this technique has been the basis for the assessment of estrogen receptor (ER), progesterone receptor (PR), and HER2 status in breast cancer. These 3 biomarkers constitute the minimal data set required for prognostication and management of all newly diagnosed cases of breast cancer. Other immunohistochemical markers beyond the minimal data set, such as Ki67 (2), have been proposed as additional tools for predicting prognosis and responsiveness to adjuvant systemic treatment.

Assessment of hormone receptors and HER2 determines eligibility of patients with breast cancer for receiving endocrine and anti-HER2 therapies, respectively. Given this crucial role in the management of a patient with breast cancer, pathology laboratories offering those assays must ensure accuracy of their results and follow available guideline recommendations (3–6). In addition to their predictive role, assessment of the minimal data set delineates 3 distinct categories of breast cancer (ER+/HER2−, HER2+ and ER−/HER2−), which differ not only in their response to targeted treatment agents but also in their clinicopathological, transcriptomic, and genetic features (7,8).

In the last decade, microarray-based gene expression analysis demonstrated objectively the molecular heterogeneity of breast cancer, revealing that breast carcinomas can be classified according to their transcriptome into at least 5 distinct molecular subtypes, which have distinctive clinical and biological characteristics, namely, luminal A, luminal B, normal breast-like, HER2, and basal-like (9,10). This molecular classification, which is significantly associated with outcome and has a potential role for clinical decision making (11), raised great interest among the scientific and medical communities. Given that the methodologies for the assignment of patients into the molecular subtypes by microarray-based methods still need further optimization (12,13), immunohistochemical surrogate panels have been proposed for the assignment of individual breast tumors into these molecular subtypes (14–17). In fact, there is evidence to suggest a good correlation between the distinct subgroups of breast cancer identified using the minimal data set (ER+/HER2−, HER2+, and ER−/HER2−) and the main microarray-defined subtypes (luminal, HER2, and basal-like) (18,19). Nevertheless, several limitations including the stability of the molecular subtypes must be taken into account before the introduction of this molecular taxonomy in daily practice (12,13).

In this chapter, we will first review the use of immunohistochemical markers for the differential diagnosis of some breast lesions that may raise difficulties at the morphological level. Second, we will discuss the role of IHC in the prediction of prognosis and response to treatment in breast cancer, with an emphasis on the assessment of the minimal data set and the use of IHC for molecular subtyping breast cancers.

■ DIAGNOSTIC MARKERS

Proliferative and Precursor Lesions

The spectrum of proliferative and precursor lesions of the breast has been well characterized at the morphological and molecular levels (20). Although several experts have defined the histological criteria for these entities, the distinction between some of these lesions, in particular between atypical ductal hyperplasia (ADH)/low-grade ductal carcinoma in situ (DCIS) and hyperplasia of usual type (HUT), is a daily challenge in breast pathology practice. Immunohistochemistry may assist in the differential diagnosis between these entities (Table 10.1).

Hyperplasia of usual type, a polyclonal lesion involving cells with luminal and "basal"/myoepithelial

■ **Table 10.1** Expression of immunohistochemical markers in proliferative and precursor lesions of the breast

Marker	HUT	Apocrine Metaplasia	Columnar Cell Change	ADH	Low-Grade DCIS	High-Grade DCIS
ER	+ mosaic	–	+ diffuse	+ diffuse	+ diffuse	–/+
PR	+ mosaic	–	+ diffuse	+ diffuse	+ diffuse	–/+
HMW-CKs (CK5/6, CK14, 34bE12)	+ mosaic	–	–	–	–	–/+
LMW-CKs (CK8/18, CK19, 35bE11)	+ mosaic	+	+ diffuse	+ diffuse	+ diffuse	+/–

LMW-CKs indicates low molecular weight CKs.

differentiation, displays a mosaic pattern of expression of ER and PR. In contrast, ADH, which has been proven to be clonal and similar to low-grade DCIS at the molecular level, typically shows strong positivity for ER and PR in most, if not all, cells (20). In addition to hormone receptors, a panel of cytokeratins (CKs) may be of help. Atypical ductal hyperplasia and low-grade DCIS homogeneously express low-molecular-weight CKs (ie, CK8/18, CK19, 35βE11 cocktail) and lack expression of high-molecular-weight CKs (HMW-CKs) (ie, CK5/6, CK14, CK17, and 34βE12 cocktail) (21). On the other hand, HUT is composed of heterogeneous epithelial cells with expression of both low-molecular-weight CK and HMW-CKs (21). This panel combining hormone receptors and CKs, in particular CK5/6, has also proven to be of practical value for distinguishing between nonatypical and atypical proliferations in papillary lesions (22). It should be emphasised that the availability of these immunohistochemical markers is not an excuse for less detailed and thorough histological analysis of preinvasive lesions. In fact, one should interpret these immunostainings in conjunction with well-defined histological criteria and be aware of potential pitfalls, such as apocrine metaplasia, columnar cell change, and high nuclear-grade features (Table 10.1).

Detection of Invasion

The morphological distinction between benign and malignant lesions of the breast is relatively straightforward in most breast biopsies and excision specimens. Nevertheless, a considerable interobserver disagreement has been documented (23). For a lesion to be classified as invasive, the lack of a myoepithelial cell (MEC) layer is required in most cases. To help determine the disappearance of MECs in breast tumors, a gamut of MEC markers (Table 10.2 and Figure 10.1) is available for IHC. An ideal marker would have absolute specificity and sensitivity for MECs of the breast. Although progress has been made in this area, such

a marker is yet to be identified. The traditional markers including S-100 protein, basement membrane proteins (laminin and type IV collagen), HMW-CKs, and smooth muscle actin (SMA) have been show to display suboptimal sensitivity and specificity (23). For instance, SMA strongly cross-reacts with fibroblasts, myofibroblasts, and pericytes, whereas HMW-CKs can also be expressed in luminal epithelial cells. Several studies have compared new markers and suggested that p63, calponin, and smooth muscle myosin heavy chain (SMM-HC) provide good sensitivity and increased specificity for MEC detection (23). Other recent markers include CD10 (24), maspin (25), and p75[ntr]/NGFR (neurotrophin receptor) (26,27) (Table 10.2). Several limitations must be taken into account when selecting a marker. p63 as compared with calponin and SMM-HC seems to have the best myoepithelial specificity in relation to cross-reactivity with stromal cells and near-perfect sensitivity; however, up to 11% of invasive breast cancers display at least focal p63 expression in neoplastic cells, and gaps in the MEC layer can be more evident and misleading with a nuclear marker such as p63 (23,28). Furthermore, neoplasms with squamous metaplasia consistently express p63. Albeit not perfect, MEC markers have been proven to be useful not only in diagnostic histopathology but also in cytological specimens (29,30).

Recent studies have demonstrated phenotypic alterations in MECs associated with either complex sclerosing lesions of the breast or DCIS (31,32). Myoepithelial cells surrounding sclerosing adenosis, radial scars, and DCIS tend to show a decreased expression of MEC markers as compared with the ones surrounding normal breast ducts and lobules. This is especially true for SMM-HC, CD10, and CK5/6, which display reduced expression in 15.2% to 76.5% of the cases. Conversely, SMA, p75[ntr]/NGFR, and p63 show more consistent expression levels, being reduced in 1%, 4.2%, and 12.6% of DCIS cases, respectively (31,32). These phenotypic alterations in MECs are more prominent in DCIS, in particular in high-grade lesions, which is consistent with the concept that MECs may have

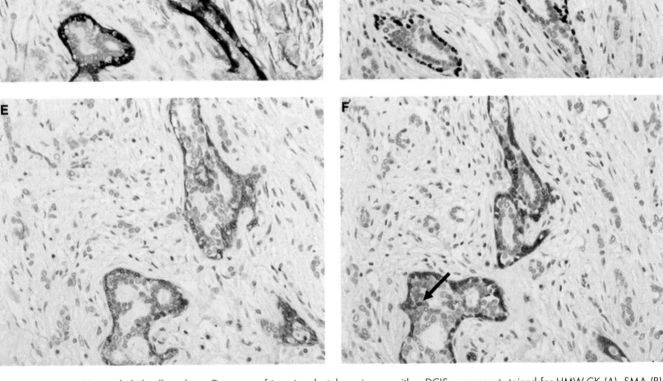

FIGURE 10.1 Myoepithelial cell markers. One case of invasive ductal carcinoma with a DCIS component stained for HMW-CK (A), SMA (B), calponin (C), p63 (D), p75ntr/NGFR (E), and maspin (F). Note that interpretation caveats must be considered when evaluating MEC markers. For instance, luminal residual or tumor cells can be positive for some markers, including HMW-CKs (A, arrows) and maspin (F, arrow). Conversely, cross-reactivity with stromal cells is observed with SMA (B) and less evidently with calponin (C). p63 displays good specificity, but its positivity may be discontinuous (D), which can accentuated in high-grade in situ lesions.

■ Table 10.2 Expression of MEC markers in the distinct compartments/cells of the breast

Marker	Subcellular Localization	MEC	Fibroblast/ Myofibroblast	Vascular Smooth Muscle	Luminal Epithelial Cell	Other	Reference
S-100 protein	Cytoplasm and/ or nucleus	+	–	–	–/+	Neural cells, adipocytes	(23,67)
SMA	Cytoplasm	+	–/+	+	–/+		(23,67)
HMW-CKs	Cytoplasm	+	–	–	–/+		(23,67)
p63	Nucleus	+	–	–	–/+		(23,67)
Calponin	Cytoplasm	+	–/+	+	–		(23,67)
Maspin	Cytoplasm and/ or nucleus	+	–	–	–/+		(23,67)
CD10	Cytoplasm	+	–/+	–	–/+	Lymphocytes	(26,27,67)
SMM-HC	Cytoplasm	+	–/+	+	–		(23,67)
p75NTR/NGFR	Cytoplasm and/ or membrane	+	–/+	–	–/+	Endothelial cells, pericytes, neural cells	(26,27,67)
CD29	Membrane	+			–/+		67
14-3-3σ	Cytoplasm	+			–/+		67

tumor suppressor functions and work as a barrier against tumor cell invasion (33) and should be taken into consideration when selecting and evaluating MEC markers for distinguishing noninvasive from invasive lesions.

Taken together, IHC for MEC detection is a reliable method for determining invasion in breast tumors provided that pathologists are aware of interpretation pitfalls and technical caveats. The selection of a marker should be based on specificity and sensitivity of the markers and on the type of the lesion being analyzed; however, personal and technical experience should also be taken into account. In addition, a panel including at least 2 markers is strongly recommended in problematic cases. These authors recommend the use of p63 in conjunction with a marker that identifies the myoid apparatus of MECs (eg, SMM-HC).

Lobular Versus Ductal Carcinoma

Although broadly accepted histological criteria allow one to distinguish lobular from ductal carcinomas, this differential diagnosis can raise difficulties in some instances. This is particularly true in invasive poorly differentiated lesions with a diffuse infiltrative pattern, in the pleomorphic variant of lobular carcinomas, and also in the solid forms of in situ neoplasia of the breast. With the identification of CDH1 (the E-cadherin protein–coding gene) inactivation as a molecular driver of lobular lesions (34-38), immunohistochemical detection of the expression of E-cadherin and other membrane-associated molecules has been introduced in pathology laboratories as an ancillary tool for the differential diagnosis between lobular and ductal neoplasms (Table 10.3 and Figure 10.2) (39,40).

E-cadherin is a transmembrane glycoprotein implicated in cell-to-cell adhesion and cell motility via interaction with catenins and cytoskeleton. E-cadherin is encoded by the CDH1 gene, which is inactivated in most lobular carcinomas by a combination of genetic and epigenetic events leading to loss of E-cadherin protein expression in most of the cases (34–38,40). In the context of tumor progression, E-cadherin down-regulation has been suggested to play a role in tumor cell infiltration and metastasis (41). Animal model studies have demonstrated that inactivation of Cdh1 and Tp53 in the cells of mouse mammary gland leads to the development of invasive carcinomas that display not only the histological features of invasive lobular carcinomas but also their pattern of metastatic dissemination (42).

■ **Table 10.3** Expression of E-cadherin, β-catenin, and p120 catenin in lobular, ductal, and tubulolobular carcinomas of the breast

Marker	Subcellular Localization	Lobular (%)	Ductal (%)	Tubulolobular (%)	Reference
E-cadherin	Normal membranous	0–16	44–100	75–100	
	Reduced membranous	0–12	54–38	14	
	Negative membrane	80–100	2–14	0–25	34,40,43,45,47,48,50,53,55–57
	Cytoplasmic	9–55	0	0	
	Complete loss	52–100	2	0	
β-Catenin	Normal membranous	6–16	47–81	63–94	
	Reduced membranous	0–8	9–52	6	
	Negative membrane	82–96	0–10	0–37	
	Cytoplasmic	0–100	2	0	34,43,45,48,50,55,56
	Nuclear	6	13	0	
	Complete loss	88–96	2	0	
p120 catenin	Normal membranous	0–9	31–100	100	
	Reduced membranous	0–3	57	0	
	Negative membrane	91–100	0–12	0	
	Cytoplasmic	88–100	10	0	43,47,50,55
	Nuclear	2	NA	0	
	Complete loss	0	2	0	

Several studies have documented the aberrant expression of E-cadherin in lobular lesions and addressed whether it can be used in the differential diagnosis between lobular and ductal carcinomas (34,39,40,43–46). In contrast to invasive ductal lesions, which usually display moderate to strong membranous E-cadherin positivity (Figure 10.2E), complete lack of membranous staining is typically observed in invasive lobular carcinomas (Table 10.3 and Figure 10.2B) (34,40,43,45,47–50). Weak to moderate cytoplasmic reactivity is reported in 9% to 55% of invasive lobular carcinomas and may display a diffuse or a Golgi pattern (Table 10.3) (34,40,43,45).

A similar pattern of E-cadherin expression is observed in the in situ counterparts of ductal and lobular lesions. In

fact, E-cadherin IHC has proven most useful in the diagnosis of solid, low-grade, intraepithelial lesions of the breast. Multiple studies have highlighted the role of E-cadherin IHC in correctly categorizing a subset of in situ breast proliferations (39,46) that show overlapping features between DCIS and lobular carcinoma in situ (LCIS) and therefore have been termed *carcinomas in situ with indeterminate histological features* (39). The latter lesions include low-grade tumors with a solid growth pattern where the distinction is extremely important given that treatment of DCIS is substantially different from that of LCIS (surgery vs clinical follow-up). In addition, E-cadherin IHC has helped in the characterization of in situ lesions displaying high-grade features historically thought to be restricted to

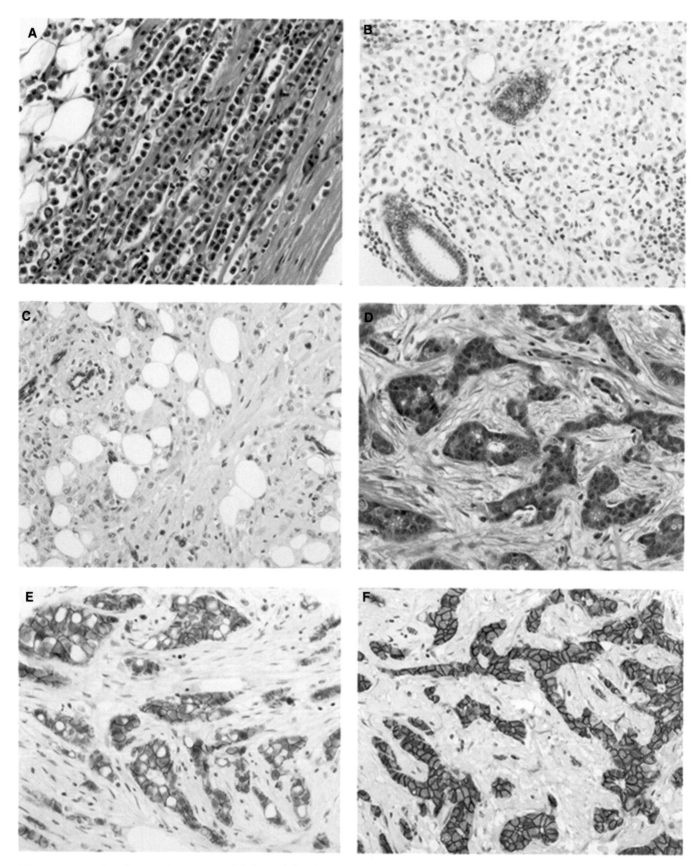

FIGURE 10.2 E-cadherin and β-catenin in lobular and ductal carcinomas. Typically, lobular carcinomas (A) lack membranous expression of E-cadherin (B) and β-catenin (C), whereas ductal carcinomas (D) display preserved membranous reactivity to E-cadherin (E) and β-catenin (F).

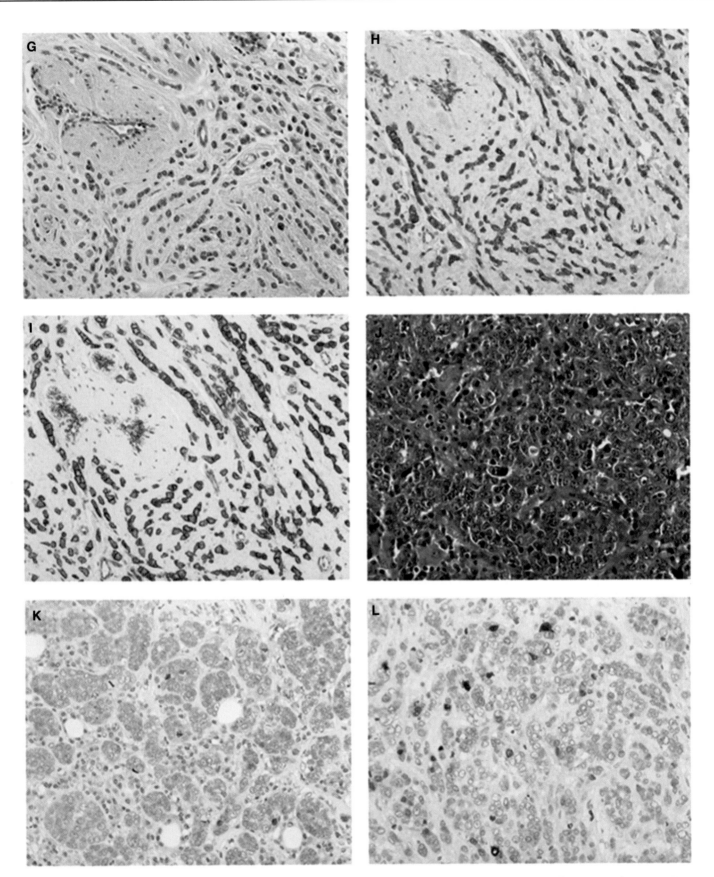

FIGURE 10.2 (*Continued*) However, a small but significant proportion of lobular carcinomas (G) can express E-cadherin (H) and β-catenin (I) at the membrane, whereas some ductal carcinomas (J), in particular those of high grade, can display reduction of membranous expression of both E-cadherin (K) and β-catenin (L) and nuclear accumulation of β-catenin (L).

DCIS, such as comedonecrosis and nuclear pleomorphism (39). Although doubts on the correct terminology and management of these lesions are still raised, the existence of a pleomorphic variant of LCIS, which lacks E-cadherin expression, is now well documented (51,52).

Although most invasive and in situ lobular carcinomas lack E-cadherin expression, it should be pointed out that most studies addressing E-cadherin expression in morphologically defined lobular lesions describe E-cadherin membranous expression, either diffuse or focal, in a subset of them (8%-16%; Figure 10.2H) (34,40,44,45). Interestingly, there is evidence to suggest that in those cases with E-cadherin–positive expression, the protein is dysfunctional, not associating normally with the catenin complex (34). Conversely, it has been demonstrated that decreased or lack of membranous expression of E-cadherin can also be observed in invasive ductal carcinomas (Figure 10.2K) and other special types of breast cancer (eg, metaplastic breast carcinomas) (43,49,53,54). Of note, reduction of E-cadherin expression in ductal carcinomas is associated with tumors of high histological grade and of triple negative and basal-like phenotype (53), and, within triple negative tumors, it has been suggested to be an independent prognostic marker (54). Therefore, to distinguish lobular from ductal lesions based solely on the immunohistochemical expression of E-cadherin can lead to inaccurate interpretation and to mismanagement of patients, given that lobular and ductal lesions are managed in different ways. Taken together, these data indicate that the use of E-cadherin immunostaining should always be coupled with thorough morphological assessment and, perhaps, limited to few situations. One should not stain a bona fide classic invasive lobular carcinoma to "confirm its lobular phenotype." Although extremely helpful in categorizing some in situ breast lesions, it is best avoided in lesions with a typical lobular morphology (34), in particular because some anti–E-cadherin antibodies may stain the membranes of entrapped MECs and residual luminal cells, creating a rather misleading pattern.

The regulation of cell-to-cell adhesion involves interaction between E-cadherin and several other membrane-associated proteins, known as the E-cadherin–catenin complex, of which β-catenin and p120 catenin are major components. Several studies have shown that lobular lesions lacking E-cadherin staining also show aberrant β-catenin and p120 catenin expression (Table 10.3) and suggested that IHC for these molecules might be useful in making the distinction between lobular and ductal carcinomas (43,45,47,50). Lobular cells usually display complete lack of β-catenin expression (Figure 10.2C) (43,45) and cytoplasmic, rather than membranous, expression of p120 catenin (43,47,50). However, in a way akin to E-cadherin, there is a considerable overlap in the pattern of expression of these molecules between lobular and ductal lesions (Table 10.3 and Figure 10.2I, L), limiting its use

for a diagnostic purpose. One advantage of β-catenin over E-cadherin is the presence of positive control in most, if not all, breast samples, given that β-catenin is expressed on the membranes of endothelial cells.

Tubulolobular carcinomas constitute a rare special histological type of breast cancer, composed of a mixture of low-grade tubular-like glands and dyscohesive lobular-like cells arranged in Indian files. Although recognized as a variant of lobular carcinoma in the last edition of the World Health Organization classification of breast cancer, most of these tumors display the membranous E-cadherin/catenin complex characteristic of the ductal immunophenotype (Table 10.3) (55–57). These observations have led to the suggestion that tubulolobular carcinomas may be better classified as variants of ductal/tubular rather than lobular carcinomas.

Spindle Cell Lesions

Spindle cell lesions of the breast constitute a complex group of rare tumors, encompassing a spectrum of lesions with varied clinicopathological and therapeutic implications (58,59). An accurate diagnosis of these lesions is often needed in an early stage of patient management when surgical decision is made. In this setting, IHC plays an important role, in particular when dealing with specimens of small size such as core needle biopsies. Importantly, no single marker can accurately discriminate within this wide spectrum of differential diagnoses, which include fibromatosis, fibroepithelial lesions, reactive spindle cell nodules (60), pseudoangiomatous stromal hyperplasia, spindle cell metaplastic carcinomas, sarcomas, and multiple benign stromal lesions, which have been recently catalogued under the term *benign spindle cell tumors of the mammary stroma* (61). Antibodies that may be included in an IHC panel for the elucidation of the nature of these lesions are summarized in Table 10.4 and shown in Figure 10.3.

As a rule of thumb, pathologists must be aware of the multiple histological and immunophenotypical features of spindle cell metaplastic carcinomas (Figure 10.3A, C, E, G, and I), which are far more commonly encountered than are primary spindle cell sarcomas of the breast. In fact, the first differential diagnosis that needs to be ruled out in the case of spindle cell lesions of the breast is metaplastic breast cancer. Not all spindle cell metaplastic carcinomas are high-grade tumors, but some can have a strikingly bland morphology, with little nuclear pleomorphism and low mitotic activity, resembling fibromatosis or nodular fasciitis (62,63). Therefore, when confronted with a spindle cell lesion of the breast, it is always crucial to search diligently for epithelial elements (Figure 10.3A) and/or differentiation. In this context, a battery of epithelial cell markers should be used and include those that detect HMW-CKs (64) (Figure 10.3C). Another useful

■ **Table 10.4** Expression of immunohistochemcial markers in spindle cell lesions of the breast

Marker	Fibro-adenoma*	Phyllodes Tumor*	PASH	Reactive Spindle Cell Nodule**	Fibromatosis	Nodular Fasciitis	Adenomyo-epithelioma	Myofibroblastoma	Solitary Fibrous Tumor	Metaplastic Carcinoma	Angiosarcoma
Pan-CKs	−	−	−	−	−	−	+	−	−	+	−/+
HMW-CKs	−	−	−	−	−	−	+	−	−	+	−
LMW-CKs	−	−	−	−	−	−	+	−	−	+/−	−
EMA	−	−	−	−	−	−	+	−	−	+/−	
β-Catenin											
Membranous	−	−			−					+/−	
Nuclear	+	+		+	+					−/+	
p63							+			+/−	
SMA	+	+	+	+	+	+/−	+	+	−	+/−	+/−
CD10							+			+/−	
S-100 protein	−		−		+/−		+			−/+	

Continued

■ **Table 10.4** Expression of immunohistochemical markers in spindle cell lesions of the breast (*Continued*)

Marker	Fibro-adenoma*	Phyllodes Tumor*	PASH	Reactive Spindle Cell Nodule**	Fibromatosis	Nodular Fasciitis	Adenomyo-epithelioma	Myofibroblastoma	Solitary Fibrous Tumor	Metaplastic Carcinoma	Angiosarcoma
Desmin					-/+	+/-	+	+/-	-	-	
Factor VIII											+
CD34	+	+/-	+		-	-		+	+	-	+
CD31			-								+
Bcl-2			+					+	+		
Vimentin	+	+	+	+	+	+	+	+	+	+	+
ER			-/+		-			+		-	
PR			+		-			+		-	
HER2										-	
Reference	58	58,70,71	58,59,150	60	58,69,70	58,61	151	58,61,72	61,72	58,59,62–67,70	58,59,61

+ indicates majority positive; +/-, usually positive but may be negative; -/+, usually negative but may be positive; -, majority negative. EMA, epithelial membrane antigen; LMW-CKs, low-molecular-weight CKs; PASH, pseudoangiomatous stromal hyperplasia.
*In fibroepithelial biphasic lesions, expression in the stromal component is here reported.
**Normal entrapped glands may be present and stain for epithelial markers.

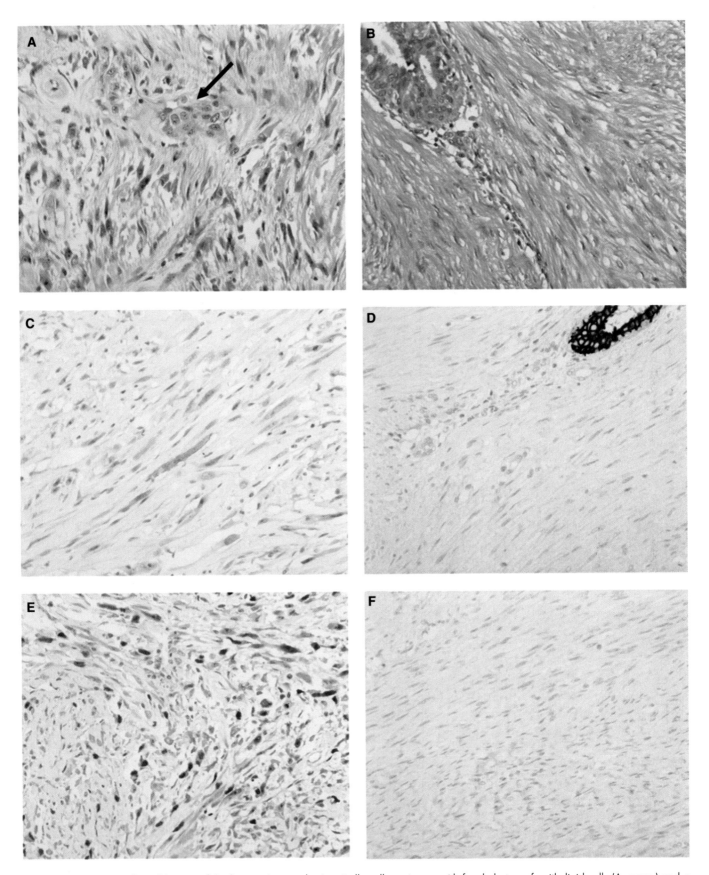

FIGURE 10.3 Spindle cell lesions of the breast. A metaplastic spindle cell carcinoma with focal clusters of epithelioid cells (A, arrow) and a fibromatosis (B) of the breast stained for pan-CK (C and D), p63 (E and F), SMA (G and H), and β-catenin (I and J). Note that the immunophenotype of these 2 differential diagnoses for a spindle cell lesion of the breast can overlap considerably. Expression of CKs can be focal and weak (C) or even negative in spindle cell carcinomas; however, in this case, positivity for p63 (E) supports an epithelial differentiation.

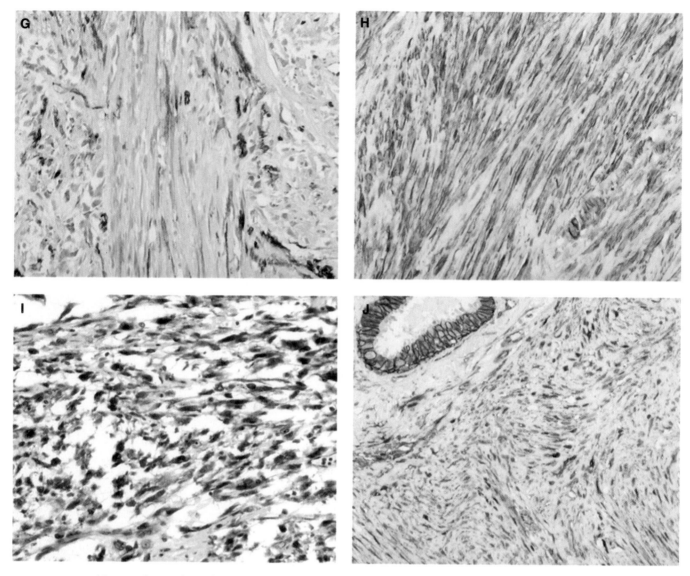

FIGURE 10.3 (Continued) Smooth muscle actin is strongly positive in fibromatosis (H) but can also be positive in metaplastic carcinomas (G). Although β-catenin nuclear expression is helpful to confirm a diagnosis of fibromatosis (J), spindle cell carcinomas often lack β-catenin membranous expression and may show β-catenin nuclear accumulation (I).

marker of epithelial differentiation is p63 (Figure 10.3E), which has been reported to be expressed in up to 100% of metaplastic carcinomas with spindle cell morphology (65,66). It should be noted that expression of CKs may be weak and focal (30% in Leibl et al (67)) or even negative (10% in Leibl et al (67)) in a subset of metaplastic carcinomas. In addition, it has been suggested that the diagnosis of a primary sarcoma of the breast should only be done after exclusion of a MEC phenotype (67); therefore, inclusion of MEC markers in the panel other than CKs is advised.

A controversial topic is how to distinguish spindle cell metaplastic breast carcinomas and myoepithelial carcinomas of the breast. We believe that this distinction is only a matter of semantics, given that the overlap in terms of morphological and immunohistochemical features between these lesions is almost complete. However, some have

suggested that rather subtle histological features (eg, "neoplastic MECs emanating from the MEC layer of entrapped ductules" (68)) may be useful to differentiate these lesions. However, direct evidence in support of these diagnostic criteria for the differentiation between myoepithelial carcinoma and metaplastic spindle cell carcinoma is yet to be provided, and the clinical importance of the distinction between myoepithelial carcinoma and spindle cell carcinoma of the breast is yet to be established.

Once the possibility of an epithelial or myoepithelial malignancy has been excluded, a diagnosis of malignant phyllodes tumor with stromal overgrowth needs to be ruled out. CD34 has been shown to be a useful marker to distinguish between a malignant phyllodes tumor predominantly composed of spindle cells and metaplastic breast cancer (58). The interpretation of this marker should be made in conjunction with the histological features of the lesion (58). After exclusion of the above differential diagnoses, a diagnosis of benign or malignant mesenchymal lesions needs to be addressed. It is important to consider the diagnosis of an angiosarcoma, which is the most common primary breast sarcoma and can display bland morphology (58). Vascular markers such as CD31, CD34, and factor VIII must therefore be included in the IHC panel (Table 10.4). Other sarcomas are exceedingly rare and display an immunophenotype similar to those occurring in other parts of the body (58).

As for benign stromal proliferations, some immunohistochemical markers are of immense value in the elucidation of their nature. β-Catenin has been advocated by some as a marker of fibromatosis, a spindle cell tumor that displays β-catenin nuclear accumulation (Figure 10.3J), often due to *CTNNB1* (β-catenin protein coding gene) or *APC* gene mutations (69). However, nuclear β-catenin expression is also found in the stromal component of most phyllodes tumors and in a subset of metaplastic carcinomas (Figure 10.3I), indicating that β-catenin should not be used as a single marker for the distinction between these entities (70,71).

In addition to angiosarcomas and phyllodes tumors, CD34 is commonly expressed in several spindle cell proliferations of the breast (Table 10.4) (58,59). Together with Bcl2, it can be used for the identification of a spectrum of lesions including myofibroblastoma, solitary fibrous tumor, and other mesenchymal entities less well characterized when occurring in the breast. These lesions often display overlapping morphological features and have a common immunophenotype (vimentin+/CD34+/Bcl2+/CD99+) (61,72). Following this line of reasoning, Magro et al (61,72) have postulated that these lesions are not only morphologically and immunophenotypically related but may also all originate from uncommitted vimentin+/CD34+ fibroblasts present in the mammary stroma and coined the term *benign spindle cell tumor of the mammary stroma* to address this group of tumors.

■ MINIMAL DATA SET

The assessment of ER, PR, and HER2 status is mandatory in all newly diagnosed invasive breast cancers and epitomizes the role of immunohistochemical markers as predictive markers. It should be emphasised that hormone receptors and HER2 are predictive markers with high negative predictive values (ie, they identify the group of patients that will not derive benefit from endocrine therapy or anti-HER2 agents, respectively). The positive predictive value of these markers is only modest. In fact, only a proportion of patients with hormone receptor–positive cancers do respond to endocrine therapy, and a substantial proportion of patients with HER2-positive disease are either de novo resistant or develop resistance over time to anti-HER2 agents.

Given that this evaluation determines patient eligibility for endocrine and anti-HER2 therapies, in the last decade, there has been great debate on the immunohistochemical evaluation of these markers and, in particular, the testing accuracy and the interlaboratory variation. In an attempt to improve the accuracy and reproducibility of ER, PR, and HER2 testing in breast cancer, groups of experts (American Society of Clinical Oncology/College of American Pathologists and the National Comprehensive Cancer Network Task Force) have recently published guideline recommendations that provide guidance on preanalytic/technical parameters and interpretation procedures that must be controlled by laboratories performing those tests (3–6). Furthermore, they emphasized the role of pathologists in this process and that initial validation of assays (73) and quality assurance of ongoing assays must be strictly followed by pathology laboratories. Although not regulatory required, adherence to those guidelines has been strongly advised, as it is estimated that currently up to 20% of ER, PR, and HER2 status determinations worldwide may be inaccurate (either false negative or false positive).

The readers are referred to the guidelines published elsewhere for a complete set of recommendations (5,6). In brief, as a rule, preanalytical variables must be carefully controlled for optimal determination of both hormone receptors and HER2 status (3–6). These include standardization of fixation procedures, which must be described in the pathological report: delay of fixation (ie, time between tissue removal and initiation of fixation, optimally as short as possible and not >1 hour), duration of fixation (optimally >6 hours and <48 hours), and type of fixative. The optimal fixative is 10% neutral buffered formalin; when using other fixatives, the laboratory must validate results against neutral buffered formalin fixation.

Estrogen and Progesterone Receptor

Initially, hormone receptor status in breast cancer was assessed by ligand-binding assays. In the 1990s, IHC began to be commonly used (Figure 10.4), and currently, it is the method of choice for this purpose due to its low cost, applicability to archival tissue specimens, and importantly, because it ensures that invasive tumor cells are being evaluated, even in small samples. Studies have shown that IHC is equivalent or superior to ligand-binding assays in predicting benefit from hormonal therapy (3,5,74,75) and that ER levels as determined by IHC positively correlate with survival (75).

The antibody selection should be restricted to the clinically validated clones that have well-established sensitivity and specificity. The ER clones 1D5, 6F11, SP1, 1D5+ER.2.123 and the PR clones 1A6, 1294, and 312

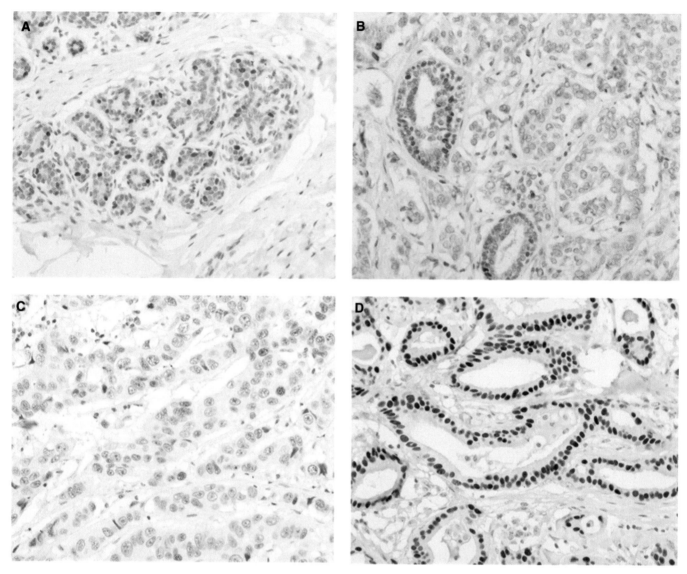

FIGURE 10.4 Estrogen receptor expression in breast cancer. Estrogen receptor expression as defined by IHC in a normal breast lobule (A) and in negative (B), weakly positive (C), and strongly positive (D) invasive breast carcinomas. Note the heterogeneous pattern of ER expression in the normal breast lobule with negative cells and positive cells with varying intensity (A) and a positive internal control required for the correct interpretation of a case lacking ER expression (B).

have been recommended (3,5). Before interpreting any ER or PR immunostainings, it is imperative to ensure adequate negative and positive controls. Of note, external controls should include not only a highly positive case but also intermediate levels of hormone receptor expression. Small tissue microarrays with negative, intermediate, and strongly positive tumors or cell lines represent good alternatives as batch run controls. Internal normal epithelial elements should be present in the paraffin block selected for analysis and display a heterogeneous staining pattern in the luminal cells (Figure 10.4A-B). If controls do not display the anticipated results, the test should not be interpreted and must be repeated. In addition, the correlation between immunophenotype and other histological features of the tumors, including histological type and grade, should be considered when reporting ER and PR results,

for example, tubular, classic lobular, cribriform, and mucinous carcinomas are unlikely to be ER- and PR-negative; on the other hand, metaplastic breast carcinomas (76) and bona fide medullary cancers are unlikely to be ER- and PR-positive (77,78).

Despite the lack of an universal cutoff for distinguishing "negative" from "positive" cases, available data suggest that tumors harboring as few as 1% of positive cells are associated with a significant clinical response to tamoxifen and/or other endocrine agents (79). Therefore, according to recent guidelines (3,5), cases with 1% or more of positive cells should be reported as positive. Given that multiple studies have shown a positive correlation between levels of hormone receptor expression and patient outcome, the percentage and an average intensity of cells with nuclear positivity should also be recorded in the pathological report (3,5). Composite scoring systems such as Allred, quickscore, and H-score (Table 10.5), combining percentage and staining intensity, may also be provided in addition to the final interpretation of the IHC analysis.

Recent guidelines have reviewed whether PR expression in breast cancer correlates with or influences the choice of endocrine therapy and reinforced the inclusion of PR in the minimal data set for breast cancer (3,5). There is evidence to suggest that response to antiestrogen treatment is increased in patients with tumors expressing both ER and PR as compared with those with tumors that are only ER-positive (75); however, this is contentious. In fact, data from Dowsett et al (80) suggest that PR is

a prognostic rather than a predictive marker, given that patients with ER+/PR+ cancers have a better outcome than patients with ER+/PR– cancers regardless of the use of endocrine therapy. In addition, oncologists may preferentially treat patients with ER+/PR– tumors with aromatase inhibitors such as Anastrozole (80); however, this is controversial with regard to other antiaromatase inhibitors such as letrozole (79). Because PR expression is strongly dependent on the presence of functional ER, a pathologist when confronted with a PR+/ER– tumor (less than 1% of invasive breast cancers in large series (79)) should request a retesting of the ER assay to eliminate a false-negative status for ER. In fact, there is evidence to suggest that the PR epitope may be more resistant to variations in the

■ **Table 10.5** Immunohistochemical scoring systems

Method	Main Application	Percentage of Stained Cells Score	Staining Intensity Score	Combination Score	Result Range	Reference
Allred	ER PR	0 = 0 1 = <1% 2 = 1%–10% 3 = 11%–33% 4 = 34%–66% 5 = 67%–100%	0 = no staining 1 = weak staining 2 = moderate staining 3 = intense staining	% score (0–5) + intensity score (0–3)	0–8	74
Quick score	ER PR	0 = 0 1 = 1%–4% 2 = 5%–19% 3 = 20%–39% 4 = 40%–59% 5 = 60%–79% 6 = 80–100%	0 = no staining 1 = weak staining 2 = moderate staining 3 = intense staining	% score (0–6) × intensity score (0–3)	0–18	152
H-score	ER PR	% of stained cells assessed for each staining intensity category	0 = no staining 1 = weak staining 2 = moderate staining 3 = intense staining	(% of stained cells at intensity category 1 × 1) + (% of stained cells at intensity category 2 × 2) + (% of stained cells at intensity category 3 × 3)	0–300	152
HER2 ASCO/ CAP guidelines	HER2	% of stained cells with membrane staining either incomplete or complete (ie, circumferential)	0 = no staining 1 = weak staining 2 = moderate staining 3 = intense staining	Score 0 = no staining; score 1+ = weak incomplete membrane staining in any proportion of tumor cells Score 2+ = >10% of stained cells with complete weak to moderate membrane staining or less than 30% of cells with complete and strong membrane staining Score 3+ = >30% of tumor cells with complete and strong membrane staining	0–3+	6

ASCO indicates the American Society of Clinical Oncology; CAP, College of American Pathologists.

preanalytical parameters than the ER epitope; therefore, cases of ER–/PR+ cancers should be considered as false ER-negative results unless proven otherwise.

Human Epidermal Growth Factor Receptor 2

HER2 gene amplification is found in approximately 11% to 20% of breast cancers and almost invariably (>95% of cases) leads to HER2 protein overexpression (17,81). Both *HER2* gene amplification and overexpression have been shown to predict response to anti-HER2 agents, such as Trastuzumab and Lapatinib (82,83). In the past 5 years, a drastic improvement in the survival of patients with HER2+ breast cancer has been observed with the introduction of this targeted therapy, which has become a standard of care for this subgroup of patients with breast cancer. Considering the cost and risk of ineffectual treatment, an accurate HER2 status assessment is of utmost importance.

HER2 status can be assessed by IHC or in situ hybridization (ISH) techniques (fluorescence, chromogenic, and silver), which are concordant and equivalent in predicting benefit from anti-HER2 therapy. Published guidelines have provided an algorithm defining positive, equivocal, and negative values for both methods (Figures 10.5A and 10.6 and Table 10.5) (4,6). Given the differences in cost, in most institutions and laboratories, IHC is performed as a first screening followed by ISH techniques in equivocal (2+) cases.

In a way akin to IHC for hormone receptors, several technical aspects must be considered. Approved commercially available kits include HercepTest (A085 polyclonal antibody, Dako), and Pathway (clone CB11, Ventana), but one can develop and offer an in-house/homebrew assay provided that it has been thoroughly validated against ISH techniques. Optimization with external and internal controls is fundamental. As for ER and PR, external controls must include tissues with varying levels of HER2 expression and *HER2* gene amplification. Normal ducts and lobules serve as an adequate internal control and must not display positivity, otherwise the test should be rejected and repeated.

Following the last the American Society of Clinical Oncology/College of American Pathologists guideline recommendations (6), HER2-positive carcinomas (ie, 3+) are defined as displaying uniform, intense, and circumferential membrane staining in greater than 30% of invasive tumor cells (Figure 10.5A and 10.6 and Table 10.5) (4,6). The 30% criteria (rather than the originally specified 10%) for a positive HER2 status reflect the experience that true IHC 3+ tumors show usually a high percentage of positive cells and are aimed to decrease the incidence of false-positive 3+ scores. Those with a lower percentage or weaker intensity will then fall into the equivocal range (2+ score) and must be subjected to ISH analysis to ascertain the definitive HER2 status (Figure 10.5A). Published studies report a prevalence of approximately 10% of 2+

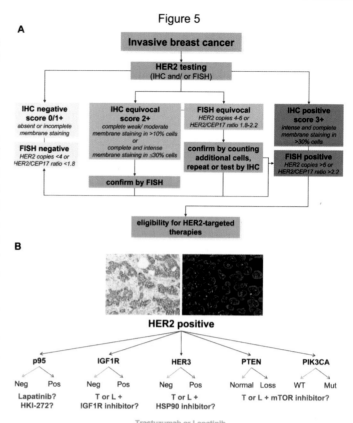

FIGURE 10.5 HER2 status assessment in breast cancer. A, Algorithms for HER2 status assessment using IHC and/or fluorescent in situ hybridization according to guideline recommendations (4,6). B, Hypothetical model of testing for patients with HER2-positive disease. Additional molecular tests addressing markers of resistance to anti-HER2-targeted therapy may be required in the near future to increase the positive predictive value of response to anti-HER2 agents and influence the choice of therapy. Preclinical data suggest that different types of combinatorial therapies, and anti-HER2 agents may be required for patients whose tumors harbor molecular aberrations that lead to de novo resistance to anti-HER2 therapy (red arrows). For instance, patients with p95 (truncated isoform of HER2 that lack the extracellular domain) may not benefit from anti-HER2 humanized monoclonal antibodies; in this case, HER2 small molecule inhibitors may be more efficacious. Other examples include those tumors that express IGF1R or alterations of the PI3K/mTOR pathway, where a combination of anti-HER2 agents with either IGF1R inhibitors or inhibitors of PI3K/mTOR pathway may provide a way of overcoming de novo resistance. Other mechanisms of resistance involving HER3 and alternative combinatorial therapies including anti-HER2 agents with HSP90 inhibitors may also play a role in the therapy of patients with HER2-positive tumors in the near future (153). L indicates lapatinib; mut, mutant; neg, negative; pos, positive; T, trastuzumab; WT, wild type.

cases, and, within 2+ cases, around 10% to 50% display *HER2* gene amplification as defined by the ISH analysis (84–86).

Recently, new assays based on modified IHC techniques using proximity-based technology were developed for HER2 testing (87). This highly sensitive and specific method allows quantitative assessment of HER2 protein expression and HER2 hetero/homodimers in formalin-fixed, paraffin-embedded samples. Retrospective analyses have suggested that a subset of *HER2*-amplified cases as

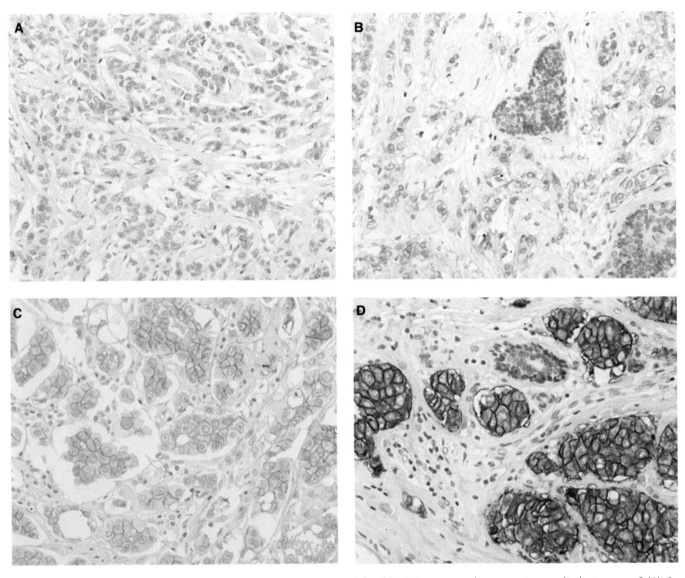

FIGURE 10.6 HER2 expression in breast cancer. HER2 expression as defined by IHC in invasive breast carcinomas displaying score 0 (A), 1+ (B), 2+ (C), and 3+ (D). Note that normal glands should not display HER2 expression (B and D). In addition, in micropapillary carcinomas (C), complete membranous expression is not required as the apical membrane in glands with the typical inside-out morphological pattern may not express HER2.

defined by ISH analysis display low levels of HER2 protein expression as defined by this new technology and have reduced response to Trastuzumab-containing therapy (88). Those results need to be validated in larger cohorts but may provide partial explanation for heterogeneous response to anti-HER2 agents and are consistent with the views that measurements made at the protein level (ie, the actual target) may offer advantage over measurements at the DNA level. On the other hand, lately, much attention has been given to quantitative reverse transcriptase polymerase chain reaction (PCR) assays to determine HER2, as well as hormone receptors mRNA levels of expression (89,90). A high degree of concordance between qRT-PCR and IHC and/or fluorescent in situ hybridization (FISH) has been reported, and those assays provide the advantage of a continuous quantitative measurement; however, it should

be pointed out that, as they are not associated with morphological analysis, that applicability may be limited by tumor size, cellularity (eg, tumor sample contamination by normal cells), and composition (eg, DCIS and invasive components intimately admixed).

■ MARKERS BEYOND MINIMAL DATA SET

Ki67 Labeling Index

Tumor proliferation is a significant prognostic factor in breast cancer (91), and markers of proliferation were recommended as ancillary tools by the St Gallen International Expert Consensus for the selection of the appropriate systemic treatment (92). Mitotic index is a histological marker of tumor proliferation; although routinely performed as one of the components of Nottingham histological grade, it is affected by fixation artifacts and its analysis suffers from interobserver variability. Furthermore, it requires at least 10 high-power fields of invasive tumor. Ki67 immunohistochemical labeling index, which detects cycling cells (ie, cells in all cell cycle phases except G0), has been proposed as an alternative and perhaps a more reliable tool to assess proliferation in breast carcinomas (2).

It has been demonstrated that Ki67 labeling index correlates with mitotic activity and is significantly associated with the outcome of a patient with breast cancer (93). Indeed, it has been suggested that an equation including Ki67 and ER, PR, HER2, and/or histological variables may predict the OncotypeDx Recurrence Score (94,95). It should be emphasized, however, that several lines of evidence indicate that the impact of proliferation on outcome is restricted to ER-positive tumors (8,96).

Apart from being a prognostic marker, Ki67 labeling index also has potential as a predictor of response to treatment and distinct treatment modalities (2). There is evidence to suggest that tumors with high proliferation rates are more sensitive to chemotherapy, as several studies have demonstrated that high Ki67 levels are associated with higher frequencies of pathological complete response in the neoadjuvant setting (2,97). Of note, Ki67 labeling index measured in postneoadjuvant chemotherapy samples has also been shown to be an independent prognostic factor for those patients not achieving a pathological complete response (98). When addressing response to chemotherapy in the adjuvant setting, Viale et al (2,99), however, could not find a benefit from chemotherapy (CMF-based) over endocrine therapy alone in patients with high Ki67 levels. On the other hand, an independent group stated that Ki67 expression identifies a subset of patients with ER-positive tumors who could be sensitive to taxane-based chemotherapy as compared with anthracycline-based chemotherapy (100). With regard to endocrine treatment modality, a reanalysis of 2685 ER-positive samples of patients enrolled in a clinical trial comparing aromatase inhibitor letrozole versus tamoxifen revealed that high Ki67 levels may identity a subgroup of ER-positive patients who particularly benefits from initial letrozole adjuvant therapy (101).

Discrepancies in the predictive role of Ki67 may be explained by distinct treatment regimens, different end points in neoadjuvant versus adjuvant settings, different scoring systems, and different cutoffs for analysis of Ki67 IHC. In fact, there is no consensus on how Ki67 immunostaining should be evaluated and which cutoffs should be used to discrimininate low from high proliferation rates. In general, scoring systems are based in the percentage of cells stained by Ki67 antibody; however, it is not established whether one should estimate the percentage of

stained nuclei in "hot spots" or count several hundreds of nuclei in different areas of the tumor and give an overall average index (2). Estimation may be less reproducible and accurate, whereas manual counting is time consuming and labor intensive. Automated readers provide an alternative method for Ki67 scoring (102), but these systems have the disadvantage that stained nonmalignant nuclei may also be counted. Cutoffs to define low and high Ki67 levels ranged from 10% to 20% in most studies (2); however, it is unclear at this moment what the ideal cutoff should be and if one cutoff will be applicable to all clinical scenarios. Noteworthy, apart from MIB1 clone, other antibodies have been raised against the Ki67 protein, including SP6, which may better suit to automated image analysis (102).

In summary, the role of Ki67 labeling index as a prognostic marker is well established; however, there is no consensus for scoring systems and cutoffs to be used. Its prognostic power, however, may be limited to ER-positive tumors. It seems that Ki67 labeling index also has a potential role as a predictive marker of response to treatment, but retrospective analyses of clinical trials are still controversial. Once standardization of Ki67 evaluation and prospective analysis are achieved, it is likely that this marker will be included in the minimal data set for breast cancer. Guidelines for the assessment of Ki67 are eagerly awaited.

Topoisomerase IIα

Topoisomerase IIα, whose function is to separate the strands of the DNA double helical structure during processes such as transcription, recombination, and replication, is the direct molecular target of anthracyclines. Anthracyclines bind covalently with topoisomerase IIα after double-strand breaks have occurred, inducing lethal cellular damage by inhibition of relegation. Topoisomerase IIα is encoded by *TOP2A* gene, which maps to 17q12 near the *HER2* gene, is coamplified in 22% to 55% of *HER2*-amplified tumors, and its amplification seems to be limited to *HER2*-amplified tumors (103–105). Patients with HER2-positive tumors are reported to particularly benefit from anthracycline-based chemotherapy; however, based on the fact that topoisomerase IIα is the molecular target of anthracyclines, it has been hypothesized that *TOP2A* gene amplification and/or overexpression, rather than HER2-positive status itself, predict response to anthracycline-based chemotherapy. Most of the studies have focused on *TOP2A* gene status, and although data are still contradictory, there is evidence to suggest that patients harboring *TOP2A* amplification may have a greater benefit with anthracyclines-based therapies (103–105). Fewer studies have addressed the correlation between topoisomerase IIα expression as defined by IHC and *TOP2A* gene amplification and whether its overexpression could predict response to anthracycline-based chemotherapy. Conflicting results and conclusions in relation to both issues were described (105–109); however, the use of different antibodies (clones 3F6, Zymed; KiS1, M7186 Dako; NCL-TOPOIIA, Novocastra), technical methods, scoring systems, and cutoffs to determine over-expression render direct comparisons between the distinct studies challenging. Nevertheless, the available data suggest that topoisomerase IIα expression, albeit significantly correlated with *TOP2A* gene amplification in some studies, is more pervasive than *TOP2A* gene amplification and is strongly associated with proliferation, possibly limiting the use of topoisomerase IIα IHC as a specific predictive marker for anthracycline-based chemotherapy benefit.

Resistance to Anti-HER2 Therapy

As discussed above, *HER2* gene copy number assessment has high negative predictive value (ie, patients lacking *HER2* gene amplification are very unlikely to benefit from anti-HER2 agents); however, its positive predictive value is limited. In the last years, several mechanisms of de novo and acquired resistance to trastuzumab have been identified. It is currently accepted that *PIK3CA*-activating mutations, phosphatase and tensin homolog (PTEN) loss of function, IGF1R overexpression, or expression of p95 HER2 isoform may all play a role in both de novo or acquired resistance to therapies that target HER2 (83). Immunohistochemistry may assist in the assessment of some of these markers of resistance to anti-HER2 agents, such as PTEN (110), IGF1R (111), and p95 isoform. Despite the substantial interest in this topic, novel diagnostic molecular approaches for testing HER2-positive cancers to increase the positive predictive value of predictors of response to anti-HER2 agents are yet to be prospectively validated (Figure 10.5B). The emerging assay above-described using proximity-based technology (87) may provide increased predictive power but is technically more challenging than routine IHC.

Cyclooxygenase-2

Cyclooxygenase-2 (COX-2) is a molecule primarily involved in inflammatory reaction, mediates production of prostaglandins and thromboxane from arachidonic acid, and is a target of nonsteroidal anti-inflammatory drugs (112,113). There are several lines of evidence to suggest that inflammation plays a role in cancer development and progression through interaction with tumor microenvironment. Multiple studies have explored the relationship between COX-2 expression as assessed by IHC and clinical outcome in breast cancer. Lucci et al (113) described a strong association between COX-2 immunostaining in primary breast tumors and bone marrow metastasis, suggesting a potential role for COX-2 inhibitors in patients with breast cancer. It has also been recently suggested that a multivariable model combining p16, COX-2, and Ki67

may indicate risk of progression in patients with DCIS (114); those results, however, must be interpreted with caution as the study design has several limitations (115). Other groups failed to find a significant and independent association between COX-2 expression and outcome of patients with breast cancer (97,112). The impact of COX-2 increased expression may be restricted to patients with hormone receptor–positive tumors who did not receive endocrine therapy (112), precluding its use as a prognostic marker in the current daily practice.

Phosphatase and Tensin Homolog

PTEN is a tumor suppressor gene, whose germ-line mutations cause Cowden syndrome. This gene plays a pivotal role in the negative regulation of the PI3K/mTOR pathway and is often inactivated in several types of human malignancies (116), although *PTEN* somatic mutations appear to be relatively rare in breast cancers (117). Recent studies have demonstrated that PTEN loss of function also leads to lack of homologous recombination DNA repair defects (118) and could be used as a predictive marker of response to platinum salts and inhibitors of the poly(ADP-Ribose) polymerase (PARP) (119). Despite the great interest in PTEN expression and function in breast cancer, there is a paucity of reliable protocols for IHC analysis of this protein and IHC with several antibodies appearing not to correlate with *PTEN* mutations and gene status (120). A recent study provided a protocol based on the 6H2.1 monoclonal antibody, which seems to be reliable for the analysis of this tumor suppressor gene in formalin-fixed paraffin-embedded tissue sections (121); however, it remains to be independently validated.

■ MOLECULAR SUBTYPING

In the last decade, seminal studies by the Stanford group (9,10) have brought to the forefront of breast cancer research the molecular heterogeneity of breast tumors. These studies have demonstrated that breast cancer is not a single disease but rather a collection of diseases with distinct clinicopathological features and biological behavior that affect the same anatomical organ. Microarray-based gene expression analysis revealed that breast cancer can be classified according to their transcriptomes into at least 5 distinct molecular subtypes that have both biological and clinical significance. These include (i) 2 groups of luminal tumors (luminal A and luminal B), which are characterized by the expression of ER and ER-regulated genes and differ according to the expression of proliferation-related genes; (ii) normal-like subtype, which is poorly characterized and believed to be an artifact of gene expression profiling due to low tumor cell content in the samples

■ **Table 10.6** Immunohistochemical surrogate panel for molecular subtyping of breast cancer

Surrogate Panel	ER	PR	HER2	CK5/6	EGFR	Ki67	No.	Prevalence %
Criteria for positive result*	>1% of stained tumor nuclei	>1% of stained tumor nuclei	IHC 3+ or 2+ and FISH positive	Any cytoplasmic or membranous staining	Any cytoplasmic or membranous staining	≥14% of stained tumor nuclei		
Nielsen et al[16]							663	
Luminal	Positive	NI	Negative	Any	Any	NI		40
HER2	Any	NI	Positive	Any	Any	NI		23
Basal-like	Negative	NI	Negative	Either CK5/6 and/or EGFR positive		NI		15
ER-/HER2- nonbasal	Negative	NI	Negative	Negative	Negative	NI		22
Cheang et al[123]							3738	
Luminal	ER and/or PR positive		Negative	Any	Any	NI		70
Luminal HER2+	ER and/or PR positive		Positive	Any	Any	NI		6
HER2+/ER-/PR-	Any	Any	Positive					7
Basal-like	Negative	Negative	Negative	Either CK5/6 and/or EGFR positive		NI		9
Triple-negative nonbasal	Negative	Negative	Negative	Negative	Negative	NI		8
Carey et al[14]							496	
Luminal A	ER and/or PR positive		Negative	Any	Any	NI		51
Luminal B	ER and/or PR positive		Positive	Any	Any	NI		16
HER2	Negative	Negative	Positive	Any	Any	NI		7
Basal-like	Negative	Negative	Negative	Either CK5/6 and/or EGFR positive		NI		20
Triple-negative nonbasal	Negative	Negative	Negative	Negative	Negative	NI		6
Voduc et al[17]							1281	
Luminal A	ER and/or PR positive		Negative	Any	Any	Negative		46
Luminal B	ER and/or PR positive		Negative	Any	Any	Positive		23
Luminal HER2	ER and/or PR positive		Positive	Any	Any	Any		5

Continued

■ **Table 10.6** Immunohistochemical surrogate panel for molecular subtyping of breast cancer (*Continued*)

Surrogate Panel	ER	PR	HER2	CK5/6	EGFR	Ki67	No	Prevalence %
HER2-enriched	Negative	Negative	Positive	Any	Any	Any		70
Basal-like	Negative	Negative	Negative	Either CK5/6 and/or EGFR positive		Any		10
Triple-negative nonbasal	Negative	Negative	Negative	Negative	Negative	Any		9
Kennecke et al[15]							1357	
Luminal A	ER and/or PR positive		Negative	Any	Any	Negative		34
Luminal B	ER and/or PR positive		Negative	Any	Any	Positive		28
Luminal HER2	ER and/or PR positive		Positive	Any	Any	Any		8
HER2-enriched	Negative	Negative	Positive	Any	Any	Any		10
Basal-like	Negative	Negative	Negative	Either CK5/6 and/or EGFR positive		Any		12
Triple-negative nonbasal	Negative	Negative	Negative	Negative	Negative	Any		8
Blows et al[122]							10,159	
Luminal 1	ER and/or PR positive		Negative	Any	Any	NI		71
Luminal 2	ER and/or PR positive		Positive	Any	Any	NI		6
Nonluminal HER2+	Negative	Negative	Positive	Any	Any	NI		6
Basal-like	Negative	Negative	Negative	Either CK5/6 and/or EGFR positive		NI		9
Triple-negative nonbasal	Negative	Negative	Negative	Negative	Negative	NI		7

NI indicates not included in the panel.

*Criteria for positive results are valid for all references quoted in this table except Blows et al (meta-analysis).

subjected to analysis; (iii) HER2 tumors, which display overexpression of HER2 and of other genes mapping to the 17q12-q21 region of the genome; and (iv) basal-like cancers, which in general lack ER, PR, and HER2 expression but express a significant number of genes usually associated with normal breast basal/MEC cells (9,10,18). Importantly, this classification was shown to be significantly associated with prognosis; luminal A tumors have a good prognosis, whereas luminal B, HER2, and basal-like cancers display a poor outcome. Given this clinical significance, proponents of this classification advocated that molecular subtyping of breast cancer would be of use for clinical decision making (11).

Following those reports, not only has the research community embraced this molecular taxonomy as a working model, but clinicians also have attempted to incorporate it in their daily practice and in clinical trial design (18). Given the technical issues limiting microarray-based gene expression profiling to be performed in large scale in formalin-fixed, paraffin-embedded samples, immunohistochemical surrogate markers for the distinct molecular subtypes have been proposed (Table 10.6) (14–17,122,123). In fact, the clinical categories identified with the minimal data set above described (ie, ER+/HER2-, HER2+, ER-/HER2-) to some extent correlate with the main molecular subtypes identified by microarrays (ie, luminal, HER2, and basal-like) (8,18,19,96). However, 2 main questions have been consistently raised: (1) how to identify basal-like carcinomas and (2) how to distinguish luminal A from luminal B tumors.

Most basal-like carcinomas display a triple-negative phenotype (ie, ER-, PR-, and HER2-negative); however, these 2 terms should not be used interchangeably (124). A significant number of triple-negative cancers do not express basal markers, and a small, but still significant, subgroup of basal-like cancers express either hormone receptors or HER2. Bertucci et al (125) have addressed this issue directly and confirmed that not all triple-negative tumors when analyzed by gene expression profiling were classified as basal-like cancers (ie, only 71% were of basal-like phenotype), and not all basal-like breast carcinomas classified by expression arrays displayed a triple-negative phenotype (ie, 77% were of triple-negative phenotype). Taken together, these results are in accord with the concept that the triple-negative phenotype is not an ideal surrogate marker for basal-like breast cancers (124–126) (Figure 10.6).

Several studies have extensively characterized the basal-like subtype of breast cancer and provided a list of immunohistochemical markers for its identification, including CK5/6 (16,127), epidermal growth factor receptor (EGFR) (16,127), c-kit (16), vimentin (127), caveolin-1 (128), caveolin-2 (129), and nestin (130) (Figure 10.7). Nielsen et al (16) were among the first to describe an immunohistochemical surrogate panel validated against microarray-based gene expression data and able to robustly identify basal-like carcinomas with prognostic significance. This panel composed of ER, HER2, CK5/6, and EGFR was shown to identify basal-like tumors with a sensitivity of 76% and a specificity of 100%. Basal-like cancers were defined as ER-negative HER2-negative tumors with any neoplastic cell displaying weak or strong membranous and/or cytoplasmic CK5/6 and/or EGFR expression. Of note, further refinement of this panel by the same group (123) has demonstrated that expression of CK5/6 and/or EGFR in ER-, PR-, and HER2-negative cases identifies a subgroup of triple-negative cancers with a significantly worse outcome than patients with triple-negative carcinomas that are negative for basal markers, providing support to the view that effort should be done to identify basal-like carcinomas in clinical practice. In an independent study, Rakha et al (131) confirmed these observations, as it was demonstrated that triple-negative breast cancers that express basal keratins and/or EGFR have a worse outcome than triple-negative tumors that lack these markers.

EGFR and c-KIT have been shown to be "overexpressed" in a subgroup of triple-negative and basal-like breast cancers (Figure 10.7G-H); however, these cancers appear not to harbor recurrent activating mutations of these genes (77,78,132). Despite the initial interest in

these tyrosine kinases as potential targets for subgroups of triple-negative breast cancers, the initial results of clinical trials with anti-EGFR agents and imatinib mesylate were disappointing (77,78,132). Furthermore, detailed molecular analysis of these genes and pathways suggests that EGFR and c-KIT may not constitute ideal targets in triple-negative cancers, given (i) the lack of EGFR- and KIT-activating gene mutations and the rarity of EGFR gene amplification (133,134), which have been associated with response to agents targeting these tyrosine kinases (77,78,132), and (ii) the frequent loss of expression of PTEN in triple-negative cancers (ie, a negative predictor of response to some tyrosine kinase inhibitors) (135).

Despite the interest in basal-like breast cancers, at the moment, a diagnosis of basal-like breast cancer does not carry any clinical implication, as the expression of basal keratins and EGFR does not alter the therapy of patients with triple-negative breast cancer. The association between BRCA1 germ-line mutations and expression of CK5/6 and CK14(136) also holds true for BRCA1 germ-line mutations and triple-negative phenotype (137). Furthermore, from a biological perspective, the term basal-like is a misnomer, given that these tumors have now been shown to originate from ER-negative luminal progenitor cells rather than basal cells (138,139). Therefore, at this stage, we would not advocate the use of the term basal-like in pathology reports.

Although the panel above robustly identifies basal-like carcinomas, it does not discriminate luminal A from luminal B tumors, which are associated with significantly different outcomes. To address this shortcoming, Carey et al (14) proposed a panel to distinguish luminal A from luminal B cancers based on the expression of HER2. ER-positive HER2-negative tumors were classified as luminal A, whereas ER-positive HER2-positive tumors were considered luminal B. Only HER2-positive ER-negative tumors were classified as of HER2 subtype. Although this definition can be easily applied and does not require additional markers, it is perhaps not sensitive enough for the identification of the luminal B subgroup, which overexpress HER2 in only 30% to 50% of the cases, and also not specific enough for the luminal A subtype, as ER-positive tumors with high proliferation rates will be misclassified as of luminal A. In fact, in the study of Carey et al (14), no significant differences in outcome were detected between luminal A and luminal B tumors using this definition.

More recently, effort has been done to stratify luminal tumors not only based on HER2 expression but also according to proliferation rates, including Ki67 to the panel composed of ER, PR, HER2, CK5/6, and EGFR (15,17). Using a cutoff of 14% for Ki67 labeling index, ER-positive HER2-negative tumors were classified as luminal A (<14%) or B (≥4%). In total, 6 molecular subtype categories were defined (Table 10.6). Applying this surrogate panel to a

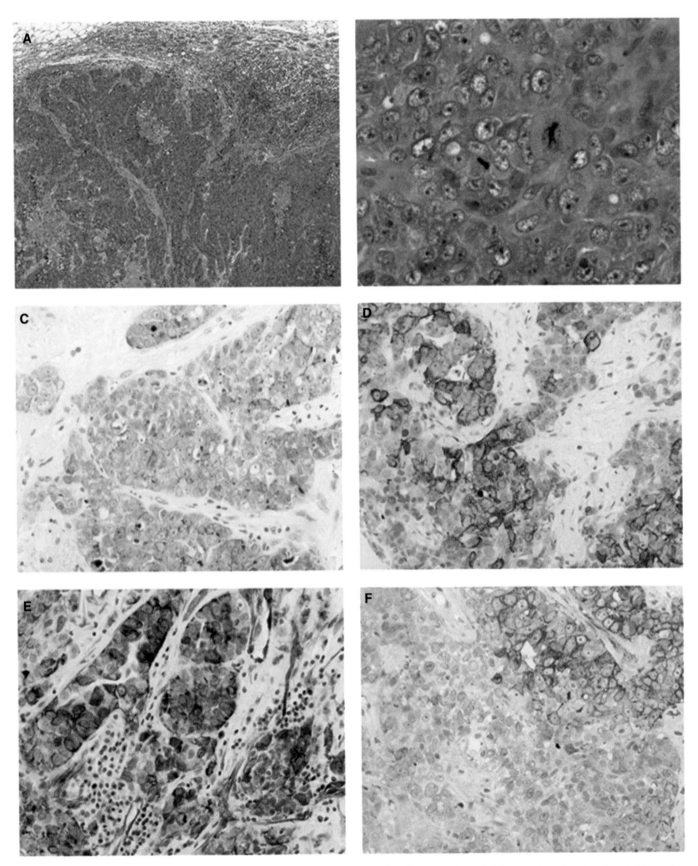

FIGURE 10.7 Basal-like markers. A high-grade invasive breast carcinoma with cells arranged in solid sheets with pushing borders, brisk lymphocytic infiltrate (A), conspicuous pleomorphism, and high mitotic activity (B) displaying positivity for CK5/6 (C), CK14 (D), nestin (E), caveolin-1 (F).

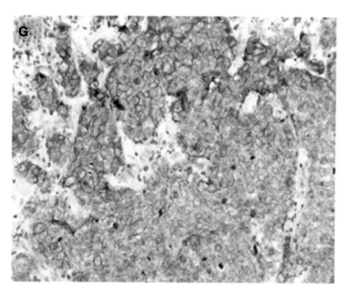
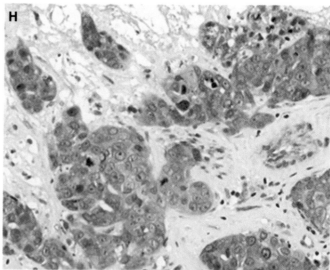

FIGURE 10.7   Basal-like markers. A high-grade invasive breast carcinoma displaying positivity for EGFR (G), and c-kit (H).

large series of archival breast cancer samples, Voduc et al (17) and Kenennecke et al (15) have, respectively, confirmed that the luminal A subtype is associated with a better outcome with a low risk of local or regional recurrence and that the molecular subtypes of breast cancer have distinct patterns of metastatic behavior.

It should be emphasised that there are several lines of evidence to suggest that the allocation of ER-positive tumors into the luminal A or B subtypes might be arbitrary. Meta-analyses of gene expression data including more than 2100 samples have shown that only 3 subgroups of breast cancer can be robustly identified: (1) ER+/HER2−, (2) HER2+, and (3) ER−/HER− (8,96). Proliferation was indeed the strongest parameter predicting clinical outcome in the former subgroup; however, proliferation rates in ER+/HER2− tumors formed a continuum rather than 2 separate clusters. Furthermore, Ki67-labeling indices also form a continuum in ER+/HER2− cancers. Therefore, the distinction between luminal A and B cancers based on proliferation may be arbitrary, as no natural cutoffs appear to exist.

Furthermore, several other considerations must be made before the introduction of this molecular taxonomy in clinical practice for clinical decision making (12,13,18,140). Recently, Weigelt et al (12) by performing a retrospective analysis of gene expression data compared the distinct methods for single sample prediction previously published by the proponents of the molecular classification and raised concern on the stability of the methods for the identification of molecular subtypes other than basal-like breast cancers. The authors demonstrated that different single sample predictors do not reliably assign the same patients to the same molecular subtype, except for the basal-like subtype. Because the assignment of a tumor using criterion standard methodologies (ie,

microarray gene expression data) is still not fully standardized and has only modest levels of reproducibility, caution needs to be exercised when using immunohistochemical surrogates for subgroups whose microarray definitions are still unclear.

The lack of stability of this molecular taxonomy is also emphasized by the fact that a recently developed qRT-PCR based assay (ie, PAM50) for classification of archival samples into the molecular subtypes aimed to be clinically applicable does not assign all HER2-positive cases (as ascertained by IHC and FISH) into the HER2 subtype (12,141,142). Conversely, not all cases classified as HER2 subtype by gene expression profiling display HER2 overexpression and/or *HER2* gene amplification. Given that patients with HER2-positive tumors are eligible for HER2-targeted treatment, such a misclassification calls into question the potential role of this molecular taxonomy to define treatment for patients with breast cancer.

Although the identification of the basal-like subtype seems to be reproducible and can be achieved with relative accuracy using immunohistochemical surrogates, there is not yet any international consensus about how this subtype should be defined by IHC. In addition, no targeted therapy is currently available for this subset of patients, thus limiting the impact of the identification of this subtype in daily practice. There is evidence to suggest that basal-like tumors may be more sensitive to platinum-salts and PARP inhibitors, but the biological mechanism underlying this responsiveness seems to be the homologous recombination DNA repair defect frequently found in those cancers and intrinsically associated with BRCA1 pathway down-regulation (143,144). Therefore, it is likely that testing biomarkers that indicate the capacity of tumor cells to elicit homologous recombination DNA repair in the presence of double-strand breaks (eg, RAD51 foci formation (145)) may better predict response to those agents and be introduced in clinical practice (146). BRCA1 IHC analysis may not constitute an ideal predictor for the use of these agents, given (i) the cross-reactivity of antibodies with other ring finger proteins (147,148), (ii) the lack of a strict correlation between BRCA1 IHC results and *BRCA1* gene status (149), and (iii) the fact that alterations of genes other than *BRCA1* (eg, *PTEN*) may also constitute markers of sensitivity to platinum salts and PARP inhibitors (119).

In summary, despite the considerable progress in our understanding of the biology of breast cancer and its molecular heterogeneity, it is perhaps still premature to recommend its routine use. Incorporation of immunohistochemical markers beyond the minimal data set aiming to assign invasive breast tumors into the microarray-defined molecular subtypes may not be justified at this stage.

■ KEY POINTS

- Advantages of IHC: low cost, optimal for archival material, allows morphological analysis ensuring only neoplastic cells are scored.
- Disadvantages of IHC: not quantitative, influenced by preanalytical parameters, subjected to technical variability, suboptimal interobserver and interlaboratory reproducibility.
- Validation, standardization, and participation to quality assurance programs are mandatory when using IHC for the diagnosis/management of breast lesions.
- Hormone receptors and CK5/6 are useful for distinguishing HUT from ADH/low-grade DCIS.
- P63, calponin, and SMM-HC are currently the MEC markers with better sensitivity and specificity; the use of a combination of at least 2 markers is recommended in a diagnostic setting, when MECs need to be identified.
- The use of E-cadherin and β-catenin immunostaining for distinction between lobular and ductal neoplasia should be limited to few situations and is not recommended in lesions with typical lobular morphology.
- In spindle cell lesions, the diagnosis of metaplastic carcinoma must be ruled out morphologically or by an immunohistochemical panel with CKs and p63.
- Guideline recommendations for ER, PR, and HER2 assessment are available and must be followed to improve accuracy and interlaboratory reproducibility.
- Minimal data set (ER, PR, and HER2) identify 3 subtypes of breast cancers with distinct clinicopathological features, biological behaviour, and response to

treatment: (i) ER+/HER–, (ii) HER2+, and (iii) ER–/HER2–.
- Assessment of proliferation using Ki67 IHC might provide valuable additional information, but standardization of methodologies and cutoff is still required.

■ CONCLUSION

In conclusion, IHC is one of the most valuable techniques to be used in breast pathology, either for assisting histological diagnosis or providing prognostic and predictive markers that guide the oncologist in breast cancer patient management. It has advantages of low cost, ready application to archival samples, and morphological analysis and is a broadly available technique; however, standardization of preanalytical and analytical technical aspects, interpretation, and scoring systems is strictly necessary. Accuracy of IHC results, in particular in relation to ER, PR, and HER2, must be a top priority in all pathology laboratories. In addition to their predictive role, these markers delineate 3 molecular subtypes of breast cancer that have distinct clinicopathological features, important differences in their biological behavior, and distinct repertoires of systemic therapies.

■ REFERENCES

1. Moriya T, Kozuka Y, Kanomata N, Tse GM, Tan PH. The role of immunohistochemistry in the differential diagnosis of breast lesions. *Pathology*. 2009;41:68–76.
2. Yerushalmi R, Woods R, Ravdin PM, Hayes MM, Gelmon KA. Ki67 in breast cancer: prognostic and predictive potential. *Lancet Oncol*. 2010;11:174–183.
3. Allred DC, Carlson RW, Berry DA, et al. NCCN Task Force Report: estrogen receptor and progesterone receptor testing in breast cancer by immunohistochemistry. *J Natl Compr Canc Netw*. 2009;7(suppl 6):S1-S21;quiz S22–S23.
4. Carlson RW, Moench SJ, Hammond ME, et al. HER2 testing in breast cancer: NCCN Task Force report and recommendations. *J Natl Compr Canc Netw*. 2006;4(suppl 3):S1-22;quiz S23–S24.
5. Hammond ME, Hayes DF, Dowsett M, et al. American Society of Clinical Oncology/College Of American Pathologists guideline recommendations for immunohistochemical testing of estrogen and progesterone receptors in breast cancer. *J Clin Oncol*. 2010;28:2784–2795.
6. Wolff AC, Hammond ME, Schwartz JN, et al. American Society of Clinical Oncology/College of American Pathologists guideline recommendations for human epidermal growth factor receptor 2 testing in breast cancer. *J Clin Oncol*. 2007;25:118–145.
7. Shiu KK, Natrajan R, Geyer FC, Ashworth A, Reis-Filho JS. DNA amplifications in breast cancer: genotypic-phenotypic correlations. *Future Oncol*. 2010;6:967–984.

8. Wirapati P, Sotiriou C, Kunkel S, et al. Meta-analysis of gene expression profiles in breast cancer: toward a unified understanding of breast cancer subtyping and prognosis signatures. *Breast Cancer Res.* 2008;10:R65.

9. Perou CM, Sorlie T, Eisen MB, et al. Molecular portraits of human breast tumours. *Nature.* 2000;406:747–752.

10. Sorlie T, Perou CM, Tibshirani R, et al. Gene expression patterns of breast carcinomas distinguish tumor subclasses with clinical implications. *Proc Natl Acad Sci U S A.* 2001;98:10869–10874.

11. Sorlie T. Introducing molecular subtyping of breast cancer into the clinic? *J Clin Oncol.* 2009;27:1153–1154.

12. Weigelt B, Mackay A, A'Hern R, et al. Breast cancer molecular profiling with single sample predictors: a retrospective analysis. *Lancet Oncol.* 2010;11:339–349.

13. Lusa L, McShane LM, Reid JF, et al. Challenges in projecting clustering results across gene expression-profiling datasets. *J Natl Cancer Inst.* 2007;99:1715–1723.

14. Carey LA, Perou CM, Livasy CA, et al. Race, breast cancer subtypes, and survival in the Carolina Breast Cancer Study. *JAMA.* 2006;295:2492–2502.

15. Kennecke H, Yerushalmi R, Woods R, et al. Metastatic behavior of breast cancer subtypes. *J Clin Oncol.* 2010;28:3271–3277.

16. Nielsen TO, Hsu FD, Jensen K, et al. Immunohistochemical and clinical characterization of the basal-like subtype of invasive breast carcinoma. *Clin Cancer Res.* 2004;10: 5367–5374.

17. Voduc KD, Cheang MC, Tyldesley S, Gelmon K, Nielsen TO, Kennecke H. Breast cancer subtypes and the risk of local and regional relapse. *J Clin Oncol.* 2010;28: 1684–1691.

18. Weigelt B, Baehner FL, Reis-Filho JS. The contribution of gene expression profiling to breast cancer classification, prognostication and prediction: a retrospective of the last decade. *J Pathol.* 2010;220:263–280.

19. Sotiriou C, Pusztai L. Gene-expression signatures in breast cancer. *N Engl J Med.* 2009;360:790–800.

20. Lopez-Garcia MA, Geyer FC, Lacroix-Triki M, Marchio C, Reis-Filho JS. Breast cancer precursors revisited: molecular features and progression pathways. *Histopathology.* 2010;57:171–192.

21. Boecker W, Moll R, Dervan P, et al. Usual ductal hyperplasia of the breast is a committed stem (progenitor) cell lesion distinct from atypical ductal hyperplasia and ductal carcinoma in situ. *J Pathol.* 2002;198:458–467.

22. Grin A, O'Malley FP, Mulligan AM. Cytokeratin 5 and estrogen receptor immunohistochemistry as a useful adjunct in identifying atypical papillary lesions on breast needle core biopsy. *Am J Surg Pathol.* 2009;33:1615–1623.

23. Werling RW, Hwang H, Yaziji H, Gown AM. Immunohistochemical distinction of invasive from noninvasive breast lesions: a comparative study of p63 versus calponin and smooth muscle myosin heavy chain. *Am J Surg Pathol.* 2003;27:82–90.

24. Kalof AN, Tam D, Beatty B, Cooper K. Immunostaining patterns of myoepithelial cells in breast lesions: a comparison of CD10 and smooth muscle myosin heavy chain. *J Clin Pathol.* 2004;57:625–629.

25. Reis-Filho JS, Milanezi F, Silva P, Schmitt FC. Maspin expression in myoepithelial tumors of the breast. *Pathol Res Pract.* 2001;197:817–821.

26. Popnikolov NK, Cavone SM, Schultz PM, Garcia FU. Diagnostic utility of p75 neurotrophin receptor (p75NTR) as a marker of breast myoepithelial cells. *Mod Pathol.* 2005;18:1535–1541.

27. Reis-Filho JS, Steele D, Di Palma S, et al. Distribution and significance of nerve growth factor receptor (NGFR/p75NTR) in normal, benign and malignant breast tissue. *Mod Pathol.* 2006;19:307–319.

28. Barbareschi M, Pecciarini L, Cangi MG, et al. p63, a p53 homologue, is a selective nuclear marker of myoepithelial cells of the human breast. *Am J Surg Pathol.* 2001;25:1054–1060.

29. Dabbs DJ, Gown AM. Distribution of calponin and smooth muscle myosin heavy chain in fine-needle aspiration biopsies of the breast. *Diagn Cytopathol.* 1999;20:203–207.

30. Reis-Filho JS, Milanezi F, Amendoeira I, Albergaria A, Schmitt FC. Distribution of p63, a novel myoepithelial marker, in fine-needle aspiration biopsies of the breast: an analysis of 82 samples. *Cancer.* 2003;99:172–179.

31. Hilson JB, Schnitt SJ, Collins LC. Phenotypic alterations in ductal carcinoma in situ-associated myoepithelial cells: biologic and diagnostic implications. *Am J Surg Pathol.* 2009;33:227–232.

32. Hilson JB, Schnitt SJ, Collins LC. Phenotypic alterations in myoepithelial cells associated with benign sclerosing lesions of the breast. *Am J Surg Pathol.* 2010;34:896–900.

33. Hu M, Yao J, Carroll DK, et al. Regulation of in situ to invasive breast carcinoma transition. *Cancer Cell.* 2008;13:394–406.

34. Da Silva L, Parry S, Reid L, et al. Aberrant expression of E-cadherin in lobular carcinomas of the breast. *Am J Surg Pathol.* 2008;32:773–783.

35. Cleton-Jansen AM. E-cadherin and loss of heterozygosity at chromosome 16 in breast carcinogenesis: different genetic pathways in ductal and lobular breast cancer? *Breast Cancer Res.* 2002;4:5–8.

36. Vos CB, Cleton-Jansen AM, Berx G, et al. E-cadherin inactivation in lobular carcinoma in situ of the breast: an early event in tumorigenesis. *Br J Cancer.* 1997;76:1131–1133.

37. Sarrio D, Moreno-Bueno G, Hardisson D, et al. Epigenetic and genetic alterations of APC and CDH1 genes in lobular breast cancer: relationships with abnormal E-cadherin and catenin expression and microsatellite instability. *Int J Cancer.* 2003;106:208–215.

38. Droufakou S, Deshmane V, Roylance R, Hanby A, Tomlinson I, Hart IR. Multiple ways of silencing E-cadherin gene expression in lobular carcinoma of the breast. *Int J Cancer.* 2001;92:404–408.

39. Jacobs TW, Pliss N, Kouria G, Schnitt SJ. Carcinomas in situ of the breast with indeterminate features: role of E-cadherin staining in categorization. *Am J Surg Pathol.* 2001;25:229–236.

40. Acs G, Lawton TJ, Rebbeck TR, LiVolsi VA, Zhang PJ. Differential expression of E-cadherin in lobular and ductal neoplasms of the breast and its biologic and diagnostic implications. *Am J Clin Pathol.* 2001;115:85–98.

41. Behrens J. The role of cell adhesion molecules in cancer invasion and metastasis. *Breast Cancer Res Treat.* 1993;24:175–184.

42. Derksen PW, Liu X, Saridin F, et al. Somatic inactivation of E-cadherin and p53 in mice leads to metastatic lobular mammary carcinoma through induction of anoikis resistance and angiogenesis. *Cancer Cell.* 2006;10:437–449.

43. Sarrio D, Perez-Mies B, Hardisson D, et al. Cytoplasmic localization of p120ctn and E-cadherin loss characterize lobular breast carcinoma from preinvasive to metastatic lesions. *Oncogene.* 2004;23:3272–3283.

44. Moll R, Mitze M, Frixen UH, Birchmeier W. Differential loss of E-cadherin expression in infiltrating ductal and lobular breast carcinomas. *Am J Pathol.* 1993;143:1731–1742.

45. De Leeuw WJ, Berx G, Vos CB, et al. Simultaneous loss of E-cadherin and catenins in invasive lobular breast cancer and lobular carcinoma in situ. *J Pathol.* 1997;183:404–411.

46. Maluf HM, Swanson PE, Koerner FC. Solid low-grade in situ carcinoma of the breast: role of associated lesions and E-cadherin in differential diagnosis. *Am J Surg Pathol.* 2001;25:237–244.

47. Dabbs DJ, Bhargava R, Chivukula M. Lobular versus ductal breast neoplasms: the diagnostic utility of p120 catenin. *Am J Surg Pathol.* 2007;31:427–437.

48. Geyer FC, Lacroix-Triki M, Savage K, et al. Beta-catenin pathway activation in breast cancer is associated with triple negative phenotype but not with CTNNB1 mutation. *Mod Pathol.* 2011;24:209–231.

49. Harigopal M, Shin SJ, Murray MP, Tickoo SK, Brogi E, Rosen PP. Aberrant E-cadherin staining patterns in invasive mammary carcinoma. *World J Surg Oncol.* 2005;3:73.

50. Mastracci TL, Tjan S, Bane AL, O'Malley FP, Andrulis IL. E-cadherin alterations in atypical lobular hyperplasia and lobular carcinoma in situ of the breast. *Mod Pathol.* 2005;18:741–751.

51. Reis-Filho JS, Simpson PT, Jones C, et al. Pleomorphic lobular carcinoma of the breast: role of comprehensive molecular pathology in characterization of an entity. *J Pathol.* 2005;207:1–13.

52. Simpson P, Reis-Filho J, Lambros M, et al. Molecular profiling pleomorphic lobular carcinomas of the breast: evidence for a common molecular genetic pathway with classic lobular carcinomas. *J Pathol.* 2008;215:231–244.

53. Mahler-Araujo B, Savage K, Parry S, Reis-Filho JS. Reduction of E-cadherin expression is associated with non-lobular breast carcinomas of basal-like and triple negative phenotype. *J Clin Pathol.* 2008;61:615–620.

54. Kashiwagi S, Yashiro M, Takashima T, et al. Significance of E-cadherin expression in triple-negative breast cancer. *Br J Cancer.* 2010;103:249–255.

55. Esposito NN, Chivukula M, Dabbs DJ. The ductal phenotypic expression of the E-cadherin/catenin complex in tubulolobular carcinoma of the breast: an immunohistochemical and clinicopathologic study. *Mod Pathol.* 2007;20:130–138.

56. Kuroda H, Tamaru J, Takeuchi I, et al. Expression of E-cadherin, alpha-catenin, and beta-catenin in tubulolobular carcinoma of the breast. *Virchows Arch.* 2006;448:500–505.

57. Wheeler DT, Tai LH, Bratthauer GL, Waldner DL, Tavassoli FA. Tubulolobular carcinoma of the breast: an analysis of 27 cases of a tumor with a hybrid morphology and immunoprofile. *Am J Surg Pathol.* 2004;28:1587–1593.

58. Lee AH. Recent developments in the histological diagnosis of spindle cell carcinoma, fibromatosis and phyllodes tumour of the breast. *Histopathology.* 2008;52:45–57.

59. Tse GM, Tan PH, Lui PC, Putti TC. Spindle cell lesions of the breast—the pathologic differential diagnosis. *Breast Cancer Res Treat.* 2008;109:199–207.

60. Gobbi H, Tse G, Page DL, Olson SJ, Jensen RA, Simpson JF. Reactive spindle cell nodules of the breast after core biopsy or fine-needle aspiration. *Am J Clin Pathol.* 2000;113:288–294.

61. Magro G, Michal M, Bisceglia M. Benign spindle cell tumors of the mammary stroma: diagnostic criteria, classification, and histogenesis. *Pathol Res Pract.* 2001;197:453–466.

62. Sneige N, Yaziji H, Mandavilli SR, et al. Low-grade (fibromatosis-like) spindle cell carcinoma of the breast. *Am J Surg Pathol.* 2001;25:1009–1016.

63. Gobbi H, Simpson JF, Borowsky A, Jensen RA, Page DL. Metaplastic breast tumors with a dominant fibromatosis-like phenotype have a high risk of local recurrence. *Cancer.* 1999;85:2170–2182.

64. Carter MR, Hornick JL, Lester S, Fletcher CD. Spindle cell (sarcomatoid) carcinoma of the breast: a clinicopathologic and immunohistochemical analysis of 29 cases. *Am J Surg Pathol.* 2006;30:300–309.

65. Koker MM, Kleer CG. p63 expression in breast cancer: a highly sensitive and specific marker of metaplastic carcinoma. *Am J Surg Pathol.* 2004;28:1506–1512.

66. Tse GM, Tan PH, Chaiwun B, et al. p63 is useful in the diagnosis of mammary metaplastic carcinomas. *Pathology.* 2006;38:16–20.

67. Leibl S, Gogg-Kammerer M, Sommersacher A, Denk H, Moinfar F. Metaplastic breast carcinomas: are they of myoepithelial differentiation?: immunohistochemical profile of the sarcomatoid subtype using novel myoepithelial markers. *Am J Surg Pathol.* 2005;29:347–353.

68. Buza N, Zekry N, Charpin C, Tavassoli FA. Myoepithelial carcinoma of the breast: a clinicopathological and immunohistochemical study of 15 diagnostically challenging cases. *Virchows Arch.* 2010;457:337–345.

69. Abraham SC, Reynolds C, Lee JH, et al. Fibromatosis of the breast and mutations involving the APC/beta-catenin pathway. *Hum Pathol.* 2002;33:39–46.

70. Lacroix-Triki M, Geyer FC, Lambros MB, et al. Beta-catenin/Wnt signalling pathway in fibromatosis, metaplastic carcinomas and phyllodes tumours of the breast. *Mod Pathol.* 2010;23:1438–1448.

71. Sawyer EJ, Hanby AM, Rowan AJ, et al. The Wnt pathway, epithelial-stromal interactions, and malignant progression in phyllodes tumours. *J Pathol.* 2002;196:437–444.

72. Magro G, Bisceglia M, Michal M, Eusebi V. Spindle cell lipoma-like tumor, solitary fibrous tumor and myofibroblastoma of the breast: a clinico-pathological analysis of 13 cases in favor of a unifying histogenetic concept. *Virchows Arch.* 2002;440:249–260.

73. Fitzgibbons PL, Murphy DA, Hammond ME, Allred DC, Valenstein PN. Recommendations for validating estrogen and progesterone receptor immunohistochemistry assays. *Arch Pathol Lab Med.* 2010;134:930–935.

74. Harvey JM, Clark GM, Osborne CK, Allred DC. Estrogen receptor status by immunohistochemistry is superior to the ligand-binding assay for predicting response to adjuvant endocrine therapy in breast cancer. *J Clin Oncol.* 1999;17:1474–1481.

75. Elledge RM, Green S, Pugh R, et al. Estrogen receptor (ER) and progesterone receptor (PgR), by ligand-binding assay compared with ER, PgR and pS2, by immuno-histochemistry in predicting response to tamoxifen in metastatic breast

cancer: a Southwest Oncology Group Study. *Int J Cancer.* 2000;89:111–117.

76. Reis-Filho JS, Milanezi F, Steele D, et al. Metaplastic breast carcinomas are basal-like tumours. *Histopathology.* 2006;49:10–21.

77. Reis-Filho JS, Tutt AN. Triple negative tumours: a critical review. *Histopathology.* 2008;52:108–118.

78. Rakha EA, Reis-Filho JS, Ellis IO. Basal-like breast cancer: a critical review. *J Clin Oncol.* 2008;26:2568–2581.

79. Viale G, Regan MM, Maiorano E, et al. Prognostic and predictive value of centrally reviewed expression of estrogen and progesterone receptors in a randomized trial comparing letrozole and tamoxifen adjuvant therapy for postmenopausal early breast cancer: BIG 1-98. *J Clin Oncol.* 2007;25:3846–3852.

80. Dowsett M, Cuzick J, Wale C, Howell T, Houghton J, Baum M. Retrospective analysis of time to recurrence in the ATAC trial according to hormone receptor status: an hypothesis-generating study. *J Clin Oncol.* 2005;23:7512–7517.

81. Yaziji H, Goldstein LC, Barry TS, et al. HER-2 testing in breast cancer using parallel tissue-based methods. *JAMA.* 2004;291: 1972–1977.

82. Romond EH, Perez EA, Bryant J, et al. Trastuzumab plus adjuvant chemotherapy for operable HER2-positive breast cancer. *N Engl J Med.* 2005;353:1673–1684.

83. Esteva FJ, Yu D, Hung MC, Hortobagyi GN. Molecular predictors of response to trastuzumab and lapatinib in breast cancer. *Nat Rev Clin Oncol.* 2010;7:98–107.

84. Gong Y, Sweet W, Duh YJ, et al. Performance of chromogenic in situ hybridization on testing HER2 Status in breast carcinomas with chromosome 17 polysomy and equivocal (2+) herceptest results: a study of two institutions using the conventional and new ASCO/CAP scoring criteria. *Am J Clin Pathol.* 2009;132:228–236.

85. Shah SS, Ketterling RP, Goetz MP, et al. Impact of American Society of Clinical Oncology/College of American Pathologists guideline recommendations on HER2 interpretation in breast cancer. *Hum Pathol.* 2010;41:103–106.

86. Chibon F, de Mascarel I, Sierankowski G, et al. Prediction of HER2 gene status in Her2 2+ invasive breast cancer: a study of 108 cases comparing ASCO/CAP and FDA recommendations. *Mod Pathol.* 2009;22:403–409.

87. Shi Y, Huang W, Tan Y, et al. A novel proximity assay for the detection of proteins and protein complexes: quantitation of HER1 and HER2 total protein expression and homodimerization in formalin-fixed, paraffin-embedded cell lines and breast cancer tissue. *Diagn Mol Pathol.* 2009;18:11–21.

88. Lipton A, Kostler WJ, Leitzel K, et al. Quantitative HER2 protein levels predict outcome in fluorescence in situ hybridization-positive patients with metastatic breast cancer treated with trastuzumab. *Cancer.* 2010;116:5168–5178.

89. Badve SS, Baehner FL, Gray RP, et al. Estrogen- and progesterone-receptor status in ECOG 2197: comparison of immunohistochemistry by local and central laboratories and quantitative reverse transcription polymerase chain reaction by central laboratory. *J Clin Oncol.* 2008;26: 2473–2481.

90. Baehner FL, Achacoso N, Maddala T, et al. Human epidermal growth factor receptor 2 assessment in a case-control study: Comparison of fluorescence in situ hybridization

and quantitative reverse transcription polymerase chain reaction performed by central laboratories. *J Clin Oncol.* 2010;28:4300–4306.

91. Desmedt C, Sotiriou C. Proliferation: the most prominent predictor of clinical outcome in breast cancer. *Cell Cycle.* 2006;5:2198–2202.

92. Goldhirsch A, Ingle JN, Gelber RD, Coates AS, Thurlimann B, Senn HJ. Thresholds for therapies: highlights of the St Gallen International Expert Consensus on the primary therapy of early breast cancer 2009. *Ann Oncol.* 2009;20:1319–1329.

93. de Azambuja E, Cardoso F, de Castro G Jr, et al. Ki-67 as prognostic marker in early breast cancer: a meta-analysis of published studies involving 12,155 patients. *Br J Cancer.* 2007;96:1504–1513.

94. Cuzick J. Prognostic value of a combined ER, PgR, Ki67, HER2 immunohistochemical (IHC4) score and comparison with the GHI recurrence score—results from TransATAC. *Cancer Res.* 2009;69:74.

95. Flanagan MB, Dabbs DJ, Brufsky AM, Beriwal S, Bhargava R. Histopathologic variables predict Oncotype DX recurrence score. *Mod Pathol.* 2008;21:1255–1261.

96. Desmedt C, Haibe-Kains B, Wirapati P, et al. Biological processes associated with breast cancer clinical outcome depend on the molecular subtypes. *Clin Cancer Res.* 2008;14:5158–5165.

97. Penault-Llorca F, Abrial C, Raoelfils I, et al. Changes and predictive and prognostic value of the mitotic index, Ki-67, cyclin D1, and cyclo-oxygenase-2 in 710 operable breast cancer patients treated with neoadjuvant chemotherapy. *Oncologist.* 2008;13:1235–1245.

98. Jones RL, Salter J, A'Hern R, et al. The prognostic significance of Ki67 before and after neoadjuvant chemotherapy in breast cancer. *Breast Cancer Res Treat.* 2009;116:53–68.

99. Viale G, Regan MM, Mastropasqua MG, et al. Predictive value of tumor Ki-67 expression in two randomized trials of adjuvant chemoendocrine therapy for node-negative breast cancer. *J Natl Cancer Inst.* 2008;100:207–212.

100. Penault-Llorca F, Andre F, Sagan C, et al. Ki67 expression and docetaxel efficacy in patients with estrogen receptor-positive breast cancer. *J Clin Oncol.* 2009;27:2809–2815.

101. Viale G, Giobbie-Hurder A, Regan MM, et al. Prognostic and predictive value of centrally reviewed Ki-67 labeling index in postmenopausal women with endocrine-responsive breast cancer: results from Breast International Group Trial 1-98 comparing adjuvant tamoxifen with letrozole. *J Clin Oncol.* 2008;26:5569–5575.

102. Zabaglo L, Salter J, Anderson H, et al. Comparative validation of the SP6 antibody to Ki67 in breast cancer. *J Clin Pathol.* 2010;63:800–804.

103. Slamon DJ, Press MF. Alterations in the TOP2A and HER2 genes: association with adjuvant anthracycline sensitivity in human breast cancers. *J Natl Cancer Inst.* 2009;101:615–618.

104. Konecny GE, Pauletti G, Untch M, et al. Association between HER2, TOP2A, and response to anthracycline-based preoperative chemotherapy in high-risk primary breast cancer. *Breast Cancer Res Treat.* 2010;120:481–489.

105. Arriola E, Rodriguez-Pinilla SM, Lambros MB, et al. Topoisomerase II alpha amplification may predict benefit from adjuvant anthracyclines in HER2 positive early breast cancer. *Breast Cancer Res Treat.* 2007;106:181–189.

106. Bhargava R, Lal P, Chen B. HER-2/neu and topoisomerase IIa gene amplification and protein expression in invasive breast carcinomas: chromogenic in situ hybridization and immunohistochemical analyses. *Am J Clin Pathol.* 2005;123:889–895.

107. Coon JS, Marcus E, Gupta-Burt S, et al. Amplification and overexpression of topoisomerase IIalpha predict response to anthracycline-based therapy in locally advanced breast cancer. *Clin Cancer Res.* 2002;8:1061–1067.

108. Mueller RE, Parkes RK, Andrulis I, O'Malley FP. Amplification of the TOP2A gene does not predict high levels of topoisomerase II alpha protein in human breast tumor samples. *Genes Chromosomes Cancer.* 2004;39:288–297.

109. Schindlbeck C, Mayr D, Olivier C, et al. Topoisomerase IIalpha expression rather than gene amplification predicts responsiveness of adjuvant anthracycline-based chemotherapy in women with primary breast cancer. *J Cancer Res Clin Oncol.* 2010;136:1029–1037.

110. Nagata Y, Lan KH, Zhou X, et al. PTEN activation contributes to tumor inhibition by trastuzumab, and loss of PTEN predicts trastuzumab resistance in patients. *Cancer Cell.* 2004;6:117–127.

111. Harris LN, You F, Schnitt SJ, et al. Predictors of resistance to preoperative trastuzumab and vinorelbine for HER2-positive early breast cancer. *Clin Cancer Res.* 2007;13:1198–1207.

112. van Nes JG, de Kruijf EM, Faratian D, et al. COX2 expression in prognosis and in prediction to endocrine therapy in early breast cancer patients. *Breast Cancer Res Treat.* 2011;125:671–685.

113. Lucci A, Krishnamurthy S, Singh B, et al. Cyclooxygenase-2 expression in primary breast cancers predicts dissemination of cancer cells to the bone marrow. *Breast Cancer Res Treat.* 2009;117:61–68.

114. Kerlikowske K, Molinaro AM, Gauthier ML, et al. Biomarker expression and risk of subsequent tumors after initial ductal carcinoma in situ diagnosis. *J Natl Cancer Inst.* 2010;102:627–637.

115. Allred DC. Biomarkers predicting recurrence and progression of ductal carcinoma in situ treated by lumpectomy alone. *J Natl Cancer Inst.* 2010;102:585–587.

116. Cully M, You H, Levine AJ, Mak TW. Beyond PTEN mutations: the PI3K pathway as an integrator of multiple inputs during tumorigenesis. *Nat Rev Cancer.* 2006;6:184–192.

117. Miller TW, Perez-Torres M, Narasanna A, et al. Loss of phosphatase and tensin homologue deleted on chromosome 10 engages ErbB3 and insulin-like growth factor-I receptor signaling to promote antiestrogen resistance in breast cancer. *Cancer Res.* 2009;69:4192–4201.

118. Shen WH, Balajee AS, Wang J, et al. Essential role for nuclear PTEN in maintaining chromosomal integrity. *Cell.* 2007;128: 157–170.

119. Mendes-Pereira AM, Martin SA, Brough R, et al. Synthetic lethal targeting of PTEN mutant cells with PARP inhibitors. *EMBO Mol Med.* 2009;1:315–322.

120. Pallares J, Bussaglia E, Martinez-Guitarte JL, et al. Immunohistochemical analysis of PTEN in endometrial carcinoma: a tissue microarray study with a comparison of four commercial antibodies in correlation with molecular abnormalities. *Mod Pathol.* 2005;18:719–727.

121. Sakr RA, Barbashina V, Morrogh M, et al. Protocol for PTEN expression by immunohistochemistry in formalin-fixed paraffin-embedded human breast carcinoma. *Appl Immunohistochem Mol Morphol.* 2010;18:371–374.

122. Blows FM, Driver KE, Schmidt MK, et al. Subtyping of breast cancer by immunohistochemistry to investigate a relationship between subtype and short and long term survival: a collaborative analysis of data for 10,159 cases from 12 studies. *PLoS Med.* 2010;7:e1000279.

123. Cheang MC, Voduc D, Bajdik C, et al. Basal-like breast cancer defined by five biomarkers has superior prognostic value than triple-negative phenotype. *Clin Cancer Res.* 2008;14:1368–1376.

124. Rakha EA, Tan DS, Foulkes WD, et al. Are triple-negative tumours and basal-like breast cancer synonymous? *Breast Cancer Res.* 2007;9:404;author reply 405.

125. Bertucci F, Finetti P, Cervera N, et al. How basal are triple-negative breast cancers? *Int J Cancer.* 2008;123:236–240.

126. Tan DS, Marchio C, Jones RL, et al. Triple negative breast cancer: molecular profiling and prognostic impact in adjuvant anthracycline-treated patients. *Breast Cancer Res Treat.* 2008;111:27–44.

127. Livasy CA, Karaca G, Nanda R, et al. Phenotypic evaluation of the basal-like subtype of invasive breast carcinoma. *Mod Pathol.* 2006;19:264–271.

128. Savage K, Lambros MB, Robertson D, et al. Caveolin 1 is overexpressed and amplified in a subset of basal-like and metaplastic breast carcinomas: a morphologic, ultrastructural, immunohistochemical, and in situ hybridization analysis. *Clin Cancer Res.* 2007;13:90–101.

129. Savage K, Leung S, Todd SK, et al. Distribution and significance of caveolin 2 expression in normal breast and invasive breast cancer: an immunofluorescence and immunohistochemical analysis. *Breast Cancer Res Treat.* 2008;110:245–256.

130. Parry S, Savage K, Marchio C, Reis-Filho JS. Nestin is expressed in basal-like and triple negative breast cancers. *J Clin Pathol.* 2008;61:1045–1050.

131. Rakha EA, Elsheikh SE, Aleskandarany MA, et al. Triple-negative breast cancer: distinguishing between basal and nonbasal subtypes. *Clin Cancer Res.* 2009;15:2302–2310.

132. Constantinidou A, Jones RL, Reis-Filho JS. Beyond triple-negative breast cancer: the need to define new subtypes. *Expert Rev Anticancer Ther.* 2010;10:1197–1213.

133. Reis-Filho JS, Pinheiro C, Lambros MB, et al. EGFR amplification and lack of activating mutations in metaplastic breast carcinomas. *J Pathol.* 2006;209:445–453.

134. Miettinen M, Lasota J. KIT (CD117): a review on expression in normal and neoplastic tissues, and mutations and their clinicopathologic correlation. *Appl Immunohistochem Mol Morphol.* 2005;13:205–220.

135. Marty B, Maire V, Gravier E, et al. Frequent PTEN genomic alterations and activated phosphatidylinositol 3-kinase pathway in basal-like breast cancer cells. *Breast Cancer Res.* 2008;10:R101.

136. Lakhani SR, Reis-Filho JS, Fulford L, et al. Prediction of BRCA1 status in patients with breast cancer using estrogen receptor and basal phenotype. *Clin Cancer Res.* 2005;11:5175–5180.

137. Collins LC, Martyniak A, Kandel MJ, et al. Basal cytokeratin and epidermal growth factor receptor expression are not predictive of BRCA1 mutation status in women with triple-negative breast cancers. *Am J Surg Pathol.* 2009;33:1093–1097.

138. Molyneux G, Geyer FC, Magnay FA, et al. BRCA1 Basal-like breast cancers originate from luminal epithelial progenitors and not from basal stem cells. *Cell Stem Cell.* 2010;7:403–417.

139. Lim E, Vaillant F, Wu D, et al. Aberrant luminal progenitors as the candidate target population for basal tumor development in BRCA1 mutation carriers. *Nat Med.* 2009;15:907–913.

140. Pusztai L, Mazouni C, Anderson K, Wu Y, Symmans WF. Molecular classification of breast cancer: limitations and potential. *Oncologist.* 2006;11:868-877.

141. Parker JS, Mullins M, Cheang MC, et al. Supervised risk predictor of breast cancer based on intrinsic subtypes. *J Clin Oncol.* 2009;27:1160–1167.

142. de Ronde JJ, Hannemann J, Halfwerk H, et al. Concordance of clinical and molecular breast cancer subtyping in the context of preoperative chemotherapy response. *Breast Cancer Res Treat.* 2010;119:119–126.

143. Ashworth A. A synthetic lethal therapeutic approach: poly(ADP) ribose polymerase inhibitors for the treatment of cancers deficient in DNA double-strand break repair. *J Clin Oncol.* 2008;26:3785–3790.

144. Turner N, Tutt A, Ashworth A. Hallmarks of 'BRCAness' in sporadic cancers. *Nat Rev Cancer.* 2004;4:814–819.

145. Graeser MK, McCarthy A, Lord CJ, et al. A marker of homologous recombination predicts pathological complete response to neoadjuvant chemotherapy in primary breast cancer. *Clin Cancer Res.* 2010;16:61596168.

146. Geyer FC, Lopez-Garcia MA, Lambros MB, Reis-Filho JS. Genetic characterization of breast cancer and implications for clinical management. *J Cell Mol Med.* 2009;13:4090–4103.

147. Perez-Valles A, Martorell-Cebollada M, Nogueira-Vazquez E, Garcia-Garcia JA, Fuster-Diana E. The usefulness of antibodies to the BRCA1 protein in detecting the mutated BRCA1 gene. An immunohistochemical study. *J Clin Pathol.* 2001;54:476–480.

148. Wilson CA, Ramos L, Villasenor MR, et al. Localization of human BRCA1 and its loss in high-grade, non-inherited breast carcinomas. *Nat Genet.* 1999;21:236–240.

149. Turner NC, Reis-Filho JS, Russell AM, et al. BRCA1 dysfunction in sporadic basal-like breast cancer. *Oncogene.* 2007;26:2126–2132.

150. Virk RK, Khan A. Pseudoangiomatous stromal hyperplasia: an overview. *Arch Pathol Lab Med.* 2010;134:1070–1074.

151. McLaren BK, Smith J, Schuyler PA, Dupont WD, Page DL. Adenomyoepithelioma: clinical, histologic, and immunohistologic evaluation of a series of related lesions. *Am J Surg Pathol.* 2005;29:1294–1299.

152. Detre S, Saclani Jotti G, Dowsett M. A "quickscore" method for immunohistochemical semiquantitation: validation for oestrogen receptor in breast carcinomas. *J Clin Pathol.* 1995;48:876–878.

153. Baselga J, Swain SM. Novel anticancer targets: revisiting ERBB2 and discovering ERBB3. *Nat Rev Cancer.* 2009;9:463–475.

Index

Page numbers followed by *f or t* indicate figures or tables, respectively.